LESS TIME TO DO MORE

PSYCHOTHERAPY ON THE SHORT-TERM INPATIENT UNIT

LESS TIME TO DO MORE

PSYCHOTHERAPY ON THE SHORT-TERM INPATIENT UNIT

Edited by

Ellen Leibenluft, M.D.
Medical Officer, Clinical Psychobiology Branch
National Institute of Mental Health, Bethesda, Maryland;
Clinical Associate Professor of Psychiatry,
Georgetown University School of Medicine, Washington, DC

Allan Tasman, M.D.
Professor and Chair, Department of Psychiatry,
University of Louisville, Louisville, Kentucky

and

Stephen A. Green, M.D.
Clinical Professor, Department of Psychiatry,
Georgetown University School of Medicine;
Senior Scholar, Center for Clinical Bioethics,
Georgetown University, Washington, DC

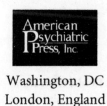

American Psychiatric Press, Inc.

Washington, DC
London, England

Note: The authors have worked to ensure that all information in this book concerning drug dosages, schedules, and routes of administration is accurate as of the time of publication and consistent with standards set by the U.S. Food and Drug Administration and the general medical community. As medical research and practice advance, however, therapeutic standards may change. For this reason and because human and mechanical errors sometimes occur, we recommend that readers follow the advice of a physician who is directly involved in their care or the care of a member of their family.

Copyright © 1993 American Psychiatric Press, Inc.
ALL RIGHTS RESERVED
Manufactured in the United States of America on acid-free paper
96 95 94 93   4 3 2 1
First Edition

American Psychiatric Press, Inc.
1400 K Street, N.W., Washington, DC   20005

Library of Congress Cataloging-in-Publication Data
Less time to do more : psychotherapy on the short-term inpatient unit
  /   edited by Ellen Leibenluft, Allan Tasman, and Stephen A. Green.
      p.   cm.
  Includes bibliographical references and index.
  ISBN 0-88048-512-4 (alk. paper)
  1. Psychiatric hospital care.   2. Brief psychotherapy.
I. Leibenluft, Ellen, 1953–   . II. Tasman, Allan, 1947–
III. Green, Stephen A., 1945–   .
  [DNLM: 1. Psychotherapy, Brief.   2. Hospital Units.
3. Inpatients.   WM 420 L638 1993]
RC439.L467   1993
616.89'14—dc20
DNLM/DLC
for Library of Congress   93-20081
                                                                  CIP

British Library Cataloguing in Publication Data
A CIP record is available from the British Library.

CONTENTS

I
THE MODALITIES

II
SPECIAL POPULATIONS

CONTRIBUTORS

Gerald Adler, M.D.
Training and Supervising Analyst, Boston Psychoanalytic Society and Institute; Lecturer on Psychiatry, Harvard Medical School, Boston, Massachusetts

David Bienenfeld, M.D.
Associate Professor, Vice-Chair, and Director of Residency Training, Department of Psychiatry, Wright State University, Dayton, Ohio

Lisa Borg, M.D.
Assistant Professor of Clinical Psychiatry, New Jersey Medical School, University of Medicine and Dentistry, Newark, New Jersey; Chief of Addictive Services, Department of Veterans Affairs Medical Center, East Orange, New Jersey

Stephen A. Cole, M.D.
Director, St. Vincent's Partial Hospitalization Program; Clinical Associate, Professor of Psychiatry, New York University, New York, New York

Francine Cournos, M.D.
Associate Clinical Professor of Psychiatry, Columbia University College of Physicians and Surgeons; Director, Washington Heights Community Service, New York State Psychiatric Institute, New York, New York

Richard J. Frances, M.D.
Professor of Clinical Psychiatry, New Jersey Medical School,
University of Medicine and Dentistry, Newark, New Jersey; Director
of Psychiatry, Hackensack Hospital, Hackensack, New Jersey

Richard L. Goldberg, M.D.
Professor and Chair, Department of Psychiatry,
Georgetown University School of Medicine, Washington, DC

Stephen A. Green, M.D.
Clinical Professor, Department of Psychiatry,
Georgetown University School of Medicine,
and Senior Scholar, Center for Clinical Bioethics,
Georgetown University, Washington, DC

Ewald Horwath, M.D.
Associate Clinical Professor of Psychiatry, Columbia University
College of Physicians and Surgeons, New York, New York;
Director, Community Service Inpatient Unit, New York State
Psychiatric Institute, New York, New York

Howard D. Kibel, M.D.
Associate Professor of Clinical Psychiatry, Cornell University
Medical College, New York, New York; Coordinator of Group
Psychotherapy, New York Hospital-Cornell Medical Center,
Westchester Division, White Plains, New York

Ellen Leibenluft, M.D.
Medical Officer, Clinical Psychobiology Branch,
National Institute of Mental Health, Bethesda, Maryland;
Clinical Associate Professor of Psychiatry,
Georgetown University School of Medicine, Washington, DC

John M. Oldham, M.D.
Professor and Associate Chair, Department of Psychiatry,
Columbia University College of Physicians and Surgeons;
Director, New York State Psychiatric Institute, New York, New York

Michelle Riba, M.D.
Assistant Professor of Psychiatry and Associate Director of
Residency Training, Department of Psychiatry,
University of Connecticut School of Medicine,
Farmington, Connecticut

Bruce S. Rothschild, M.D.
Assistant Professor of Psychiatry, University of Connecticut
School of Medicine, Farmington, Connecticut;
Head, Eating Disorders Day Hospital, The Institute of Living,
Hartford, Connecticut

Paul A. Silver, M.D.
Assistant Professor of Psychiatry, Georgetown University
School of Medicine, Washington, DC

Andrew E. Skodol II, M.D.
Associate Professor of Clinical Psychiatry,
Department of Psychiatry, Columbia University
College of Physicians and Surgeons; Director, Unit for Personality
Studies, New York State Psychiatric Institute, New York, New York

Marcia Slomowitz, M.D.
Assistant Professor of Psychiatry, Department of Psychiatry and
Behavioral Sciences, and Director, Clinical Inpatient Services,
Northwestern University Medical School, Chicago, Illinois

Allan Tasman, M.D.
Professor and Chair, Department of Psychiatry,
University of Louisville, Louisville, Kentucky

Michael E. Thase, M.D.
Associate Professor of Psychiatry, University of Pittsburgh
School of Medicine; Director, Cognitive Therapy Clinic;
Director, Mood Disorders Module; and Associate Director,
Mental Health Clinical Research Center, Western Psychiatric
Institute and Clinic, Pittsburgh, Pennsylvania

PREFACE

Few would argue that the practice of inpatient psychiatry has undergone a virtual revolution within the last 10 years. The most striking characteristic of this upheaval is the dramatically decreased length of stay. In addition, contemporary inpatient units differ from their forebears in that patients have a greater variety of psychiatric, medical, and substance abuse problems; are more likely to be treated with psychotropic medications; and often have more limited access to family and community support. The implications of these changes for the practice of inpatient psychotherapy form the central question of this book.

The causes of the revolution in inpatient psychiatry are multiple. Most observers agree that the driving forces have been economic, as American society has become increasingly concerned about the high costs of health care. Pressure to decrease costs focused first on the hospital setting, which traditionally accounted for nearly three-quarters of mental health costs (Kiesler 1982). Deinstitutionalization of patients from state mental hospitals occurred for both philosophical and economic reasons (Asch 1987). The growth of managed care and concurrent utilization review also brought economic constraints to the private sector (Mirin and Namerow 1991; Sederer 1987). All of these factors contributed to decreased length of stay and stricter control over access to hospitalization.

Other forces contributed to the inpatient revolution. Sociologists wrote of the detrimental effects of institutionalization, and the American public became more concerned about the protection of individual rights (Goffman 1961). Stricter criteria for involuntary commitment—and shorter stays for voluntary patients—reflect these philosophical trends. Several studies demonstrated that, at least for certain patient populations, more time in the hospital did not necessarily mean a better clinical result

(Cournos 1987; Glick et al. 1976; Herz et al. 1979). The increased efficacy of antipsychotic and thymoleptic medications made shortened stays more feasible, and physicians under pressure to discharge patients rapidly prescribed medications more readily (Klerman 1982).

These profound events brought changes to an inpatient environment that had been dominated first by the tenets of psychoanalytic psychotherapy, and then by the philosophy of the therapeutic community (Gutheil 1985). Both of these psychotherapeutic approaches, at least in their original forms, employed regressive techniques and required lengthy hospital stays. It is easier to delineate the models that we've lost than the models that we use. In fact, one might wonder if the psychiatric unit is a treatment setting in search of a model. Perhaps it is difficult to conceptualize a model for all psychiatric inpatients because the patients themselves are such a varied lot—patients with concurrent psychiatric and medical illness, previously well-functioning patients with an acute Axis I disorder, patients with chronic mental illness (who in times past might have had lengthy stays in state hospitals), patients with severe Axis II pathology, and patients with acute or chronic sequelae of substance abuse. Under either of the previous two treatment models, many of these individuals would have been denied admission to the typical acute psychiatric unit; now they are the primary recipients of its care.

Most psychiatric units now subscribe to a biopsychosocial model, with varying admixtures of a modified therapeutic community. How has the advent of the biopsychosocial model changed the practice of inpatient treatment and, in particular, inpatient psychotherapy? The "bio" portion of the biopsychosocial model has brought the most dramatic changes, because previous models eschewed, or minimized, the use of medications. Now, most inpatients are on medication, and a common goal of inpatient psychotherapy is to increase compliance with somatic treatments. In addition, the increased emphasis on systematic diagnosis and somatic interventions has changed the role of the psychiatrist, with the reflective analyst giving way to the more active physician. Not only has the relationship of the physician to his or her patient changed, but also the physician's relationship with other staff members has been modified. The consensus decision making of the therapeutic community has been replaced—with great difficulty, in some instances—with a more hierarchical structure. Third-party payors now require that psychiatrists be involved in, and accountable for, all major clinical decisions. In many inpatient settings, psychiatrists prescribe medication and supervise psychotherapy conducted by other mental health professionals, but no longer do psychotherapy themselves. Many units now have "rounds" modeled on those that occur on medical units; their psychotherapeutic implications have received little attention.

Although previous inpatient models also emphasized psychological processes, the "psycho" aspect of the contemporary unit's biopsychosocial model has still brought changes. Inpatient psychotherapists continue to use psychodynamic principles, but the most commonly used techniques have changed. Supportive interventions (including psychoeducation) have supplanted more regressive, exploratory approaches. There is an increased emphasis on conscious cognitions and phenomenology, rather than unconscious psychology. Just as the inpatient psychiatrist is more likely to be active in prescribing medication, the inpatient psychotherapist is more likely to take an active, directive stance with his or her patient. On many units, brief, frequent sessions of individual psychotherapy have replaced more infrequent, longer sessions. Or, patients may be seen for brief sessions early in the hospitalization, with longer sessions being introduced as recompensation occurs. In fact, this book will clearly demonstrate that a hallmark of inpatient psychotherapy is the need for the therapist to be flexible, pragmatic, and eclectic.

Social interventions on inpatient units have also changed over the last 10 years. The therapeutic community emphasized the importance of social interactions, but it included only those members of society who were on the unit. Today's inpatient units have more fluid boundaries. Now, units charged with discharging patients rapidly strive to involve the patient's family and community supports throughout the hospitalization. However, in many instances these social supports are insufficient, or even absent, and the inpatient staff must struggle to try to fill in the gaps.

Thus, hapless inpatient clinicians are often left trying to do more with less—less time, fewer resources. To meet this challenge, the inpatient psychotherapist often plays several roles simultaneously, prescribing medications, meeting with the patient individually and in group, intervening with the patient's family, and consulting with the patient's internist or group home supervisor. In this context, the boundary between psychotherapy and management becomes blurred. Because the inpatient clinician must fulfill multiple roles, we have defined psychotherapy broadly, as any interaction between staff and patients, or between staff and members of the patient's support system, that is conducted by the staff with an aim of accomplishing specific therapeutic goals. Psychotherapy can be guided by one or more theoretical orientations, including psychodynamic or cognitive-behavioral theory. Thus, we consider the conscious management of the inpatient milieu by the professional staff to be a form of psychotherapy, as are group or family meetings conducted by staff. The psychiatrist's description of a medication's side effects may be "psychotherapy," if the explanation is made particularly relevant to patients' concerns, and if the physician uses the interaction to help patients understand their resistance to compliance.

According to our definition, mental health professionals of several disciplines may conduct psychotherapy on short-term inpatient units. In fact, on many units, psychiatrists, psychologists, social workers, and psychiatric nurses conduct most of the psychotherapy, whereas occupational therapists and trained mental health workers are involved in certain specialized therapeutic interactions. This book should be useful for any mental health professional who spends a significant amount of time interacting with inpatients. However, certain sections of the book may be most germane for practitioners from particular disciplines. For example, Chapter 2 is targeted particularly toward psychiatrists, although psychiatric nurses (who administer medication and educate patients and their families about psychotropic medications) should also find useful information in it. Chapter 4 may be most relevant for social workers, but it is also likely to be useful to psychiatrists, nurses, and other staff who interact with the distressed members of patients' families.

What characteristics of inpatient psychotherapy distinguish it from outpatient psychotherapy? The hospitalized patient and the therapist interact in the context of the inpatient milieu, where the treatment is susceptible to influence from unit events, other patients, and unit staff. The therapist meets with the unit staff routinely, to share information about the patient and collaborate on a treatment approach. As part of this process, the inpatient therapist's treatment of the patient is subjected to almost daily scrutiny and discussion by other team members, as well as by outside reviewers doing utilization review. Unlike his or her outpatient counterpart, the inpatient therapist typically has contact with the patient outside the scheduled therapeutic sessions, as well as control over concrete aspects of the patient's life, such as passes, privileges, and the discharge date. Although the goal of outpatient therapy is often negotiable between patient and therapist, the basic task of the inpatient therapist is clearly defined in concrete terms (i.e., to help the patient recompensate to the point where his or her behavior and symptoms are manageable on an outpatient basis).

Other characteristics of inpatient psychotherapy pertain to the outpatient setting, but to a much lesser degree. For example, although some outpatients participate in several forms of psychotherapy simultaneously, virtually all inpatients do so; although some outpatients enter therapy in crisis, almost all inpatients are in an acute state when they are hospitalized. Therefore, inpatients are more likely to be treated with medication in addition to psychotherapy. Finally, the relationship between the inpatient psychotherapist and the patient is more likely to be time-limited.

Many of the technical aspects of inpatient psychotherapy derive from this charge, to accomplish concrete goals within a time-limited framework, working with an acutely distressed patient who is temporarily living in the inpatient milieu. The delineation of the technical aspects of inpatient psychotherapy forms the basis for this book. The theoretical underpinnings of the book are eclectic; although many of the authors approach their task from a psychodynamic perspective, others employ a cognitive-behavioral or psychoeducational approach, and all acknowledge the importance of biological interventions. Where appropriate, the relevant research literature is reviewed. However, there is relatively little research on the efficacy of specific psychotherapeutic interventions with inpatients, so the authors generally base their recommendations on the clinical literature and their own clinical experience. In addition, although the driving force behind the decreased length of inpatient stays is economic, the focus of the book is psychotherapy, not reimbursement. Therefore, we do not describe how to maximize reimbursement under different payment systems, in part because of the large variability between these systems. Instead, we describe general principles and techniques that can be used to deliver psychotherapeutic care efficiently in a number of settings.

Although we have obviously tried to keep the repetition between chapters to a minimum, we believe that some overlap is inevitable because this overlap reflects the inpatient milieu itself, with several therapists using different techniques to work toward some shared, and some distinct, therapeutic goals. Thus, several common themes pervade the chapters. The time-limited nature of inpatient work means that a therapeutic alliance must be established as rapidly as possible. This alliance must include not only the patient, but also his or her family, to whose care the patient will be discharged soon. The therapist's task, to make the patient "dischargeable" quickly, means that he or she must focus on clearly defined behavioral goals. Furthermore, the therapist must accept the fact that the patient will often be discharged with significant symptoms, and will certainly be discharged with his or her underlying conflicts unresolved. Several authors describe the inpatient stay as an extended assessment process; in essence, as a prelude to more definitive outpatient work. Because the patient is in crisis, the therapist must balance confrontation with support, exploration with active intervention, and talking therapies with somatic interventions. And because the therapy takes place within the context of the inpatient milieu, the therapist has more treatment options available, but he or she must be aware of the milieu's complex influences on the patient and the patient's treatment.

This book is divided into two sections. The first describes major psychotherapeutic modalities on the inpatient unit, including milieu therapy, individual psychodynamic psychotherapy, cognitive-behavioral psychotherapy, family therapy, and group therapy. In addition, a chapter describes how to combine somatic therapies and psychotherapy. The chapters in the second section discuss psychotherapeutic work with patient populations that require specialized approaches, including patients with major psychiatric and medical illness, patients with eating disorders, alcoholic patients, geriatric patients, adolescents, chronically mentally ill patients, and patients with severe personality disorders. Finally, a chapter in the second section discusses supervision and teaching on the inpatient unit.

Given the acute symptoms that hospitalized patients experience, inpatient psychotherapy has always been demanding work. Its challenges have certainly not been diminished by shorter hospital stays, stricter criteria for admission, and decreased community services. The inpatient staff now feels caught between managed care companies who ask for early discharge and the threat of a lawsuit if that early discharge results in an adverse outcome. In the ensuing chapters, we do not promise easy and clear answers to the multitude of problems that exist on the contemporary inpatient unit. Because each patient and unit (and even, it seems, each reimbursement system!) is unique, we do not propose one approach to inpatient care that can be universally applied. Our goals are much more modest: to examine the implications of shorter stays for the practice of inpatient psychotherapy, and to describe techniques that inpatient psychotherapists can employ in their attempts to remain therapeutically effective despite increased pressure and decreased resources.

Ellen Leibenluft, M.D.

REFERENCES

Asch SS: History of the general hospital psychiatric inpatient unit: 1947 to 1986. Psychiatr Clin North Am 10:155–164, 1987

Cournos F: Hospitalization outcome studies: implications for the treatment of the very ill patient. Psychiatr Clin North Am 10:165–176, 1987

Glick ID, Hargreaves WA, Drues J, et al: Short versus long hospitalization: a prospective controlled study, V: one-year follow-up results for non-schizophrenic patients. Am J Psychiatry 133:515–517, 1976

Goffman E: Asylum. New York, Doubleday, 1961

Gutheil TG: The therapeutic milieu: changing themes and theories. Hosp Community Psychiatry 36:1279–1285, 1985

Herz MI, Endicott J, Gibbon M: Brief hospitalization: two-year follow-up. Arch Gen Psychiatry 36:701–705, 1979

Kiesler CA: Public and professional myths about mental hospitalization: an empirical reassessment of policy-related beliefs. Am Psychol 37:1323–1329, 1982

Klerman GL: The psychiatric revolution of the past twenty-five years, in Deviance and Mental Illness. Edited by Gove WR. Beverly Hills, CA, Sage, 1982, pp 177–198

Mirin SM, Namerow MJ: Why study treatment outcome? Hosp Community Psychiatry 10:1007–1013, 1991

Sederer LI: Utilization review and quality assurance: staying in the black and working with the blues. Gen Hosp Psychiatry 9:210–219, 1987

I

THE MODALITIES

CHAPTER 1

Application of Therapeutic Community Principles in Short-Stay Units

Allan Tasman, M.D.

THE THERAPEUTIC COMMUNITY

The therapeutic community, a term coined by Main (1946), is a specific type of therapeutic milieu applied to psychiatric treatment. The therapeutic community was based on a concept that the nature of psychiatric illness can be understood from a social-interactional model of illness, as opposed to a medical model, and that a treatment program could be devised with specific structures and processes that would utilize this view of psychopathology for therapeutic benefit. Before this approach became popular, most psychotherapeutic intervention emphasized exploration and resolution of intrapsychic forces and conflicts, as emphasized by psychoanalytic theory. In contrast, the therapeutic community, based on a social psychology (Clark 1977; Fort 1979), emphasized the role of environment and interpersonal interactions, not intrapsychic conflict, as modifiers of behavior.

The first therapeutic community, set up by Maxwell Jones at Belmont Hospital in England, was based on four concepts of key importance to the therapeutic process (Burkitt 1975; Jones et al. 1953).

1. *Democratization.* Unlike a program based on the principles of medical treatment, the therapeutic community is viewed as a treatment setting

in which responsibility for decisions regarding treatment is shared among patients and staff. The therapeutic benefit is felt to occur as community members begin to feel more responsible for themselves and for each other.

2. *Permissiveness.* This refers to people's capacity to tolerate one another's behavior and is closely allied to the democratic principle. It is concerned with freedom of expression but should not be confused with an absence of community rules or the necessity of adhering to those rules. Permissiveness also emphasizes individual rights and responsibility in an environment where this responsibility is valued and examined.

3. *Communalism.* This reflects the importance of a tightly knit and intimate set of relationships. The flattening of the administrative hierarchy and the increased sharing of responsibilities are important aspects of this concept.

4. *Reality confrontation.* This reflects a continual confrontation and discussion, by other members of the community, of various aspects of an individual's general and specific behaviors. This sometimes occurs individually, but more often in community or smaller group interactions.

Implicit in these concepts is a view of the way behavior is shaped. Although individual responsibility for behavioral action is stressed, behavior is believed to be modified by both a sense of belonging to a larger social organization as well as the resulting responses to a shared set of beliefs and values concerning appropriate behavior. Behavioral changes are thought to reflect changes in value or belief systems to more closely coincide with those of the larger group. This phenomenon is followed by a gradual internalization of these new beliefs, which is then carried over to behavior outside of the specific group. Because interpersonal problem-solving behaviors are valued, the modeling by the staff, through their relationships with one another, helps the patient to regain or establish these skills and to develop new and more adaptive ways of taking responsibility. The ward culture (i.e., the shared set of expected values regarding behavior and social interaction) will also provide an opportunity for the patient to learn roles in a setting that resembles in some way the context outside the hospital.

PROBLEMS IN APPLICATION OF THERAPEUTIC COMMUNITY PRINCIPLES

In the late 1940s and early 1950s, therapeutic community concepts provided an innovative way of providing psychiatric treatment, without relying on individual psychotherapy or somatic therapies. Since then, however, a variety of changes in hospital psychiatry have led to a reevaluation of therapeutic community concepts (Gutheil 1985; Islam and Turner 1982; Johnson and Parker 1977; Karasu et al. 1977; Kernberg 1981; Lehman and Ritzler 1976; Moline 1976; Oldham and Russakoff 1982; Sacks and Carpenter 1974; Tucker and Maxmen 1973). One such change has been the shift in hospital admissions away from neurotic and less disturbed patients toward more severely and chronically ill patients. Although neurotic patients accounted for nearly one-half the admissions to Jones's unit (Jones et al. 1953), patients with psychotic illnesses and severe character disorders now make up a large and growing proportion of psychiatric hospital admissions, necessitating modification of traditional approaches (Kahn and White 1989).

The shift toward brief hospital stays, with increased reliance on community aftercare, also dilutes the functioning of a traditional hospital therapeutic community (Karterud 1988; Kleespies 1986). The mean length of stay in Jones's therapeutic community was approximately 80 days, and stays of up to 1 year were not uncommon (Jones et al. 1953). With general hospital stays currently averaging less than 2 weeks, most clinicians believe that there is not enough time to implement traditional therapeutic community concepts. In addition, the revolutions in psychopharmacologic treatments make democratization of treatment planning difficult to apply in the ways originally envisioned. In the traditional therapeutic community, all treatment decisions were made by the community as a whole, with staff and patients having equal responsibilities and rights. This model was based on the belief that problem solving occurs best in a large group setting. Studies in group problem solving (Moline 1976) have, however, raised questions about the validity of this assumption. These studies indicate that group problem solving is superior to individual efforts only when all of the individuals involved share the same knowledge and data base. Decisions regarding medications and passes from the hospital are two obvious areas where group decision making is deficient in an acute hospital setting.

Although many forces are operating against the utility of a traditional therapeutic community model, the continued pressure to decrease lengths of stay obliges clinicians to use every tool at their disposal to maximize the benefit from hospitalization. In fact, the use of modified therapeutic community programs for specialized populations, such as those with substance abuse problems, still enjoys support (Rosenthal 1989; Sorensen et al. 1987; Yohay and Winick 1986). There is also continuing work on long-term therapeutic community programs (Berke 1987; Miskimins 1990; Strochak 1987; Yohay 1986). However, for the reasons just reviewed, the original techniques of a therapeutic community are increasingly difficult to apply in a short-term setting.

New understanding of group processes, however, coming from an unexpected place—developments in applied psychoanalytic theory—may offer assistance. Work by Heinz Kohut (1971, 1977) and his followers provides a new way of understanding group and individual functioning and allows for the development of concepts that can describe the types of interaction between the individual and the group that are emphasized in a therapeutic community. This framework can be used to effectively implement a therapeutic community in a short-term setting.

A BRIEF REVIEW OF PERTINENT ASPECTS OF KOHUT'S PSYCHOLOGY OF THE SELF

Self psychology, the body of theoretical and clinical work growing out of Kohut's original formulations, focuses on the interaction between parent and child as development progresses. This view emphasizes the importance of the parent in providing self-regulatory functions that are not yet developed in the child. In this context, the parent serves as a "selfobject" for the child (i.e., one who is psychologically tied to and who provides significant soothing and self-regulatory functioning for the child). The parent who picks up a crying child and, through holding and gently rocking the child, calms him or her, is the paradigm for a small infant of this soothing, self-regulatory functioning to which Kohut refers. As the child gains increasing self-regulatory capacities of his or her own (i.e., increased self-cohesion), the role of the parent changes toward more reinforcement of the child's appropriate coping and regulatory capabilities, with less direct provision of self-regulatory functioning by the parent.

Self psychology envisions an ongoing balance between reinforcement of the child's autonomous functioning and provision of self-regulatory support when needed. When new developmental tasks must be learned, for example, or during times of significant stress, the balance may shift somewhat. In addition, as selfobject needs become less intense and more diffuse with maturation, various selfobject functions may be met by several people. The needs for "selfobject" support are seen as normally continuing (though in differing forms) throughout life.

This theoretical perspective provides an important framework for understanding group formation, group processes, and the role of the group leader. Once it is formed, a group can be understood as a type of selfobject matrix. This function supports group cohesion. One of the roles of the leader is to monitor the state of cohesion and to intervene when the selfobject matrix is distorted or malfunctioning.

THE ROLE OF THE THERAPEUTIC COMMUNITY FOR PATIENTS WITH SEVERE PSYCHOPATHOLOGY

It is standard practice that patients with severe character disorders, psychotic disorders, and severe mood disorders are maintained as much as possible in an ambulatory setting. Hospitalization is used only when there is a decompensation (often precipitated by as-yet incompletely understood biological processes in the brain) in the patient's ability to function outside the hospital. From a behavioral point of view, however, we can describe these individuals as having lost the capacity to function autonomously (i.e., they have lost their usual self-regulatory capacities). Especially in individuals with psychotic or borderline disorders, this self-fragmentation may also be related to the loss of, or threat to, the stability of a relationship with a person or support system that functions to fulfill the individual's cohesion-maintaining, self-regulatory needs.

It follows, therefore, that the first task in the treatment of the severely disturbed patient is to help that individual return to a state of self-cohesion in which self-regulatory functioning is maximized. In patients with severe psychopathology, the therapist and therapeutic/social support system function to provide self-regulatory functions for the individual. In the same way, the therapeutic community during a brief hospitalization can serve as an important component in a treatment program designed to help reestablish self-regulation in the decompensated individual. The milieu can function as a series of interlocking and overlapping selfobject matrices, composed of both patient and staff groups, which serve a reparative function for and foster return to more adaptive functioning in the patient.

Once self-equilibrium is reestablished, the therapeutic community can also provide a setting within which resolution of conflicts (which may have played a role in the decompensation) can begin to occur. With modifications that will be described later in this chapter, the principles of democratization, permissiveness, communalism, and reality confrontation, which were reviewed earlier, can foster the formation of a therapeutic community that functions as a selfobject matrix. This function of the therapeutic community has been found to be helpful in previous studies (Katz and Kirkland 1990; Stern et al. 1986).

Specific aspects that can foster the development and maintenance of therapeutic community functioning in a short-stay unit (e.g., staff roles and cohesion, rules and structure of the treatment program, acting-out behavior and clique formation, staff development, role of the leader, use of seclusion) are discussed in the next section. I will discuss necessary modification of the original four principles of Jones's therapeutic community where appropriate.

FOSTERING THE DEVELOPMENT OF A THERAPEUTIC COMMUNITY

Staff Roles and Cohesion

Anyone who has ever worked on an inpatient unit has experienced times when everything seems to be working like a well-oiled machine. Staff are interacting well, opportunities for resolving differences of opinion about patient care are provided, and there is minimal testing of limits or acting out among the patients. At these moments cohesion is high, and the staff can provide a relatively stable selfobject matrix for the patients.

For staff to function in this way, the staff's professional needs must be addressed in a way that enhances their sense of professional identity and self-esteem. Every individual needs to be recognized as worthwhile, to have his or her individual and particular skills and expertise recognized, and to feel that there is an opportunity to participate in planning and carrying out the individual patient's treatment. These professional needs are addressed implicitly in a traditional therapeutic community through the principle of democratization, which recognizes the benefits of a "flattening" of the administrative and leadership hierarchies compared to more traditional medical hospital settings. To some extent, however, implementation of this principle reflected the relatively leisurely pace of hospital treatment when therapeutic communities were instituted, and it is not applicable in the same ways today.

Because of the increased intensity of work concomitant with high turnover rates, differentiation of staff roles (specifically, how each individual will intervene as part of an overall treatment plan) must be delineated to a greater degree than was often the case in the traditional therapeutic community. Further, although opportunities for participation in treatment planning must be part of the overall staff responsibilities, clear-cut lines of decision-making responsibility and authority must be established. Thus, the traditional principles of democratization and communalism must be modified to meet the needs of today's inpatient units.

The phenomenon of burnout, well known among staff working with severely ill patients (Freudenberger 1986; Lamb 1979), occurs when the demands of caring for these patients far outweigh the gratifications staff receive in return. Attention to inpatient staff professional needs helps minimize the burnout phenomenon. When staff needs are not addressed, distressing affects may be stimulated in them (Searles 1968). This can cause a disturbance in staff cohesion, resulting in fragmentation of the milieu functioning. This loss of cohesive milieu functioning is often followed quickly by signs of a lack of self-regulation within individual patients and within the patient's subgroup as a whole.

Signs of patient dysregulation typically appear as increased bizarre or inappropriate behavior in more psychotic patients, increased testing of limits and rule testing, acting-out behavior, social withdrawal and decreased participation in activities, and angry questioning of the therapeutic program's values. This phenomenon was described as early as 1954 in the book *The Mental Hospital* (Stanton and Schwartz 1954) and has since come to be called the Stanton-Schwartz phenomenon. In that work, it was shown that covert problems among staff members were often reflected by similar problems in communication and behavior on an overt level within the patient group. It is easy to see how such a phenomenon would occur if one understands the staff to be functioning as a selfobject matrix. In order to avoid this, a high premium must be placed on openness of communication about the working alliances among the staff, which are necessary to maintain the selfobject matrix of the therapeutic community. This necessary interchange can be accomplished through specific scheduled opportunities for staff to meet to review the unit's functioning, and with specific and frequent opportunities for the members of the treatment team to meet and discuss individual patient treatment plans. Although staff often complain that time is at a premium and that such activities take away from necessary patient care activities, these structured meeting times actually provide a highly efficient way of monitoring intrastaff relationships and functioning and of resolving problems that come up in this area.

> On an inpatient unit with low staff turnover, the entire treatment staff were preoccupied by the pending resignation of two of the most senior (and most effective) nurses on the staff. Because of the significance of the loss of these two nurses, the rest of the staff was less available to attend to monitoring the emotional state of the patients, who were also reacting to the impending loss. During the week before the two nurses were to leave, there were several angry discharges against medical advice on the service. A review of the events in a succeeding staff meeting revealed that little attempt had been made to explore the reasons for the patients' requests to leave against medical advice. It was apparent that staff had been preoccupied by their own sense of loss and were less available to attend to the patients' needs. Airing these concerns in the staff meeting allowed staff members to step back from their own preoccupation somewhat. Although it did not resolve their distress over the impending nursing resignations, the opportunity for reflection allowed the staff to more adequately separate their own personal responses and needs from those of the patients. This fostered increased responsiveness to the

patients' requirements for emotional support during the difficult period of staff transition.

Although there are many factors that can influence staff cohesion, staff turnover is one of the most frequent stresses, particularly if the unit is a teaching service where trainees play important roles in the community but come and go at frequent intervals. Of particular importance during times of turnover is the interval following loss of important staff but prior to the integration of new members into the group. It is particularly important during these periods that staff have opportunities to discuss how the changes within their own group functioning play a role in their ability to function. Staff meetings should not be seen as a time for individual or group staff psychotherapy, but should be structured in such a way that staff have an opportunity to identify factors that are interfering with carrying out their normal functions within the therapeutic community.

Patient Group Cohesion

During a community meeting, attended by all members of the inpatient unit staff and patients, a preoccupation of the meeting revolved around the impending discharge of two patients who had played strong leadership roles on the unit. Patients expressed a strong sense of loss and anxiety about the future and their ability to be cared for on the unit. Several staff members responded to these concerns by attempting to reassure the patients that the staff were aware of the patient needs and would still be there to take care of them. However, these attempts at reassurance were unsuccessful. One of the staff members then talked about how the impending discharge of the two patients had precipitated the feelings of sadness and anxiety in the patients. The staff member noted that this loss was an important one and wondered how staff and patients could work together to deal with the feelings stimulated by the loss of these important members of the community. This comment was followed by an intense discussion of the important role that other patients played for each other in helping to get well.

Even though rapid patient turnover in a unit with a relatively short length of stay results in staff cohesion playing the more significant role in milieu function, the role of the patient group is still quite important, as the clinical example demonstrates. Staff must be aware that patient turn-over in a therapeutic community setting can have a potentially disruptive effect on one level of the selfobject matrix that is present in the community (i.e., the role that patients play for each other in helping provide support in the service of increased self-regulatory capacity). When the length of stay of patients is relatively longer, the importance of the patient group in the selfobject matrix becomes more important, because individual patients in the group tend to be a more stable part of the environment.

Because of the short lengths of stay now prevalent in inpatient treatment, the original intent of the democratization principle in therapeutic communities, which was to allow patients significant roles in decision making about treatment progress of other patients, can no longer be easily applied. However, it is important not to ignore the utility of the role that the patients still play for one another in functioning as part of the stabilizing selfobject matrix on the inpatient unit. One of the benefits of specialized inpatient services (e.g., services for individuals with eating disorders or substance abuse or for special populations, such as a geriatric unit) is the enhanced cohesion of the patient group because of easier identification with each other. The success of such specialized inpatient programs fails to support the traditional conventional wisdom and theory. The old view held that when there are too many patients with the same pathology, they merely reinforce each others' pathological adaptation.

As individual patients progress in treatment and are able to function at higher levels of adaptation, their importance in the selfobject matrix increases. As in the clinical example, when well-functioning patients are discharged, there may be a temporary disruption in the patient subgroup. The traditional therapeutic community concepts of sharing responsibilities and encouraging all patients to play important roles in community governance are attempts to address this issue and to avoid disruptions in the patient subgroup following the loss of important members. It is essential that staff recognize the role patients play for one another as part of the overall therapeutic community matrix. As well as attending to the relationships between staff, the unit must be structured in a way that can provide regular opportunities to resolve concerns among patients. Staff often must play a mediator role, because severely disturbed patients may not have the capacity to negotiate solutions to interpersonal problems on their own.

At times, the patient group cohesion is threatened not only by discharge of important patients but by the admission of individuals who are particularly difficult to interact with not only for staff, but for other patients as well. Although reviewing the specific treatment issues in these types of patients is beyond the scope of our discussion, it is important to recognize that patients who have significant paranoid delusions may stir fear among the other patients because of worries about potential violent behavior from the paranoid patient. In addition, severely suicidal patients, highly manipulative patients such as those with severe borderline or antisocial disorders, patients with significant medical illness, and any other patient who may be identified by patients or staff as "special" may exert disruptive influences within patient group and milieu cohesion.

Given that lengths of stay are so short, patients must often be given specific guidance in how to deal with one another. This requires a modification of the principle of permissiveness. Because of the leisurely pace in traditional therapeutic communities, patients were more often taught the value of patience and tolerance of difficult interpersonal relations rather than assisted in developing concrete and immediate strategies for interacting with severely disturbed or disturbing patients. Originally, permissiveness emphasized individual rights and freedom of expression. The constraints of brief lengths of stay mean that greater limits must be placed on this than were originally envisioned in a therapeutic community. However, it is still possible to identify behaviors as unacceptable without labeling the patient who has those behaviors as an unacceptable member of the milieu. Staff must serve as role models for patients in dealing with these situations with difficult patients. There is also a need to modify the original principle of reality confrontation. Rather than allowing confrontation about any and all aspects of behavior to be fair game for discussion, staff and patients need to know what appropriate limits are when dealing with very disturbed or disturbing individuals. Once again, the value of good staff communication and decision making in this area will allow for smoother functioning within the milieu.

Role of the Leader and Staff Training

In addition to the typical and traditional roles of supervising individuals and providing consultation around patient care, the leader of the unit must also include, as an appropriate part of his or her role, the monitoring of the cohesive functioning of the staff within the selfobject matrix of the therapeutic community. The unit director must also model the type of communication and decision making that is felt to be optimal.

> Over a weekend, illicit drugs were found in one of the patient's rooms on the unit. The staff organized a unit search that did not reveal the presence of any other illicit substances on the unit. This was followed by an emergency community meeting that all patients and staff working at the time attended. The discovery of the drugs was discussed, with a review of the negative impact on individual patient treatment and milieu functioning that this breach of the rules of the unit entailed. Staff were apparently satisfied that appropriate action had been taken.
>
> On Monday morning during the staff meeting, the staff demanded that the unit director schedule another emergency community meeting to review the events of the weekend. The unit director explored the reasons for this request but could find no rational basis for calling an emergency meeting. In spite of his concerns that staff would react angrily, the director declined to hold an emergency community meeting. The unit nursing staff reacted to this decision with strong expressions of anger and lack of support for the director. In a staff meeting the following week, these events were reviewed. The discussion revealed that staff were feeling underappreciated by the unit director and that the call for the community meeting was an attempt to have the unit director publicly affirm the appropriateness of the treatment decisions that the staff had made over the weekend.

This clinical example illustrates that an important aspect of the director's role is to attend to the appropriate needs for professional gratification and recognition among the staff, but not to act when the needs are being expressed inappropriately. Monitoring this is often difficult for the unit director, who must find a stance that models the type of decision making that is felt to be desirable for all of the staff. This stance of emotionally neutral inquiry into treatment planning and decision making and response to patient problems, while simultaneously allowing appropriate input from all members of the staff and recognition of their contributions, is often easier said than done. It may be helpful for the unit director to have weekly opportunities to discuss the unit's functioning with the senior colleague or consultant who may not be involved with day-to-day unit functioning. It is important that the director's own professional needs also be satisfied in the performance of his or her role (Leibenluft et al. 1989).

The staff training must also emphasize the perspective that the inpatient milieu supplies important selfobject needs of the patients. At times, this may be a source of conflict in staff who may have been taught that gratification of any patient needs is antitherapeutic. Helping staff to understand psychopathology from a self-deficit perspective will help foster understanding of how the milieu is functioning and will help staff appreciate the kinds of supportive structure that helps promote a return to self-cohesion within individual patients. To gratify the selfobject needs to help a severely decompensated individual gain increased self-regulation ability is often the most therapeutic aspect of the staff's intervention.

FACTORS INFLUENCING MILIEU COHESION

Clique Formation and Pairing

> During a community meeting, it was noted that two adolescent boys were talking quietly to each other throughout the meeting. Attempts by various other patients and members of the staff to ask them to share what they were discussing with the entire group were met with derision from the two boys. The unit director then commented that the two boys seemed to be getting something from each other that was important and beneficial. This was followed by several patients commenting on the important role other patients played in their own treatment and reflecting on the unavailability of staff at certain times of stress.

In the traditional therapeutic community, the presence of a subgroup, such as in this clinical example, was actively discouraged and viewed as a violation of the basic principle of communalism within the milieu. However, it can be seen that such a response can fail to address the underlying motivation for such behavior. Clique formation among patients may be viewed as a reflection of inadequate large-group cohesion. The emergence of a clique may reflect an attempt to adapt to decreased selfobject responsiveness in the milieu by forming a smaller "mutual therapy group" (Caudill et al. 1952). Thus, rather than focusing interventions on directly discouraging clique formation, the presence of this behavior must be seen as reflecting disruptions in the larger selfobject matrix and addressed on this level.

The intense, close relationship between two or more patients within a clique on an inpatient unit can be seen as reflecting their experience of being similar and having a special ability to empathically respond to one another's needs. This experience can be therapeutic in certain instances when this phenomenon is reparative for the decompensated individual patient. For example, adolescents on inpatient services will often band together in pairs or small groups, share a great deal of information about themselves, and provide strong support to one another. In a traditional therapeutic community approach, this behavior would be seen as a violation of the need for sharing among the entire patient group—the principle of communalism. The process would be discouraged rather than empathically understood as an important part of the reestablishment of self-cohesion of the individuals involved. The unit director's comments about this phenomenon in the case example allowed for a nonpejorative understanding and attention to this process. This awareness fostered further ability to address sources of stress within the community.

Although pairing or clique formation may be helpful not only for adolescents but also for any subgroup of patients, it is important that staff continually monitor the effect of the clique on the milieu. The benefits to the individual patients involved must be weighed against the potential disruptive effect to the overall milieu functioning. When the balance tilts toward greater disruption, staff must intervene in an empathic but firm way to encourage greater participation in the overall milieu.

Idealization of the Staff

In an individual therapy session with a severely suicidal borderline patient, the patient expressed to a staff member that the staff member was the best therapist the patient had ever come across. The patient was highly complimentary of the staff member's abilities to be helpful. The staff member felt uncomfortable with these overly effusive comments and averred that, although no one could possibly live up to those high expectations, the staff member was more than willing to work with the patient to try to help solve the problems leading to the patient's hospitalization. This was met by an angry response from the patient, who stormed out of the room, leaving the staff member somewhat bewildered.

Hospitalized patients often idealize staff members, particularly during times of decompensation or when the usual selfobject supports are less available. Traditionally, the therapeutic community credo of reality confrontation would discourage such feelings with a response that every member of the community is important and equal and thus shares responsibility for helping individuals deal with their problems and then leave the hospital.

One of the basic mechanisms underlying idealization is the projection of a primitive grandiose perception of the self onto others, who are then experienced as all-protective of the self. This phenomenon may occur particularly during times when the patient is decompensated and in need of an individual to play this role. It can be seen that responses to such idealization that minimize its importance or only discourage such expressions may be experienced as anxiety provoking rather than soothing or therapeutic. It is important to accept the patient's need for an idealized caretaker, especially because there may be some reality basis in a patient who has lost significant capacity for self-regulation.

Staff must accept *some* responsibility for caretaking, while recognizing at the same time that the idealization represents a need that cannot possibly be completely gratified. Staff members often experience anxiety, anger, and frustration when they try to live up to the patient's idealization; this inevitably leads to disappointment in themselves. Part of the staff's role in situations such as this involves recognizing that they are playing a balancing role between providing needed self-regulatory functions for the patient, while at the same time encouraging the gradual development of more autonomous function in the patient. Looking toward an idealized other involves a process of inevitable disappointment, with resultant emotional upset. Staff members must recognize that an important part of their role lies not in either taking away the patient's need to idealize another or in trying to gratify the idealization, but in helping the patient deal with the disappointment that inevitably must occur. It is important not only to help the patient gain an appreciation that the staff member can provide assistance, but also to help the patient understand that the ultimate aim of this assistance is to enable him or her to provide the functions that may at the time be experienced as only available from the staff member.

Seclusion and Restraint

> During a community meeting, the patients angrily confronted the staff about a recent seclusion of an agitated patient. Staff members were somewhat mystified by this response, because the patient who had been placed in seclusion had been very disruptive on the unit. Attempts by the staff to discuss the seclusion as a response to the patient's disruption of the community were met with little support from the patients, who believed the staff members were acting punitively.

No aspects of hospital care stir stronger responses in a therapeutic community in both patients and staff than the use of seclusion or restraint (American Psychiatric Association 1985). Patients often respond as if these aspects of treatment are expressions of staff hostility and punitive intent, even though the staff may view these interventions as valuable ways of helping patients regain control. It can be seen that helping to reestablish behavioral control, or regulate stimulus input, may be important aspects of selfobject functioning that staff may utilize for severely decompensated patients.

However, it is not enough for staff to be aware of patient fears of the staff's response. Another underlying aspect of patients' response to an individual who is placed in seclusion and restraints often involves an intuitive but not quite conscious recognition that the other patient has lost control. This stirs anxiety and concerns in other patients, who often are struggling with similar difficulties regarding maintaining control or fearing loss of control. Therefore, it is important to recognize that although the patients may only be commenting on the aspect of the event related to the staff's intervention, they are also responding to the phenomenon of loss of control in the individual patient. At times, the anxiety precipitated is so great in particularly vulnerable patients that they may lose control themselves and require seclusion as well. When seclusion of an individual on a unit occurs, it is often helpful to discuss this as soon after the event as possible with the other patients on the unit. It is particularly important to allow for discussion of the experience of seeing another patient being out of control and the fears that this arouses in the other patients. Clear messages should be given by staff members to these patients that any anxieties or concerns the patients may have about loss of control can be openly discussed with the staff, either in the group or individually.

Structure, Limit Testing, and Acting Out

A hostile, hypomanic young man angrily demanded to sign out against medical advice. The primary therapist attempted to explore the patient's concerns in a quiet setting, but the patient would not leave the nursing station and angrily demanded an immediate release from the unit. The staff member assessed that the patient could not be held against his will and acceded to his request to sign out of the hospital. It was soon noticed that the tension level on the unit had significantly increased.

On another unit, it had been noted for several days that there was increased symptomatology and agitation among many of the patients. However, what was causing this could not be discerned. It was later discovered that two patients had been having sexual encounters late at night when few staff were on the unit. Once the situation was aired and the prohibitions against such behavior were openly discussed in the community meeting, the agitation and increased symptomatology on the unit abated.

A suicidal patient had been placed on precautions by the staff, which involved 15-minute checks. The patient had been discussing his suicidal intent openly among the patients, so they were well aware of his status. At 8:00 P.M., immediately following his staff contact, the patient attempted to suffocate himself by placing a plastic bag over his head. The staff member responsible for performing the checks returned to the patient's room earlier than expected and found the patient had apparently suffocated. A code blue was called. The patient was successfully resuscitated and transferred to the intensive care unit. Later that evening, several other patients approached the staff with strong concerns that they would harm themselves.

Although each of these situations involves a different set of clinical concerns, the common thread among all of them involves a patient's inability to keep from acting on impulses that may not be in his or her best interest, and the inability of staff to respond adequately to prevent this. However, each of these clinical situations also involves the need for an immediate active response by staff to the patient.

Though it is beyond our discussion to provide specific details on how to address each of these situations, several general principles can be outlined. In each case (and in other cases, such as elopement from the unit), patients behave in ways that are beyond the limits imposed by the structure and treatment guidelines on the unit. In a traditional therapeutic community, the principle of permissiveness was at times interpreted as a lack of need to adhere strictly to community rules or standards of behavior. This, however, was not the intent of this principle. Tolerance of another's behavior without rejection is not the same as absence of behavioral standards. Especially on units with brief lengths of stay, there is inadequate time to discuss all of the motivations that underlie a particular form of rule testing or acting out before a staff member needs to respond. Staff are often placed in a position in which concrete rapid interventions must be made, especially in situations where patient safety is at stake.

It is also important to recognize that in these emergency situations, the "holding" capacity of the selfobject matrix of the therapeutic community is inadequate to help the individual patient regulate his or her behavior. Often at these times, extraordinary measures must be taken to prevent either distress in the milieu or harm to individual patients. In these situations, staff time and attention is appropriately directed to resolution of the acute problem, often while temporarily directing attention away from usual responsiveness to the other patients in the milieu. Although such responses in the staff are appropriate and necessary, it is also important to recognize the impact of such responses on the other patients. It is clear that although the other patients on the unit will often be reassured by the concrete evidence of the staff's ability to respond to difficult emergency situations, they may also experience a loss of control, related both to the stimulation from the other patients' behavior as well as from the direction of staff attention away from the other patients. This lack of attention may be experienced by the other patients as a loss of the cohesion-maintaining matrix of the community.

Once the specific crisis is responded to appropriately, it is important to assess its impact on the other patients and to respond to it within group or individual sessions. In addition, further exploration with the individual patient who lost control may be helpful to discern ways in which the staff and other patients can provide greater self-regulatory help to the distressed individual.

However, it is important to reemphasize that the rules and structure of the program play a significant role in providing a stable environment within which decompensated patients can regain self-regulatory capacities. Patients will often test limits and respond in a hurt or angry way when staff do not give in to demands. It is important at such moments that staff not react angrily or punitively to the patients, but attempt to explore with them whether some aspect of self-dysregulation may be causing the acting-out or limit-testing behavior. This stance is especially important with patients who may be particularly problematic management problems (i.e., patients with medical illness or those with borderline disorders), who by the nature of their problems require a greater amount of staff attention than might usually be deemed appropriate.

SUMMARY

Although many forces impinge on the clinician's ability to utilize traditional therapeutic community principles, attention to the milieu still has an essential place in brief hospital treatment. This discussion has emphasized the ways in which a milieu can play an important role in providing self-regulation for patients who have lost the ability to regulate their own affects or interpersonal interactions. The nature of the patient population and the recent changes in focus of inpatient treatment require that the original principles of a therapeutic community—democratization, permissiveness, communalism, and reality confrontation—be modified. This discussion has outlined a way in which these principles can be modified to take into account the changing role of hospitalization in a system that increasingly emphasizes continuity of care and decreased lengths of hospital stay.

Although this chapter focuses on certain aspects of staff responsiveness based on principles of self psychology, this is not the only way that a therapeutic community can be structured to provide a cohesive, selfobject matrix. The principles of self psychology do provide a valuable framework for understanding staff roles and interventions as part of an overall treatment approach in brief hospitalization; some units are also structuring a therapeutic community based on principles of cognitive-behavioral theory and therapy. Whatever model is used to structure the milieu, a key aspect of its success involves continued monitoring of the milieu's functioning by the unit leadership and staff. Attention to these aspects of the inpatient experience will maximize the benefit to the patients from the milieu aspect of hospitalization.

REFERENCES

American Psychiatric Association: Task Force Report on Seclusion and Restraint. Washington, DC, American Psychiatric Association, 1985

Berke JH: Arriving, settling-in, settling-down, leaving and following-up: stages of stay at the Arbours Centre. Br J Med Psychol 60:181–188, 1987

Burkitt PA: The concept of a therapeutic community. Nursing Times, January 9, 1975, pp 75–78

Caudill W, Redlich FC, Gilmor HR, et al: Social structure and interaction processes on a psychiatric ward. Am J Orthopsychiatry 22:314–334, 1952

Clark DH: The therapeutic community. Br J Psychiatry 131:553–564, 1977

Fort JP: Milieu therapy. National Association of Private Psychiatric Hospitals Journal 10(3):12–16, 1979

Freudenberger HJ: The issues of staff burnout in therapeutic communities. J Psychoactive Drugs 18(3):247–251, 1986

Gutheil TG: The therapeutic milieu: changing themes and theories. Hosp Community Psychiatry 36(12):1279–1285, 1985

Islam A, Turner DL: The therapeutic community: a critical reappraisal. Hosp Community Psychiatry 33(8):651–653, 1982

Johnson JM, Parker KE: Some antitherapeutic effects of a therapeutic community. Hosp Community Psychiatry 28(6):436–440, 1977

Jones M, Baker A, Freeman T, et al: The Therapeutic Community: A New Treatment Method in Psychiatry. New York, Basic Books, 1953

Kahn EM, White EM: Adapting milieu approaches to acute inpatient care for schizophrenic patients. Hosp Community Psychiatry 40(6):609–614, 1989

Karasu TB, Plutchik R, Conte HR, et al: The therapeutic community in theory and practice. Hosp Community Psychiatry 28(6):436–440, 1977

Karterud S: What are the prerequisites and indications of the therapeutic community proper? a comparative study. Acta Psychiatr Scand 77:658–669, 1988

Katz P, Kirkland FR: Violence and social structure on mental hospital wards. Psychiatry 53:262–277, 1990

Kernberg OF: The therapeutic community: a re-evaluation. National Association of Private Psychiatric Hospitals Journal 12(2):46–55, 1981

Kleespies PM: Hospital milieu treatment and optimal length of stay. Hosp Community Psychiatry 37(5):509–510, 1986

Kohut H: The Analysis of the Self. New York, International Universities Press, 1971

Kohut H: The Restoration of the Self. New York, International Universities Press, 1977

Lamb HR: Staff burnout in work with long-term patients. Hosp Community Psychiatry 30(6):396–398, 1979

Lehman A, Ritzler B: The therapeutic community inpatient ward: does it really work? Compr Psychiatry 17(6):755–761, 1976

Leibenluft E, Summergrad P, Tasman A: The academic dilemma of the inpatient unit director. Am J Psychiatry 146(1):73–76, 1989

Main TF: The hospital as a therapeutic institution. Bull Menninger Clin 10:66–70, 1946

Miskimins RW: A theoretical model for the practice of residential treatment. Adolescence 25(100):867–890, 1990

Moline RA: Hospital psychiatry in transition. Arch Gen Psychiatry 33:1234–1238, 1976

Oldham JM, Russakoff LM: The medical-therapeutic community. Journal of Psychiatric Treatment and Evaluation 4:337–343, 1982

Rosenthal MS: The therapeutic community: exploring the boundaries. Br J Addict 84:141–150, 1989

Sacks MH, Carpenter WT: The pseudotherapeutic community: an examination of antitherapeutic forces on psychiatric units. Hosp Community Psychiatry 25(5):315–318, 1974

Searles HF: Paranoid processes among members of the therapeutic team in psychotherapy in the designed therapeutic milieu. Edited by Eldrid SH, Vanderpol M. Boston, MA, Little, Brown, 1968, pp 95–113

Sorensen JL, Acampora A, Trier M, et al: From maintenance to abstinence in a therapeutic community: follow-up outcomes. J Psychoactive Drugs 19(4):345–351, 1987

Stanton AH, Schwartz MS: The Mental Hospital. New York, Basic Books, 1954

Stern DA, Fromm G, Sacksteder JL: From coercion to collaboration: two weeks in the life of a therapeutic community. Psychiatry 49:18–32, 1986

Strochak RD: Developing alternate models for long-term care: the "family model" and the therapeutic community. Am J Psychother 41(4):580–592, 1987

Tucker GJ, Maxmen JS: The practice of hospital psychiatry: a formulation. Am J Psychiatry 130(8):887–891, 1973

Yohay S: ACI: a therapeutic community. J Subst Abuse Treat 3:219–221, 1986

Yohay S, Winick C: AREBA-Casriel Institute: a third-generation therapeutic community. J Psychoactive Drugs 18(3):231–237, 1986

Integrating Somatic and Psychological Treatment in Inpatient Settings

Paul A. Silver, M.D.
Richard L. Goldberg, M.D.

INTRODUCTION

In recent years, the trend has been for most long-term, psychologically based treatment to be carried out in outpatient settings. Hospitalization is reserved for the most seriously ill, often in times of crisis. The majority of those hospitalized patients have a significant biological component to their illnesses and require pharmacotherapy. Nonetheless, even the most biologically based illnesses (e.g., bipolar disorder or schizophrenia) require concomitant psychological treatment if patients are to accrue full benefit. Consequently, combined psychological and pharmacological interventions are the mainstay of treatment for the typical inpatient (Klerman 1984), as illustrated by the following case.

> Charles D., a 41-year-old attorney with bipolar disorder, was hospitalized during his fifth manic episode in 3 years. His psychotic behavior had driven away many of his clients, caused estrangement from his family, and plunged him into debt. Over the first 10 days in the hospital, his

The authors would like to thank Stephen A. Green, M.D., and Rochelle Silver for their assistance in the preparation of this chapter.

hyperactivity, pressured speech, and grandiosity responded to lorazepam and lithium carbonate. Though his mania was not followed by a major depression, Mr. D. was greatly concerned and upset about the impact of his illness on his day-to-day life, and this became the focus of his individual and group psychotherapeutic work.

In recent years, providing such complete, multimodal treatment has been complicated by shortened lengths of stay and the pervasive influences of managed care and utilization review. In this chapter, we discuss the indications for integrating somatic and psychosocial treatments with inpatients and use case material to highlight the efficacy, as well as the difficulties, of this comprehensive treatment approach.

COMBINED TREATMENT

Though combining treatment modalities makes eminent sense, there had been much controversy as to whether pharmacotherapy and psychotherapy could be used effectively together (Karasu 1982; Klerman 1984; Rousaville et al. 1981). However, over the past two decades, clinical experience and widespread research have successfully argued for the utility of combining modalities (Conte et al. 1986; DiMascio et al. 1979; Klerman 1984; Rousaville et al. 1981).

EFFECTS OF SOMATIC TREATMENTS ON THE THERAPEUTIC RELATIONSHIP

Clinicians must be wary concerning some potential pitfalls of integrating psychotherapy and pharmacotherapy. Although concerns regarding gratification within the transference may have been somewhat overstated by certain psychoanalytic writers, clinicians must carefully attend to the patient's interpretation of receiving medication as well as to the process of prescribing. Some patients will view any sort of somatic treatment as an intrusion or invasion. Paranoid patients may experience the use of medication as evidence of a plot to harm or poison them. Such fears may be exacerbated with the onset of disturbing side effects, such as dystonia or akathisia, during treatment. Patients may view medication use as a loss of control or autonomy and will struggle for independence against it.

Upon being brought to the emergency room by the police, Howard A., a man diagnosed as having paranoid schizophrenia, was resistant to taking the antipsychotic offered him. The physician was able to calm him, and he eventually accepted a dose of haloperidol. Two hours later, he developed an acute dystonic reaction. Believing that the staff was intentionally trying to harm him with the medication, Mr. A. refused further doses.

Admission to the inpatient unit may provide an opportunity during which focused but intensive psychotherapeutic work can be undertaken. Pressures for shortened stays make it necessary to proceed expediently and to concentrate on those issues that prevented successful outpatient management.

Despite Ellie L.'s years of severe depression and her primary care physician's repeated recommendation that she take antidepressant medication, Ms. L. refused psychiatric treatment and eventually required admission after a suicide attempt. Through careful exploration, her psychiatrist was able to discern that this reluctance to enter treatment was part of her struggle against dependency needs. Accepting medication would mean that she would have to rely on the prescribing physician for her well-being. Ms. L. became willing to take medication and agreed to follow-up treatment upon discharge the week following admission.

For patients attempting to minimize the reality or seriousness of their illness, the administration of medication may confront their denial in a manner that causes considerable distress. Similarly, some patients view the need to take medication as a severe narcissistic injury. Our culture still views psychiatric distress as a moral failing, and the need for biological intervention is often seen as further condemnation that one is unable to overcome emotional difficulties exclusively by self-reliance. Families can also take part in this denial process and attempt to undermine treatment.

Donald F., a senior corporate executive, was initially puzzled when he developed symptoms of depression. For months he attempted to "pull [himself] out of this rut." It was with reluctance that he finally consulted a psychiatrist. Mr. F.'s hope was that the psychiatrist would tell him that his mood disturbance was transient and would soon improve. But he became enraged, and then even more depressed, when the physician told Mr. F. that he had a major depression and would require treatment with antidepressant medication. The onset of suicidal ideation led to admission. Exploration revealed that Mr. F. was shaken by the thought that he had an illness and was therefore vulnerable. The recommendation of medication reinforced the idea that the malady was beyond his direct control.

The administration of medication can gratify and stimulate dependency needs of some patients, causing them to develop the belief that the therapist is an omnipotent force who can produce magical effects. Other patients will view the medication as a transitional object connecting them with the therapist.

During one of his several admissions, Jack D., a 45-year-old man with schizophrenia, developed a psychotic transference to the treating psychiatric resident. He became convinced that the medication prescribed by the resident would cure him of his disease and would completely protect him against "the fates." Mr. D. continued to comply with the medication after discharge, and he resisted any attempt to modify "[his] doctor's" regime.

The potential benefits and facilitating effects of mediation far outweigh the risks. As with any intervention or act on the part of therapist in a psychotherapeutic relationship, the symbolic meaning that patients attribute to this activity, reflected in transference reactions, must be constantly monitored and dealt with. Conversely, the physician must ensure that he or she does not prescribe medication as a form of acting out his or her countertransference. For example, some therapists utilize medication as an attempt to either overtly nurture or control the patient. This is particularly true if the patient's lack of response to psychotherapeutic intervention results in a narcissistic injury to the therapist. Main (1957) has even raised the spectre of sadistic acting-out behavior toward frustrating patients. It is possible that this sadism may take the form of inappropriate prescription of medication.

Yale S., a young man with antisocial personality disorder, was admitted to the inpatient unit after a trivial overdose. He had no signs of psychosis or depression, but he had just been thrown out of his boarding home and had no place to stay. Mr. S. engaged in a variety of provocative behaviors on the unit that led the staff to insist that the physician do something to control him. Large doses of a high potency antipsychotic were ordered, which resulted in Mr. S. developing severe akathisia and extrapyramidal side effects. In response to requests that his medication be reduced, Mr. S. was told that no change in medication would be made until his acting-out behavior ceased.

The patient's response to medication may provoke other countertransference reactions. Just as lack of improvement from psychotherapy can evoke anger and frustration in the therapist, so can a lack of a favorable medication response, particularly in conjunction with pronounced side effects. Noncompliance by a patient can also provoke an destructive countertransference, unless the therapist appropriately views such behavior as a resistance to treatment that requires active interpretation and/or limit setting. A patient's repeated complaints about side effects can evoke similar feelings of anger or hopelessness in the therapist. In these ways, the use of medication may provide an arena for projective identification, as the patient's angry, helpless, and hopeless feelings are induced in the therapist, who must then guard against subsequent antitherapeutic reactions.

Thus, the clinician must be carefully attuned to the transferential implications of the prescription of medication, as well as countertransference motivations. The indications for pharmacotherapy must be carefully assessed, particularly as to their *medical* need. Similarly, an untoward reaction must be carefully evaluated, so that physical phenomena are not misinterpreted as psychological in origin, or vice versa—circumstances that do great damage to the patient and the therapeutic alliance.

Despite the unfortunate current schism between biological and psychodynamic psychiatry, it is imperative that all psychiatrists have some common skills in order to best serve their patients. The effective pharmacotherapist must have a working knowledge of psychodynamics so as to address the issues outlined previously, whereas psychiatrists primarily engaged in psychotherapeutic work must know when medication is indicated and how to monitor the effects of a wide spectrum of psychoactive agents—even if their patients are referred to psychopharmacologists for the actual prescriptions. One would hope that a psychopharmacologist would at least have the skills in the psychosocial aspects of care expected of a competent primary care nonpsychiatric physician, and a psychiatrist-psychotherapist the pharmacologic knowledge of a sophisticated psychologist. That some specialized psychiatrists devalue the worth of the knowledge and techniques outside their purview, and then pass these prejudices on to their trainees, does harm to our field as well as to our patients.

However, having sufficient knowledge is not enough. One must constantly move between different therapeutic models to intelligently and competently treat patients. In the process of prescribing medication and checking side effects, it is difficult to simultaneously engage in the listening and free-floating attention required of a psychotherapist. Conversely, it may be difficult for the clinician during a therapy hour to switch gears and concretely explore such issues as compliance, side effects, and therapeutic efficacy. It is important to structure therapy sessions and ward rounds in such a way that both areas can be surveyed, though the techniques of inquiry may actually be similar. Good physicians in all specialties recognize that they get much more clinical data when they question patients in a nondirective, open-ended manner as opposed to asking questions with a limited focus and scope. Being open to both biological and psychological explanations for any given statement by the patient, while constantly and vigilantly monitoring transferential and countertransferential phenomena, is the key to effectively combining biologic and psychosocial treatment interventions.

During morning rounds, Karl E., who had chronic schizophrenia, informed the treatment team that he was not feeling well. The resident physician took a detailed medical history, which included a review of a list of potential medication side effects, but was unable to determine the cause of Mr. E.'s complaints. Later that day, a member of the nursing staff asked Mr. E. what was bothering him without asking specific questions. He soon related that he was upset and anxious because his family had not come to visit over the weekend. He was afraid that they were going to abandon him in the hospital.

Problem Areas and Their Treatment

Just as the use of appropriate pharmacotherapy can enhance the psycho-therapeutic process, psychotherapy can augment the effects of psychoactive medication. The most carefully chosen medication has no effect if the patient fails to take it, and noncompliance significantly contributes to psychiatric morbidity—25%–50% of patients treated for affective disorders fail to take their medications as prescribed (Prien and Caffey 1977). By engaging the patient in psychotherapy, forming an alliance, and identifying and working with resistances to treatment, the clinician can greatly increase medication compliance and, therefore, the efficacy of treatment. This is particularly important, because the benefits of many psychotropic medications often begin well after the patient has experienced unpleasant (and at times severe) side effects. An effective alliance between therapist and patient can help sustain the treatment during this interval and facilitate medication compliance. This is particularly important when medication is started when the patient is in the hospital, because the patient is often discharged before the medication has taken its full effect.

> Alan Y., a young man with an acute exacerbation of his schizophrenic illness, was admitted by his outpatient physician of 3 years. Increasing his high-potency antipsychotic precipitated severe extrapyramidal side effects, and there was growing concern about his worsening tardive dyskinesia. Mr. Y. asked to have his medication stopped and to be discharged. His longtime physician was able to convince him to remain in hospital, and a switch to clozapine was initiated. Because of his solid relationship with the outpatient psychiatrist, Mr. Y. was able to be discharged while his medication was being adjusted and remained compliant throughout the transition, despite some new side effects.

Families are often overtly and covertly resistant to the notion of relatives having a psychiatric illness; consequently, they will frequently attempt to sabotage treatment, including pharmacotherapy. By engaging those families in the medication process, they can be enlisted in supporting treatment rather than undermining it.

> Albert N., a 26-year-old man with chronic schizophrenia, required repeated hospitalizations, largely because of medication noncompliance.

Though distressed by his dysfunction, his family was resistant to the notion that Mr. N. had a severe mental illness. During his last hospitalization, the N.s became involved in a group on the inpatient unit and gained a better understanding of their relative's illness and ongoing need for treatment, including pharmacotherapy. As the family began to help Mr. N. with his medication regimen, his compliance improved and his decompensations became less frequent.

As noted previously, it is important to carefully explore reasons for noncompliance or adverse effects. Medication noncompliance may be due to the patient's resistance in the classic psychodynamic sense of the word, as well as lack of support by the family, reaction to the stigmatization of needing psychotropic medication, or organic impairment that leads to forgetting dosages (Sarti and Cournos 1990). Certainly a high level of adverse effects can contribute to noncompliance, but the clinician must ascertain whether the patient is truly having severe side effects or merely magnifying unpleasant symptoms as a form of resistance or acting out. Because it is sometimes difficult to accurately assess the motivations for a patient's complaints, careful exploration of all reported side effects is warranted but must be taken in the context of the patient's overall psychodynamics.

Admitted to the hospital for severe depression, Bertram P. was a 69-year-old man who had resisted his outpatient therapist's attempts to start him on an antidepressant. He would forget to take his medication, alter or reduce the dose, or only take it on an as-needed basis. When he did take it, he complained that it would slow him down to the point that he could hardly function. In helping Mr. P. explore the issue of medication, the inpatient staff made several important discoveries. These included Mr. P.'s memory of his father's starting to take cardiac medication and his observation that his father seemed to then rapidly age—indeed, his father died within 2 years of beginning the medication. Mr. P. expressed fears that this was the beginning of a similar decline for him. In addition, he had mild dementia and had difficulty understanding how to take the antidepressant properly. He believed that, like an analgesic, the antidepressant could be taken when he felt the worst and he could adjust the dose to achieve the desired effect. Mrs. P. was very concerned about her husband's depression, but because she did not know that he was being prescribed medication, she was unable to help monitor his regimen and encourage compliance.

Staff interventions included an exploration of the meaning of being medicated in regard to Mr. P.'s memories of his father. Staff met with Mr. and Mrs. P. to inform them about the antidepressant's proper use. The couple was also invited to attend the medication group. Strategies for reminding Mr. P. to take his medication were developed and implemented while he was still on the unit. Once-a-day dosing at bedtime was utilized so that Mrs. P. would be home to remind her husband to take his pills as well as to reduce daytime sedation. These strategies were markedly effective, according to the outpatient psychiatrist, leading to good compliance and the sustained remission of Mr. P.'s depression.

The therapist must always be willing to explore his or her own psychological issues when patients complain about medication. Minimizing such reports may reflect countertransferential indifference or anger. To indulge in polypharmacy, when a patient reports minimal therapeutic effectiveness, may reflect similar issues. Because psychopharmacology is, as yet, an inexact science, it is important for therapist, patient, and family to reach some general consensus as to an appropriate treatment regimen. The family must be supportive, and at times assertive, in encouraging the patient's compliance. The treating clinician must be willing to compromise and negotiate in regard to medication, as well as to set firm limits when warranted. This is particularly important when the patient has a history of abusing any type of medication or substance—another form of treatment noncompliance.

After her admission for suicidal ideation, Helen F. began complaining bitterly about insomnia and demanded something to help her sleep. Because she had other symptoms of major depression, a tricyclic antidepressant was prescribed; however, her requests for sleeping medication continued. In discussions with previous care providers and family members, the ward staff discovered Ms. F.'s significant history of substance abuse. Ms. F. was confronted with this information and told that she was not going to be started on a sedative. She agreed to be switched to a more sedating antidepressant and to wait for its therapeutic benefits regarding her insomnia. When her depression resolved, Ms. F. resumed her complaints of insomnia, though it was the staff's observation that she slept through the night. When she saw that sedatives were not forthcoming, she threatened to leave the hospital against medical advice. The treatment team determined that Ms. F. was not an immediate threat to herself or others and therefore did not attempt to commit her. She was discharged against medical advice; however, the reasonable and comprehensive assessment of Ms. F.'s insomnia had provided some insight into her addictive patterns, while simultaneously preventing the continuation of that behavior in the hospital.

Because the majority of major psychiatric illnesses have such a significant biological component, it is virtually impossible to resolve symptoms by psychotherapy alone. It is therefore a disservice to patients if they are made to feel like failures when they are unable to overcome severe depression or psychosis solely through the use of psychotherapy. By educating patients regarding the biological nature of many of these illnesses, and by helping them understand that pharmacotherapy should not be viewed as a treatment of last resort, clinicians can decrease the stigma of patients who feel like moral or psychological failures for being unable to resolve what is essentially a medical illness through nonmedical means.

Kathleen H., a 39-year-old business executive, was admitted to the hospital after taking an overdose of over-the-counter sleeping pills. She had experienced increasing depression for the previous 6 months and eventually sought treatment from a psychiatrist. Although her therapist had urged Ms. H. to consider pharmacotherapy for a month prior to admission, she resisted, believing that her continued depression was evidence of a lack of willpower. The suicide attempt was a reflection of her sense of failure and hopelessness. Once on the inpatient unit, the staff and other patients helped Ms. H. understand that, despite her efforts, her depression was primarily biological and would not resolve without medication. Learning from the experience of other patients who had shared Ms. H.'s prejudices against pharmacotherapy, she ultimately accepted and benefited from the medication.

Electroconvulsive therapy (ECT) carries an even greater sense of stigma than pharmacotherapy. Most patients have some experience taking medication; but ECT is poorly understood by most laypersons, and frequently surrounded by controversy promoted by its stereotypic image as a punitive, archaic treatment. Even for the patient knowledgeable about ECT, a recommendation for its use often evokes feelings of despair based on the belief that his or her condition is so severe it requires the use of what is perceived as an extraordinary treatment. There is also concern about long-term effects of ECT, such as memory loss. It is therefore imperative that a recommendation for ECT be accompanied by a detailed explanation of the procedure, including its technical aspects, and a discussion of the risk-benefit analysis. The patient's knowledge and feelings about ECT must be thoroughly explored. Stereotypes must be corrected via education, and the evoked dynamic issues must be worked through. Family members and significant others should be involved in this process. ECT, an extraordinarily effective, safe treatment for properly selected patients, is unfortunately underutilized because of the widespread prejudices against it that are not properly addressed in psychotherapy.

On some psychiatric units, the primary task of the psychiatrist is medical management, whereas much of the psychotherapy is done by nonphysicians. This division of responsibility, compounded by differences in professional training, necessitates careful coordination between disciplines. Lacking that attention to the treatment, the milieu is ripe for the development of splitting. A borderline patient may engage the nonphysician therapist as a good object who is nurturing and empathic, while casting the psychiatrist in the role of the cold, uncaring scientist who does nothing but "push drugs." Conversely, the physician may be seen as the omnipotent provider of magical cures, whereas those trying to work psychotherapeutically with a patient are seen as intrusive and demanding in their desire for the patient to actively engage in therapy.

Sally B. was a 54-year-old woman admitted to the psychiatric unit because her depression was not responding to outpatient treatment. Dr. Z., her psychiatrist, sensed that certain emotional issues were impeding her progress. However, he was unable to elicit them largely because of Ms. B.'s idealization of him, which made it difficult for her to discuss embarrassing material. Dr. Z. hoped that Ms. B.'s contact with various staff members might enable her to find one with whom she would be more willing to share this information. However, once on the unit, Ms. B. announced that her admission was only for an adjustment of medication, and she informed the staff that they had no business prying into personal matters that she only discussed with her therapist. Ms. B. refused to go to groups or engage in meaningful conversations with any of the staff, many of whom were unaware of Dr. Z.'s primary goal for hospitalization. As a result, several staff members were annoyed at Dr. Z. for allegedly telling Ms. B. that she did not have to participate in the unit program. When the situation was discussed at the next interdisciplinary team meeting, a coordinated treatment plan was developed and presented to Ms. B. by Dr. Z. and Ms. B.'s primary nurse.

Effective intrastaff communication has always been essential to optimize the therapeutic efficacy of an inpatient unit (Stanton and Schwartz 1954). As the orientation and goals of inpatient treatment have changed in recent years, due in large measure to greater reliance on biological treatments, such communication has taken on a broader dimension. Attention to patients' psychodynamics must be supplemented by the physician's clear understanding of the need for medication and careful assessment of the patient's medication response. Nonmedical staff must keep the physician apprised of what feelings the patient discusses regarding pharmacotherapy, and their perception of the psychological impact of the biological treatment. In addition to benefiting the patient, this collaboration provides all involved the opportunity to learn about other therapeutic approaches, ultimately enabling the staff to provide more comprehensive, integrated treatment.

McHugh (1988) wrote of the need for psychiatry to start basing treatments on a complete understanding of the pathogenesis of patients' disorders, rather than along the lines of personal theoretical persuasions. The evidence for the need to combine pharmacologic and psychotherapeutic modalities is compelling. To routinely use one to the exclusion of the other is clearly inconsistent with good medical practice. The multidisciplinary structure of most modern inpatient units makes them particularly well suited to provide such multimodal care. However, to do so effectively requires mutual respect and close collaboration between disciplines. Successful integration of biological and psychosocial treatment modalities can then lead to

an understanding of the differences among the patients we see and eventually an appreciation of the varieties of etiology and mechanism found in different psychiatric disorders. We can expect to realize preventive strategies and effective therapies based on this knowledge. But fundamentally, we can anticipate the emergence of a psychiatry identified by its subject matter, unified in its conceptual base, and no longer subdivided into camps with different "orientations." (McHugh 1988, p. 918)

REFERENCES

Conte HR, Plutchik R, Wild KU, et al: Combined psychotherapy and pharmacotherapy for depression. Arch Gen Psychiatry 43:471–479, 1986

DiMascio A, Weissman MM, Prusoff BA, et al: Differential symptom reduction by drugs and psychotherapy in acute depression. Arch Gen Psychiatry 36:1450–1456, 1979

Karasu TB: Psychotherapy and pharmacotherapy: toward an integrative model. Am J Psychiatry 139:1102–1113, 1982

Klerman GL: Ideological conflicts in combined treatment, in Combining Psychotherapy and Drug Therapy in Clinical Practice. Edited by Beitman BD, Klerman GL. New York, Spectrum Publications, 1984, pp 17–34

Main TF: The ailment. Br J Med Psychol 30:129–145, 1957

McHugh PR: William Osler and the new psychiatry. Ann Intern Med 107:914–918, 1988

Prien RF, Caffey EM: Long term maintenance drug therapy in recurrent affective illness: current status and issues. Diseases of the Nervous System 38:981–992, 1977

Rousaville BJ, Klerman GL, Weissman MM: Do psychotherapy and pharmacotherapy conflict? Arch Gen Psychiatry 38:24–29, 1981

Sarti P, Cournos F: Medication and psychotherapy in the treatment of chronic schizophrenia. Psychiatr Clin North Am 13:215–228, 1990

Stanton AH, Schwartz MS: The Mental Hospital: A Study of Institutional Participation in Psychiatric Illness and Treatment. New York, Basic Books, 1954

CHAPTER 3

Individual Psychodynamic Psychotherapy

Gerald Adler, M.D.

INTRODUCTION

Is psychotherapy possible on the short-term inpatient unit? The pressures to maintain a limited length of stay may not be conducive to thinking about a model of treatment that includes individual psychodynamic psychotherapy. This may be especially true on a unit that stresses a thorough biological and neuropsychiatric evaluation of the patient, where the staff may not utilize a framework that includes a dynamic psychotherapeutic approach. Or, if it does, the "psychotherapy" might consist of little more than a therapist meeting with the patient from the outset without a clear definition or formulation of the work to be done.

In addition, the structuring of individual psychodynamic psychotherapy on the short-term inpatient unit poses complex problems that never affect a therapist working in an outpatient setting. The inpatient therapist is not in a position to define and implement a psychotherapeutic plan on his or her own. Instead, he or she is a member of a multidisciplinary team consisting of individuals who often have different orientations in approaching the patient. The therapist's work must therefore be that of a team member who coordinates the individual psychotherapy in conjunction with the rest of the unit's professional staff. In addition to the problems that can arise in the negotiation of this aspect of the treatment, the therapist may also be faced with complex patient and staff interactions, as inevitable transference/countertransference issues appear and sometimes

39

are acted out with staff members. This is particularly true in work with certain patients (e.g., borderline and narcissistic personality disorders).

I believe it is possible to do extremely useful individual psychodynamic psychotherapy on the short-term inpatient unit if the therapist and the unit clearly define what they mean by psychotherapy and then clarify its importance to the patient, family, and the entire treatment team. If all parties understand that individual psychodynamic psychotherapy is part of a process that begins with a thorough biopsychosocial evaluation and includes a careful psychodynamic formulation, then they are in a position to use those data to benefit the patient, as well as many of the significant others in his or her life. The evaluation and formulation can then be used by the individual therapist to define the major sector or sectors of the patient's psychological difficulties that led to the hospitalization. This can facilitate significant therapeutic work even on a short-term inpatient unit, on issues responsible for the patient's current problems. If the short-term stay does not permit sufficient work on that sector, the therapist and treatment team can feel satisfied that they have effectively utilized the unit to accomplish the most important beginning aspect of individual psychodynamic psychotherapy: the careful evaluation and psychodynamic formulation of the patient's (and family's) difficulties.

In this chapter, I describe a model in which the unit (which may be a teaching unit) has total responsibility for the evaluation and treatment of the patient, while working collaboratively with the outpatient therapist. Although it differs from one in which the outpatient therapist has admitting privileges and can be largely therapeutically and administratively responsible for the patient on the inpatient unit, the basic principles to be presented are the same. However, the unit structure will differ when a unit chief has to work tactfully with an attending who is also the outside therapist. Under these circumstances, the unit chief will have to create an evaluating structure that can assess the work of the attending in ways comparable to the one that I describe here.

PSYCHODYNAMIC ASSESSMENT AND FORMULATION

Ideally, the assessment of the patient can most usefully occur in a setting of collaboration among patient, family, and treatment team. Such collaboration is present in many patients and families, because of the painful crisis that precipitated hospitalization and the relief that is desired. However, there are many situations when a patient or family will not be in a collaborative frame of mind. For example, when a patient is hospitalized against his or her will, or when a family pressures a member into the hospital because of a wish to get rid of the patient, an inevitable tension arises between the therapeutic intentions of the unit and the resistance of the patient or family. In addition, borderline patients frequently have difficulties maintaining a collaborative approach (Adler 1979). What may appear to be a therapeutic alliance at one moment can quickly disappear when some request or demand by the patient or family is not granted. At such times, anger or rage with destructive or self-destructive threats may become evident, including threats to leave the hospital.

The obvious commitment of the inpatient staff to understand and help is often all that is required to obtain the needed collaboration between patient and family. Understandably, situations in which family members have wanted to hospitalize the patient primarily as a relief from ongoing difficulties may lead to a reluctance on their part to participate in the evaluation. The active outreach by the social worker or other staff member may be necessary to collect needed data and involve them in family sessions, which is often crucial to the understanding and resolution of the crisis that resulted in hospitalization. Some inpatient units have adopted the position that the family is required to participate in data collection and a family evaluation if the patient is to be admitted; and if family cooperation is not obtained after admission, the patient is discharged. When such a stance is maintained by the unit and not confused with a sadistic countertransference response to a noncooperative or provocative family, patient discharges rarely occur. In fact, the unit's caring perseverance is often perceived by patient and family, contributing to a more solid though still tenuous therapeutic alliance. With more primitive patients and families, such active pursuit of understanding can provide the structure that leads to a positive experience of holding and containment for the participants. Upon admission, the patient usually has some sense that he or she needs help with family difficulties that are more than the patient is able to negotiate. The unit's active response provides hope that the patient will get help in an area that is beyond his or her capacity.

The data collected from patient and family are part of an assessment that attempts to understand the patient's life history (biological, psychological, and social) and its interdigitation with that of the family. To have sufficient information to arrive at a psychodynamic formulation, developmental information from childhood to adulthood is necessary from patient and family. Although the emphasis is on the patient, relevant data about family members are also important, such as the family history of mental and physical illnesses, acquired illnesses, and history of physical and emotional trauma. There are publications available that the clinician can use as an outline of the useful data to collect and ways to ask the appropriate questions (e.g., Maltsberger 1986).

It is also crucial for the inpatient staff to obtain information from any outpatient therapist, physician, or social agency working with the patient and family. As discussed later in this chapter, if the patient has been in outpatient therapy, the assessment of that treatment can be the major link in defining the patient's current difficulties.

The psychotherapist usually assumes primary responsibility for the data collection from the patient, as well as from his or her outside therapist, whereas the social worker obtains information from meetings with family members alone and together and from other outside agencies involved with the patient. Not to be minimized is the importance of information shared by the patient and his or her family with other staff members (e.g., nurses and mental health workers), either directly or through observations of patient and patient-family interactions by unit personnel. Obviously, it is important to have sufficient structured time available for team members working with patient and family to share their observations with all members of the staff.

The psychotherapist should be the prime mover in ensuring that all clinical data are effectively utilized in arriving at a psychodynamic formulation and diagnosis of the patient. He or she can work in conjunction with other staff at team meetings to bring together data about how the circumstances of the patient's current difficulties (the present illness) relate to the patient's childhood character traits, experiences, and vulnerabilities (the past history) and biological vulnerabilities and family origins (the family history). This psychodynamic formulation should be used to elaborate a treatment plan that clearly defines psychotherapeutic work that can at least be initiated during the relatively brief period the patient remains hospitalized.

ASSESSMENT OF PREVIOUS PSYCHOTHERAPY

If the patient has been in outpatient psychotherapy prior to admission, the assessment of that psychotherapy may reveal important data that help explain the current need for hospitalization. Even when psychotherapy with a capable therapist has been progressing well, it is possible that slowly or rapidly emerging transference (and countertransference) feelings could have overwhelmed the patient's (and the therapist's) capacity to tolerate the intensity of the treatment situation. Yet the assessment of that psychotherapy is one of the most difficult tasks for any psychiatric inpatient unit (Adler 1985).

The outpatient therapist almost invariably feels vulnerable, for his or her patient has been admitted to the hospital despite the therapist's efforts. Coupled with countertransference feelings that elicit shame and guilt, the outpatient therapist may have feelings or fantasies that he or she is at fault, regardless of the therapist's experience or expertise. This is especially true when working with patients with narcissistic or borderline personality disorders who are regressed and perhaps suicidal. At such intense times, the therapist's countertransference feelings may include shame and guilt for his or her own riddance or other sadistic fantasies, as well as for inevitable empathic failures. The therapist may therefore be reluctant to call the unit and volunteer knowledge about his or her work with the patient. Or counterphobically, he or she may aggressively attempt to control the unit's evaluation process, especially if the therapist has admitting privileges.

At the same time, the inpatient unit's staff may harbor a common feeling of specialness: Its work is unique and superior, and any previous outside treatment or psychotherapy, almost by definition, has to be inferior. Alternately, unit staff may feel ill equipped to carry out an evaluation of the outpatient therapy. This requires much skill, experience, and tact, and frequently, feelings of uncertainty about the problems that may be present, including the possible roles of patient or therapist in the current difficulties. It is obvious that the interdigitation of the therapist's shame and guilt (which may be largely unconscious) and the unit's omnipotent position will lead to problems with the evaluation of that treatment.

In some instances, substantive evaluation never occurs. It is not uncommon for psychiatric inpatient units to ignore ongoing outpatient psychotherapy or to speak with the therapist in the most cursory manner. In addition, the outpatient therapist may be told that he or she is not to see the patient during the hospitalization, either as a unit policy or because the staff correctly or incorrectly thinks that it was the intensity of the transference/countertransference issues (and the therapist's difficulties with those feelings) that led to the hospitalization. Such a policy reinforces the therapist's feeling of shame and of being blamed, as well as the patient's similar feelings, perhaps from recognizing on some level that the patient may have sadistically frustrated and undermined his or her therapist's efforts. The unit may also facilitate the patient's termination of a beneficial therapy by inadvertently or deliberately supporting his or her blame of the therapist.

In these circumstances, the psychiatric inpatient unit is not utilized as a resource to obtain a careful evaluation of the treatment; rather, the source of the impasse and its possible resolution are ignored. As a result, if treatment with the outpatient therapist continues after discharge, difficulties that were present before are likely to return, even though a brief respite was obtained. And if the therapy is terminated—because of acting-out behavior by the patient, therapist, or staff without the knowledge of a careful evaluation—the difficulties present in that psychotherapy are more likely to recur in the subsequent treatment.

How is the evaluation of the psychotherapy that preceded hospitalization to occur in a useful way? Ideally, the psychotherapist on the inpatient unit is in the best position to talk with the outpatient therapist, because the psychotherapist is getting to know his or her new patient and can compare the information obtained from the patient with that from the prior therapist. If he or she has the skill and experience to carry out this task, the therapist can be counted on to utilize tact and understanding of the outpatient therapist's and patient's feelings of vulnerability. If the therapist is on the unit as a trainee or as a new staff member, he or she will probably require the help of the unit director or an experienced clinician skilled in this evaluation function.

What are the data that the evaluating psychotherapist would like to obtain from the outside therapist? These must certainly include the history of the therapy from the therapist's perspective, the therapist's formulation of the patient's difficulties, and the therapist's awareness of the transference, as well as his or her own countertransference feelings and difficulties. Obtaining these data requires skill and tact, for the answers to these questions can only in part be arrived at directly. Experienced clinicians learn ways to listen to the openness or defensiveness of therapists, while optimally supporting them to elicit needed information, and ask questions concerning their feelings about the patient that are sensitive to their vulnerabilities. With experience, the clinician can obtain information about the therapist's feelings (e.g., exasperation, excitement, over-stimulation, and rage), including the therapist's wish to get rid of the patient. Experience is also required to distinguish between a therapist's destructive riddance wishes that he or she wants to act on, and the capacity to tolerate such inevitable countertransference feelings and work them through with the patient.

Ideally, an alliance between the outside therapist and the inpatient unit's therapist can lead to a series of consultations that allow such issues to be defined and partially resolved during hospitalization, or a formulation that the outside therapy should probably end. It is a particularly difficult task to help both patient and therapist terminate—if that is the appropriate clinical decision—in a way that is honest, maintains the self-esteem of both parties to the greatest possible extent, and allows them to learn as much as possible from the process. As was previously stated, until the inpatient therapist develops the skills to carry out such sophisticated and tactful work, he or she will require the help of an experienced supervisor or unit chief.

If the outpatient therapist is to continue with his or her patient, it is important that the unit support this work, both during the inpatient stay and after discharge. If the outpatient therapist feels that his or her work is valued, patient and therapist can benefit from the formulation by the unit and the unit's attempt to help them. At the same time, the inpatient therapist can keep in touch with the outpatient therapist and help the outpatient therapist and the patient carry out their work. The inpatient therapist's continuing sessions with the patient can simultaneously be used to monitor the progress of the work between patient and outpatient therapist and to clarify further difficulties in it. Any additional understanding achieved can readily and appropriately be shared with all participants.

On the occasions when the inpatient unit decides, after careful consideration, that the outpatient therapist should not continue with his or her patient, the unit has the delicate task of helping patient and outpatient therapist terminate in a way that minimizes pain and humiliation to each, while evaluating the possible increased suicidal risk to the patient. Although the concern is primarily for the safety of the patient and for the self-esteem of both patient and outpatient therapist, the unit cannot avoid being aware of the delicacy of referral relations in the current marketing climate and the tendency of inpatient units to have a low census. Thus, tact in work with the outpatient therapist includes these considerations as well as the primary clinical concerns.

An outside therapist hospitalized his seriously depressed male patient whom he had been treating in weekly psychotherapy for a year. Although the evaluating clinician on the inpatient unit had some concerns about the quality of the therapist's ongoing work, including his relatively frequent discussions with the patient's wife, he had no definite formulation about the course of the psychotherapy. It was not until a clinical conference with an experienced consulting clinician, which was also attended by the outpatient therapist, that the data became clearer. At that conference, the outpatient therapist revealed that his understanding of the patient's difficulties was similar to that of the patient's wife, which stressed the patient's ineffectual ways of handling his work situation and marital problems. In addition, the outpatient therapist interrupted the process of the conference, behaving as if he were chairing it rather than attending as an invited person.

During the patient interview, it became clear that the patient felt misunderstood by his therapist and saw both his wife and his therapist as "ganging up" on him, very much as his parents did as he was growing up. With the data collected from this conference, it was possible to conclude that the therapy was destructive to the patient; the therapist was acting out countertransference difficulties, probably part of a projective identification that recreated the patient's relationship with his parents in childhood.

Discussion with the therapist suggested he could not understand this formulation. In spite of several tactful attempts to have the therapist grasp the unit's concerns, there was no change in his perceptions or way of working with the patient. It was therefore decided that the outside therapist would not be able to continue with his patient. Although the unit's evaluator and chief both spoke to the therapist about their concerns, there was no way to help the therapist disengage from the patient without his feeling that the unit was incorrect. The patient, on the other hand, was relieved, though previously unable to acknowledge with force his wish to terminate the therapy. His work with another therapist led to a gradual resolution of his depression after discharge, probably also aided by an increase of the antidepressant medication that had been prescribed in subtherapeutic doses. At the time of the patient's discharge from the hospital, unit staff members were unhappy that they had been unsuccessful in helping the original therapist terminate with the patient in a way that felt collaborative, while allowing him to maintain his self-esteem and learn from the process. Yet the staff members believed they had no choice but to help the patient extricate himself from a harmful psychotherapy.

COORDINATION OF PSYCHOTHERAPEUTIC WORK WITH THE MILIEU

Once the formulation of the patient's difficulties and its relationship to his or her family and the past is concluded, it is shared with the rest of the treatment team. Under ideal circumstances this sharing occurs automatically, because the developing formulation is an ongoing process occurring at team meetings, involving input from all staff members. Once unit personnel are in agreement with a formulation, integrating the team's efforts to carry it out can reside with the team leader or delegated team members, including the patient's therapist. The formulation that applies to individual therapy also has a component relevant to groups in which the patient participates, as well as other milieu treatments (e.g., occupational therapy, family sessions). If the outpatient therapist is continuing with the patient as part of the unit's formulation, the unit's therapist can simultaneously continue contacts with him or her frequently enough to be certain that the work is proceeding well and that any new data from the outpatient therapist or unit are mutually shared. The alliance that is present among staff members and outside therapist can be a source of security for the patient and can facilitate the working relationship between patient and staff.

A 72-year-old woman was admitted to an inpatient unit 8 months after the death of her 75-year-old husband. He had been ill for a year, progressively requiring more care from her as his cancer spread. Although she did her best to respond to his needs, they had frequent disagreements that were increasingly upsetting to her. Two months prior to his death, their children finally urged the patient to have her husband hospitalized, and she reluctantly agreed. After his death she became depressed, but she did not respond to the antidepressants given by the family physician. At the urging of her children and physician, she was admitted to the short-term psychiatric inpatient unit.

In obtaining a history from the patient and her children, it became evident to the unit staff that the patient and her husband had had a troubled relationship for most of their almost 50 years of marriage. She had threatened to leave him on several occasions when his drinking became excessive. The last 10 years of their marriage had been characterized by intensified bickering after the husband's retirement at age 65 and his constant presence at home. She found some relief in community activities while her husband was alive, volunteering in a children's nursery school, but stopped after his death. Although the patient talked about how much she missed her husband and how guilty she was about not taking care of him well enough, she had not cried since the day he died. Further information obtained from the patient and her family revealed that the marriage in many ways replicated the marriage of the patient's own parents, with an alcoholic father and a long-suffering, passive mother. The patient's mother herself had a prolonged depression after her husband died.

It became clear to the treatment team that the patient's difficulties centered around her inability to mourn the death of her husband. Her ambivalence and guilt recapitulated similar issues that had been present with her own parents. Her problems were not about the negative aspects of her marriage, which she remembered with guilt and shame, but her inability to remember the positive aspects and the sadness that accompanied her loss. The therapist could define the task of helping her talk about her love for her husband and the happy memories of their lives, through the specific details of these events in their long marriage. The patient was also encouraged in her inpatient groups to talk about her husband and how much she missed him. Over the week available for that psychotherapeutic work, the patient began to cry in a more sustained way. Family meetings with her children aided in the process, because they too were having difficulty with their sadness. Discussions about their ability to share their tears with their mother addressed some of the tensions while also examining the family's bickering style that helped them avoid the pain of losing husband and father. At the same time, the patient's psychopharmacological evaluation led to a switch to another antidepressant, with plans for slow increases to more appropriate doses.

At the end of her 2-week admission, the patient was feeling less depressed. She continued weekly sessions with her inpatient therapist through the outpatient department and saw the psychopharmacologist at appropriate intervals. In the fourth month of weekly sessions, she began to talk about her long-standing anger at her husband and her guilt (now modified by a solid base of experience between patient and therapist) about her love for her husband. After 7 months of treatment, the patient's depression was minimal. In monthly follow-up sessions, she maintained her gains, helped by the inpatient staff's successful efforts before discharge to involve her in some volunteer programs in her community hospital. She also no longer required her antidepressant medication.

CONFIDENTIALITY ON THE PSYCHIATRIC INPATIENT UNIT

It requires thoughtfulness and tact to maintain the patient's confidentiality during a psychiatric inpatient admission, especially during the complex process of data collection, which often involves many people inside and outside the unit. The process is further complicated by some patients' wishes to keep information about important events or feelings from family members or unit personnel. Often the patient will bring in his or her own problems of distrust, compounded by the use of projective identification and splitting, to request that certain material be kept from the entire staff. With rare exception, such requests are harmful to the evaluative and therapeutic process. They reflect the patient's psychological difficulties and (usually) unconscious wish to obscure needed information. Yet the patient and his or her family have every reason to be concerned unless staff members function in a way that respects confidential material told to them, guard against destructive use of that material (e.g., scrupulously avoiding inadvertent sharing of such material with other patients unless its sharing comes directly from that patient in communication with another patient), and do not use what they have learned in any way other than to understand and work most effectively with patient, family, and all professionals involved in the patient's clinical care.

SUPPORTIVE AND INSIGHT-ORIENTED INDIVIDUAL THERAPY AND THE MILIEU

There has been a tendency in defining individual psychotherapy to make clear-cut distinctions between supportive psychotherapy and insight-oriented or expressive psychotherapy (Kernberg 1982). By implication, the latter is seen as the more valuable and reserved for "healthier" patients, whereas the former is described as most valuable for more vulnerable patients. However, in recent years, these distinctions have become less clear. Wallerstein (1986), for example, has documented that changes occurring in a supportive treatment framework can be as significant and as enduring as those that are the result of insight-oriented treatment. In addition, therapists who stress the exploratory nature of their work tend to minimize the degree of support that they give their patients (Adler 1989a). Most therapists provide a combination of both, depending upon the patient, the current status of the therapeutic alliance, and the degree of vulnerability and emotional pain.

The short-term inpatient unit can utilize similar principles to support the patient while simultaneously focusing on painful areas in an exploratory mode. In fact, optimal therapy is often a careful balance of support, so as to help the patient bear what is so painful. The formulation about the patient should include an understanding of his or her vulnerability, which defines needs for support and the capacity for insight and the ability to bear painful affects. All members of the treatment team can apply these principles to different aspects of the treatment. Awareness that the individual therapist is about to confront the patient with a particularly painful aspect of his or her difficulty that day can allow other staff members to offer more support to the patient during that period. Inpatient units can maximize this balance of support and exploration that is more difficult for an individual therapist to achieve on an outpatient basis.

The literature on short-term psychotherapy is useful in understanding the application of psychotherapeutic principles on the short-term psychiatric inpatient unit and achieving the optimal utilization of the brief time available. Although the major contributors to the psychodynamic literature (e.g., Malan, Sifneos, Mann, Davanloo) have many differences (Ursano and Hales 1986), they share a common task of using the short-term aspects of the treatment for creative advantage. They stress the need for a careful formulation as part of their work and define the degree of support, interpretation, and confrontation that each requires for the specific approach.

The fact that an inpatient unit struggles to respond thoughtfully and professionally to the patient's pain, conflicts, and provocations presents a new kind of experience for most if not all patients. Because most people who require inpatient hospitalization have had problematic histories, with parental failures and losses, the consistent, kind, caring exploratory work on the unit—with the necessary containment, limit setting, interpretation, and help in putting feelings into words—is different in many ways from their past experiences. This new experience can be an important factor in the process of change for these patients. It differs from the corrective emotional experience that Alexander (1958) described, because the staff's response is genuine and is therefore unlike Alexander's manipulative role-playing that he believed the patient needed as part of his or her treatment.

COUNTERTRANSFERENCE DIFFICULTIES FOR THE INDIVIDUAL PSYCHODYNAMIC THERAPIST ON THE SHORT-TERM INPATIENT UNIT

It is expected that countertransference difficulties that arise for the individual therapist on the short-term inpatient unit would raise more complex problems than for an individual therapist who is seeing his or her patient in an outpatient setting. In the latter situation, the therapist does not have to relate to a complex system of staff and other patients who are interacting both with the patient and with the therapist. There is a much greater tendency for the therapist's problematic countertransference feelings to lead to difficulties on the inpatient unit, as the therapist is in a position to act out these feelings toward many individuals—staff members, other patients, as well as the outpatient therapist of his or her patient, if there is one—and not confine them to his or her patient. As a general rule, the more primitive the patient, the more likely that the individual therapist's problematic countertransference feelings will be acted out.

Projective Identification and Splitting

To explain an important aspect of countertransference, especially with primitive patients, it is useful to spell out briefly the concept of projective identification and splitting. Understanding this can help illuminate many interactions between patient and therapist, as well as relationships that occur in milieu settings, such as a short-term inpatient unit.

Projective identification was first defined by Melanie Klein (1946/1952) and refined by many others (Adler 1989b; Bion 1967; Malin and Grotstein 1966; Ogden 1979). As it is currently utilized, the concept brings together the relationship between the intrapsychic or internal world of two or more people and their interpersonal connections. Projective identification is a process whereby a person "projects" part of him- or herself onto another in order to rid the self of some unacceptable part, or to preserve a valued part that might be destroyed by that individual were it not projected. The projected part consists of aspects of a previous relationship involving parts of self and other and their associated feelings. Once the projection occurs, the person projecting then interacts with the person involved in the projection in a way that attempts to provoke a response consonant with the projected part. That is, if the projected part consists of aspects of an angry relationship with a parent, the person projecting will attempt to provoke an angry response in the recipient that is very similar to that component of the earlier parental relationship.

If the provocation is to lead to the repetition of the earlier relationship through the actions of the person receiving the projection, the recipient must have a part of him- or herself that has unresolved, repressed, or split-off aspects that are similar to the projector and the aspects projected. To the extent that the person receiving the projection can "contain" the projection ([Bion 1967] i.e., not act upon the provocation even though he or she is provoked to do so), there is then the possibility of creative change within the projector. This change can occur because the projection that is modified by the person containing it can be internalized by the projector, resulting in new structure formation in that person. In this description, there is then the possibility of constructive as well as destructive projective identification (Adler 1989b). The latter occurs when the projection is not contained adequately, leading to potentially harmful responses by the recipient of the projection, in response to the projection and the provocation. Constructive projective identification results when the containment is relatively successful and is able to result in positive changes within the patient.

Splitting is related to projective identification. It tends to be seen more commonly in primitive patients and is part of their difficulties in bearing ambivalence. People who split see a relationship as either all good or all bad. At the moment that they split, they are unable to recognize the fact that the good and the bad aspects of an individual are parts of the same person. Instead, they keep those parts separate and can project one part or the other onto another person. When this is coupled with the component of interpersonal provocation, the process becomes one of projective identification.

Countertransference, Projective Identification, and Splitting: The Relationship to the Individual Psychodynamic Therapist and the Milieu

Patients on psychiatric inpatient units quickly tend to recreate the scenes of their childhood, often through the uses of splitting and projective identification. Most have an uncanny unconscious capacity to sense the strengths, personality characteristics, and vulnerabilities of others, including staff members. The processes of splitting and projective identification can be used to understand how patients can involve the individual therapist and other staff members in a process that can either be constructive or destructive. When the process consists of the patient's unconscious attempts to project unresolved, painful, and often primitive experiences, it can lead to stormy encounters on the psychiatric inpatient unit. When splitting is a major component of the process, one staff member can be "selected" for the positive aspects projected, while another receives the negative aspects. Projective identification, with its interpersonal aspect added to the splitting, often results in a struggle between the people who are recipients of different projected aspects. The individual therapist on the inpatient unit frequently finds him- or herself in the middle of such a struggle. He or she can be the idealized object for the patient, whereas other staff members are hated and devalued. Or the patient can see the therapist as cold and uncaring, a person who hates the patient, whereas others (e.g., the nurse) are viewed as truly empathic and understanding of the patient's pain. Obviously, what complicates this situation is the inter-personal provocation aspects of projective identification between the patient and a staff member, as well as among staff members whose response to the patient's projections and interpersonal behavior may resonate anti-therapeutically with their own unresolved difficulties.

The above formulation stresses the patient's use of projective identification in its constructive and destructive aspects and the unit's capacity to contain the projections. It is compatible with and complementary to the view presented in Chapter 1, in which a Kohutian model is stressed, and in which the therapeutic milieu provides selfobject functions that lead to internalization of self-esteem regulation. Although Kohut's self psychology uses a theoretical framework different from the underpinnings of the concept of projective identification, it is clinically useful to bring them together (Adler and Rhine 1988). For example, the therapist's and/or inpatient unit's capacity to contain the patient's projective identifications can be viewed as an important selfobject function of the therapist and/or unit, ultimately leading to the change in the patient's capacity for self-regulation.

The individual psychotherapist on the unit can find him- or herself angry at other staff members for not understanding or protecting the patient. The psychotherapist may also become the recipient of one or more staff members' angry charges that he or she is being too kind or empathic to a difficult patient who is acting out and who needs clearer limits and therapeutic firmness. Such potential difficulties can escalate to a point in which staff members are angry at each other in a way that is not only disruptive but is also harmful to the patient's ongoing treatment process.

The staff's capacity to understand the nature of projective identification and splitting is a step toward working creatively with the process. It requires unit leadership that ultimately provides the model of "containment" necessary for the patient's effective treatment. If that leader demonstrates his or her capacity to contain the provocation among the staff (e.g., without sadistic counterattacks), then the staff can provide a similar model for patients. Under these circumstances, the constructive aspects of projective identification and splitting can be most available for the growth of the patient.

The individual psychodynamic therapist, one hopes, is a person able to understand the nature of these complex processes. However, because he or she may be a part of the projective identification and splitting process, the therapist may not be in a sufficiently objective position to clarify it independently without seeming arrogant or authoritarian. Yet his or her own understanding of the process and tact in working with colleagues can lead to personal restraint in acting out his or her aspect of the process, thereby facilitating a developing relationship with other staff members that makes the constructive aspects more likely to occur. When staff members, including the individual therapist, know and respect one another well enough, they are in the best position to know that a patient's provocative statements about another staff member cannot be true, as they are incompatible with their knowledge of the other staff member. Such knowledge takes time to occur and requires mature unit leadership, sufficient opportunities for staff to work collaboratively over time, and adequate staff meetings where many of these experiences can be reviewed and understood. The individual psychodynamic psychotherapist on the unit can play an important role in helping this creative process grow and mature.

SUMMARY

Individual psychodynamic psychotherapy is possible on the short-term psychiatric inpatient unit if the tasks and functions of the psychotherapist are clearly defined. The need for a careful formulation and diagnosis presents the individual therapist with the task of orchestrating a thorough evaluation of the patient and family. He or she performs this function with the patient and coordinates data gathered by other staff members about the family and patient-family interaction. He or she also gathers the data of the patient's work with any current outside therapist. Once a formulation is agreed upon, the task of the individual psychotherapist consists of working with the patient (and family) on the defined sector of difficulty that led to the hospitalization. The patient and his or her family are also prepared to continue the therapeutic work after discharge.

A major role for the individual therapist on the short-term inpatient unit includes the careful exploration of the patient's treatment by the outpatient therapist; many patients require hospitalization because of impasses in that therapy, or transference/countertransference feelings that cannot be contained on an outpatient basis. The inpatient unit's sensitivity to the vulnerabilities of the outpatient therapist and the patient, as well as the staff's capacity to obtain the needed data to formulate the difficulties, often determine the success of future treatment with the therapist, or with another, if the unit's assessment defines an unresolvable impasse.

The complex mechanisms of projective identification and splitting help explain the interactions between the patient, individual inpatient psychotherapist, other staff members, and outside therapists. Constructive as well as destructive aspects of these processes are thus delineated. The patient's inevitable repetition of past relationships and the staff's response to this process often define the success or failure of the patient's hospitalization.

REFERENCES

Adler G: The myth of the alliance with borderline patients. Am J Psychiatry 136:642–645, 1979

Adler G: Borderline Psychopathology and Its Treatment. Northvale, NJ, Jason Aronson, 1985

Adler G: Psychodynamic therapies in borderline personality disorder, in Review of Psychiatry, Vol 8. Edited by Tasman A, Hales RE, Frances AJ. Washington, DC, American Psychiatric Press, 1989a, pp 49–64

Adler G: Transitional phenomena, projective identification, and the essential ambiguity of the psychoanalytic situation. Psychoanal Q 58:81–104, 1989b

Adler G, Rhine MW: The selfobject function of projective identification. Bull Menninger Foundation 52:473–491, 1988

Alexander F: Unexplored areas in psychoanalytic theory and treatment—part II, in The Scope of Psychoanalysis. New York, Basic Books, 1958

Bion WR: A theory of thinking, in Second Thoughts: Selected Papers on Psychoanalysis. New York, Jason Aronson, 1967

Kernberg OF: The psychotherapeutic treatment of borderline personalities, in Psychiatry 1982: The American Psychiatric Association Annual Review, Vol 1. Edited by Grinspoon L. Washington, DC, American Psychiatric Press, 1982, pp 470–487

Klein M: Notes on some schizoid mechanisms (1946), in Developments in Psychoanalysis. Edited by Riviere J. London, Hogarth Press, 1952

Malin A, Grotstein J: Projective identification in the therapeutic process. Int J Psychoanal 47:26–31, 1966

Maltsberger JT: Suicide Risk: The Formulation of Clinical Judgment. New York, New York University Press, 1986

Ogden TH: On projective identification. Int J Psychoanal 60:357–373, 1979

Ursano RJ, Hales RE: A review of brief individual psychotherapies. Am J Psychiatry 143:1507–1517, 1986

Wallerstein RS: Forty-Two Lives in Treatment. New York, Guilford, 1986

Family Treatment During Brief Hospitalization

Stephen A. Cole, M.D.

INTRODUCTION

Family therapy was originally developed to meet the needs of outpatients and their families. Relatively little has been written about family approaches to brief hospitalization. In this chapter, I present an inpatient family treatment model that involves engagement of the family, psychoeducation, crisis management, linkage with inpatient staff, brief family therapy, multifamily therapy, and aftercare planning. The therapists frame the patient's problem as an acute episode of a biologically based illness triggered by acute or chronic stress. They then seek to engage the family in exploring ways in which they and the patient can reduce the stress level and thereby lessen the chances of future relapse.

The work involves the modification of specific communication and problem-solving behaviors and helps the family and the inpatient staff to set realistic expectations for the patient's recovery. A survey of the family interactional correlates of schizophrenia, depression, and mania will enable practitioners to anticipate typical transactional patterns and thereby fine-tune the model to specific situations. This approach to family treatment has been validated through outcome studies of inpatients with schizophrenic and major affective disorders.

FAMILY BURDEN

Since deinstitutionalization began 20 years ago, the families of psychiatric patients have endured considerable hardships coping with the psychotic and residual symptoms of schizophrenia and bipolar disorder and the more subtle manifestations of unipolar depressive disorder (Creer and Wing 1975; Doll 1976; Fadden et al. 1987; Johnson 1990; Keitner and Miller 1990). These families frequently have become isolated from their communities and estranged from their patient-relatives (Beels et al. 1984; Kreisman and Joy 1975).

Until recently, mental health professionals tended to blame patients' families for either causing or triggering episodes of mental illness (Appleton 1974; Terkelsen 1983). This unfortunate situation has been corrected during the past 10 years in response to the emergence of an active family consumer movement. This movement has empowered families to insist that professionals provide them with a more accurate understanding of severe and persistent mental disorders, their treatments, and available community resources (Cole and Cole 1987; Hatfield 1987; Holden and Levine 1982; Lefley and Johnson 1990; Vine and Beels 1990). The efforts of the National Alliance for the Mentally Ill (NAMI) and the National Association for Research in Schizophrenia and Depression (NARSAD) support research and governmental initiatives and have stimulated a widespread effort to develop new and effective treatment strategies that enlist families as partners in health care.

FAMILY INTERACTION IN SCHIZOPHRENIA AND AFFECTIVE DISORDERS

Schizophrenia

Expressed emotion (EE), an operational measure of family criticism and emotional overinvolvement, is strongly associated with posthospital relapse rates in males with chronic schizophrenia who are returning to their parental homes (Brown et al. 1962, 1972; Kuipers and Bebbington 1988; Vaughn and Leff 1976). Studies currently in progress are helping to elucidate the clinical correlates of patient and family behavior in high- and low-EE families (see Table 4–1).

Patients in high-EE families are more likely to live at home and less likely to participate in outpatient treatment. Thus, it is important to use brief hospitalization as an opportunity to begin family treatment. Psychoeducational family interventions are tailored to reduce family burden and EE. These approaches define the patient's symptomatic behavior as caused by a disease and provide both the patient and family with cognitive, behavioral, and pharmacological strategies for coping more effectively (Cole and Jacobs 1989). Here, patients are viewed as experts in the

Table 4–1. Attitudinal and interactional correlates of expressed emotion

High-EE relatives	Low-EE relatives
See illness behavior as laziness	Accept psychosis as a disease process
Have unrealistic expectations	Understand the patient's limitations
Talk and interrupt more often	Listen to the patient
Express disagreement	Agree with the patient
Use peculiar language	Use clear language
Give intense and harsh criticism	Are emotionally neutral
Judge patient's behavior negatively	Are supportive and protective
Express personal rejections	Are accepting of the patient
Propose negative solutions to problems	Propose positive solutions to problems
Engage in negative escalations with patient	De-escalate potential conflicts
Patient's reactions	
Expresses irritability	Appears calm
Denigrates self or criticizes others	Makes neutral statements
Becomes defensive	Shows autonomous, goal-, and action-oriented behavior
Interactive pattern	
Parent attacks, patient makes excuses	Engage in problem-solving discussions

Sources. Hahlweg et al. 1987; Kuipers et al. 1983; MacCarthy and Hemsley 1986; Miklowitz et al. 1983, 1984, 1986, 1989; Strachan et al. 1986, 1989; Vaughn 1986.

subjective experience of schizophrenia (McGill et al. 1983) and relatives as potential experts in its day-to-day management. All family members are credited with doing their best to cope with the disorder (Steinglass 1987).

Depression

There have been several studies of the interactive aspects of depressive disorder.

Miller and colleagues (1986) have reported that the degree of family dysfunction in major depressive disorder exceeds that of patients with alcoholism, adjustment disorder, schizophrenia, and bipolar disorder. Whereas the schizophrenia literature focuses on interactions between patients and parents, that for depression highlights relationships of spouses with each other and of depressed parents with their children (Keitner and Miller 1990).

Depressed parents tend to have difficulty giving praise or setting limits for their children, who frequently have problems with impulsiveness and anxiety (Keitner and Miller 1990). Depressed persons have difficulty soliciting or providing positive social reinforcement, are uncomfortable with assertiveness, and may perceive others as rejecting, aloof, ungenuine, and uncaring (Janowsky et al. 1984; Youngren and Lewinsohn 1980). Interactional studies show that depressed people seem to expect others to listen to their woes without offering to reciprocate (Coyne 1976). For example, endogenously depressed wives, fearing a loss of support, express self-deprecation and are submissive to husbands who respond with reassurance and "concealed hostility" (Birtchnell 1984; Hoover and Fitzgerald 1981), whereas reactively depressed wives are openly critical of husbands who respond with disagreement or emotional distancing (Coyne 1987; Matussek and Wiegand 1985). In this manner, depressive patients may provoke the progressive withdrawal of social support and thereby increase the likelihood of further depressive episodes (Brown and Harris 1978).

As one might expect, high EE predicts relapse in cases of unipolar affective disorder (Hooley 1986; Hooley and Teasdale 1989; Hooley et al. 1986; Vaughn and Leff 1976). High-EE spouses tend to view depressive behavior as willful, and thus they are more likely than low-EE spouses to make negative and critical remarks, to argue, and to exhibit negative nonverbal behavior. In contrast, low-EE spouses tend to make more frequent accepting statements and to be more positive toward their depressed spouses in their nonverbal behavior (Hooley 1986; Hooley et al. 1987). Depressed patients appear to be highly sensitive to perceived criticism (perhaps fearing their spouses will leave them), to be passive, and to make few self-disclosures (Gotlib and Whiffen 1989; Hooley and Teasdale 1989). These studies do not clarify the extent to which hostile, destructive marital conflicts are provoked by the spouse's depression or stem from a dysfunctional marital system (Schmaling and Jacobson 1990).

Bipolar Disorder

The literature on family interaction in bipolar disorder is sparse. Clinicians have described bipolar patients as manipulative, blaming, and alienating in the manic phase and as meek and insecure in the depressive phase (Janowsky et al. 1970; Kaplan De-Nour 1980). Their spouses are described as "inadequate," viewing the manic patients as spiteful and willful (Mayo et al. 1979). Two studies (Miklowitz et al. 1988; Priebe et al. 1989) have shown that high spousal EE is predictive of relapse, whereas another study indicates that positive outcome of lithium responders is strongly correlated with social support (O'Connell et al. 1985).

Family Outcome Studies in Brief Hospitalization

Two controlled studies show that family intervention is effective for patients with schizophrenia or major affective disorder during brief hospitalization. Anderson's team (1986b) recommends that families or couples of a patient with unipolar or bipolar disorder be engaged through 4-hour psychoeducational multifamily workshops and then referred upon discharge to longer-term, process-oriented multifamily groups. Glick and colleagues (1985) found that 6 to 8 sessions of brief family crisis treatment during acute hospitalization was particularly effective for female patients with bipolar disorder and poor premorbid schizophrenic disorder. This intervention included psychoeducation, crisis management and training in communicating, problem solving, and identification of early warning signs of relapse (Clarkin et al. 1988, 1990; Glick et al. 1985, 1991; Haas et al. 1988, 1990; Spencer et al. 1988).

PRINCIPLES OF FAMILY TREATMENT IN
ACUTE HOSPITAL SETTINGS

For the family, hospitalization of a relative is often a last resort to be used only after outpatient management has failed. By the time the patient reaches the emergency room, the family is in a state of turmoil and confusion (Anderson 1977; Anderson and Reiss 1982; Bernheim and Lehman 1985; Biddle 1978; Cole and Jacobs 1989; Group for the Advancement of Psychiatry 1985; Harbin 1979). Families in crisis are often receptive to help and change, and they may welcome assistance from an understanding, empathetic, and available therapist (Hill 1965; Parad and Caplan 1965; Rabkin 1972). If it is the patient's first acute episode, spouses or families may blame themselves for the psychosis or suicide attempt and feel guilty for hospitalizing the patient. They may not understand what has happened to the patient and may have only vague notions of possible diagnoses. They may fear losing their relative forever.

Studies have shown that the presence of a relative or significant other in the emergency room and this person's continued availability during hospitalization may predict a positive patient outcome (Gould and Glick 1977; Withersty 1977). Family absence is associated with poor outcome and extended periods of inpatient care (Greenley 1982).

The goals of engagement are to establish a working alliance with the family or spouse, to educate them about the patient's disorder, and to explain the policies of the inpatient unit.

Case 1, Part 1

Michael L. was a 24-year-old man who requested an interview with his medical school dean because he could no longer tune out the voices that had been bothering him for several years. The dean referred Mr. L. to a psychiatrist who said he had a serious disorder that required immediate hospitalization for diagnosis and treatment. After obtaining Mr. L.'s permission, the psychiatrist told his parents about their son's condition and asked them to accompany him to the emergency room. There, the L.s mentioned to the psychiatrist that their son had become more reserved during his last 2 years of college. They had thought this might be normal behavior for premed students. Now, they worried that he might face the same fate as Mrs. L.'s brother, who had been in and out of state mental hospitals for years. The emergency room doctor told them, "Your son is in an acute state of psychosis. He will need to spend some time—2 to 6 weeks—in the hospital. We know that all this is difficult for you, and that you have many concerns and questions. Tomorrow, a member of our family treatment team will call you to arrange an appointment to discuss Michael, to answer your questions and to describe how things work on the inpatient service. In the meantime, you could help us by writing down all your questions."

The next day, a team composed of a social worker and a nurse met with Mr. L. and his parents. Mr. L. appeared distracted, mumbled something about the CIA, and got up to look outside the door. The nurse responded, "Michael, this meeting is so we can tell your parents what you and they can expect while you're a patient here. Now you can either stay or leave. If you leave, we will have your parents meet with you before they go home." Thus informed and given permission to leave, he left the room.

The nurse told Mr. L.'s parents that although the doors were locked, Mr. L. could earn off-ward passes once his condition had stabilized. She described the rules regarding visiting hours and the use of pay phones. Mr. L. could wear his own clothes, but he would have to store sharp objects in the nursing station. "Quiet rooms" were for patients unable to control their emotions or behavior. Each patient was assigned a primary therapist and a doctor who would join them in family meetings. The social worker described herself as the family's "advocate," and she asked that Mr. L.'s parents designate a "contact person," to avoid confusion. She then asked the parents how they were coping and whether they had any questions.

The first few meetings are often conducted without the patient, to minimize possible disruptions and to facilitate a more open discussion of the patient's immediate past behavior. The patient should be informed that family meetings are being held, given a general description of their purpose, and invited to join them once the inpatient staff and the patient's therapist agree that the patient is no longer psychotic and can participate in rational discourse. It is important for the family therapist to be available, to make the family feel welcome and let them know that the clinician understands what they are going through. The family should be told the differential diagnosis and that the patient has a chemical imbalance in the brain for which no one is to blame. Hospitalization provides a controlled environment enabling an accurate diagnostic assessment and the coordination of an individualized treatment plan for the acute episode and the aftercare period. The family therapist assumes the role of ombudsman, presenting the family's point of view to the inpatient team while advising the family regarding the patient's response to treatment. It is helpful to have the family appoint a "representative," or designated spokesperson, to simplify communications.

Families likely to resist involvement have been described by Reiss and colleagues (1980) as "distance-sensitive" (i.e., those who do not trust strangers or work together for common goals). Strategies for engaging unwilling families range from scheduling supportive and educational home visits (MacCarthy et al. 1989) to threatening premature discharge of the patient if the family does not participate in treatment (Glick and Clarkin 1982; Harbin 1979).

Case 2, Part 1

Barbara M. was brought to the emergency room by an outreach team from a homeless shelter. She was 32, had been psychotic since age 20, and was living on public assistance that was insufficient to cover her housing costs. Her 7-year-old daughter, Jessica, had been placed in temporary foster care with Ms. M.'s mother, Mrs. B., for the past 2 years. Mrs. B. was not on speaking terms with Ms. M. for several weeks, because Ms. M. had pulled the telephone cord from the wall on a mandated home visit with Jessica. After taking a brief history in the psychiatric emergency room, the nurse called Mrs. B. and succeeded in persuading her to come to the hospital, offering to drive her back and forth in the outreach team van. This intervention was crucial in recruiting Mrs. B. into treatment and for beginning the process of reuniting Ms. M. with her family.

Should the crisis be yet another of many acute episodes, the family may feel despairing and helpless over the patient's condition, as well as alienated from a health care system that has not succeeded in controlling the course of their relative's illness. These families welcome the respite and relief provided by hospitalization and often resist efforts by the inpatient staff to arrange for early discharge.

Case 3, Part 1

Robert C. was hospitalized for his third psychotic break after accidentally setting fire to his parents' home. He had become despondent and paranoid, and he had attempted to burn up his old college books in the basement. Things got out of hand when the small fire spread to an old couch with inflammable stuffing. Mr. C. was the eldest of five, the brightest of the C. offspring, but he had become psychotic while serving in Vietnam. Nowadays, he was often paranoid, and for years he had remained isolated and uninvolved in aftercare. The fire occurred several months after Mr. C. stopped taking medication. His parents loved Mr. C. very much, but they were afraid to live with him again until they were certain he would cooperate with treatment.

Realizing the gravity of the situation and the difficulty of arranging alternative housing after the fire setting, the inpatient family team resolved to work with the C. family on the following set of goals:

1. To identify the major problem as Mr. C.'s noncompliance with aftercare and medication;
2. To help Mr. C. and his family agree that his returning home would depend on his becoming actively involved in a day hospital program; and
3. To put one of Mr. C.'s parents temporarily in charge of administering medication.

It is crucial to appreciate the efforts that a patient's family and spouse have made to cope with the severe and persistent mental illness of their relative, to carefully review past programs of outpatient management, and to endeavor to design an aftercare plan that meets the current needs of both patient and family. The therapist collaborates with the family to identify problems, to recognize strengths and weaknesses, and to devise and implement strategies to help them and the patient (Epstein and Bishop 1981; Wynne et al. 1986, 1987).

All families want to know when the patient will be able to resume his or her prehospital role responsibilities, whether disability will result, and how long the rehabilitation process will last. The clinician should tell them to expect that recovery will occur several weeks or months after a first or second acute episode, and that recovery in chronic illness will follow similar patterns after each such episode. It is helpful to explain that the process of recovery is like mountain climbing: it involves at first a period of preparation during which there is no obvious progress, followed by spurts of activity that serve to "scout the terrain," when the patient may still be quite fragile before genuine improvement in functioning occurs (Strauss et al. 1985). The family should be advised to be patient. It is important for the therapist to present the patient's condition in a hopeful light, emphasizing strengths and focusing on what patient and family can do to promote healing.

In coordinating communication between the family and the ward staff, the family therapist can anticipate and prevent systemic conflicts that inevitably arise when the inpatient treatment team temporarily assumes the function of primary caretaker. The family should be informed of ward rules, policies, and procedures, including phone calls, visiting hours, and passes that provide access to the patient. This can be accomplished either in a family meeting or during a "family night," in which several families are invited to meet with the ward staff (Scharfstein and Libbey 1982).

The tendency of inpatient staff to view themselves as protectors of the patient against a family perceived as intrusive and pathological can be countered by in-service teaching of the principles of psychoeducational family treatment and by including staff in family treatment sessions (Harbin 1982; Krajewski and Harbin 1982). A similar approach may help to neutralize negative attitudes of individually oriented psychotherapists toward families (Boyd 1979).

Case 1, Part 2

Within a week of being hospitalized, Michael L., the medical student, became a favorite of the ward staff. He had confided in his primary therapist (a psychologist in training), took an active role in group therapy, and made friends with several patients who shared their experiences with psychosis. Mrs. L., his mother, would dutifully show up for the full visiting hour, and she was always asking the reasons for various ward policies. The nursing staff complained that Mrs. L. was an overprotective, high-EE mother. The social worker detected the beginnings of what might have become a divisive conflict between Mr. L.'s temporary and permanent family systems. She urged that the staff place themselves in his mother's position (i.e., her having to cope with the likelihood that her son would never become a physician). The social worker invited Mr. L.'s ward doctor, primary therapist, and nurse to the next family meeting.

The family's attitude toward hospitalization can have adverse effects on the patient's hospital treatment.

Case 2, Part 2

Even though Barbara M. had been psychotic for more than 10 years, her mother continued to believe that Ms. M. was an irresponsible drug addict whose problems were caused by marijuana and angel dust. Mrs. B. felt harassed by her daughter's angry phone calls and visits with Jessica. Mrs. B. was aware that Ms. M. had been taking lithium and antipsychotics for years, but she was convinced that only willpower could save her daughter. Hospitalization provided a temporary relief, and Mrs. B. did not intend to go out of her way to visit.

After a stormy phone call in which Mrs. B. hung up on her, Ms. M. reported that the voices were telling her she was a failure as a mother, that she would never get well, and that she should kill herself. The family therapist correctly ascertained that family treatment was imperative and developed the following goals:

1. To convince Mrs. B. that her daughter had a schizoaffective disorder, which may have been "triggered" by the drugs she took in high school;
2. To encourage Mrs. B. to attend an educational workshop led by the ward staff where she might learn more about Ms. M.'s condition and meet other families "in the same boat;"
3. To arrange for Ms. M.'s placement in a community residence rather than a public shelter;
4. To place Ms. M. in a day-care program to improve her survival and coping skills;
5. To arrange a regular schedule for Ms. M. to meet with her daughter; and
6. To enroll Ms. M. in a parent assistance program to teach her parenting skills, so that she might eventually resume her role as Jessica's mother and relieve Mrs. B. of this responsibility.

Greenman and colleagues (1989) have shown that discharges against medical advice tend to occur more often when families cannot accept the notion that the patient is genuinely ill, cannot tolerate the separation imposed by hospitalization, or feel excessively guilty in the face of the patient's anger at being hospitalized.

Case 3, Part 2

About 2 weeks after Robert C. was hospitalized, he had begun to respond to antipsychotics, and the family therapist began to discuss disposition. However, his parents were still reeling from nearly losing their home, and they were not receptive. During a heated family meeting with their son in which Mrs. C. burst into tears, Mr. C.'s father said, "We know how sick he is. We kept him at home for years when no one else would help us. You will never know what we went through. Now we are wondering what we did wrong. Maybe we didn't watch him closely enough. Our rooms are full of soot and smoke and even the insurance company is giving us trouble. And you talk about discharge?"

Later that evening, Robert C. submitted a 72-hour letter requesting discharge, saying, "I see how much pain I've caused by being so selfish. Now I have to leave, to take care of my parents and to work on the house."

The next evening, Mr. C.'s parents attended their first meeting of the multifamily support group. They told their story to four other families, who told them they could understand their plight and that they had done nothing wrong. One father suggested that perhaps their problem was that they were "too much alone" and might use their son's hospitalization to accept some new ideas. The next day in family therapy, Mrs. C. pleaded with her son not to leave the hospital, and her husband told him, "We are grateful that you want to help us with the house, but we can manage until your treatment team says you are ready to leave."

Educating the family and allowing them to unburden themselves of their distress may help to avoid premature discharge. Many families seem to undergo a natural process of emotional separation upon admission and reinvolvement during hospitalization (Stewart 1982). Drake and Sederer (1986) have reported that the patient's perception of sudden loss of family support early in the course of inpatient treatment occasionally leads to suicidal behavior. Thus the family therapist, while accepting the family's need for respite, must also foster a supportive connection to the patient by emphasizing discharge planning from the start of treatment.

The family's attitude may adversely affect both the family treatment and the patient's discharge plan. Greenley (1982) found that the family often have a major effect upon a patient's length of hospital stay.

Case 2, Part 3

Barbara M.'s mother was less than enthusiastic after her meeting with the family therapist. Mrs. B. attended the day-long workshop on schizophrenia, but she was unconvinced that the information applied to Ms. M. or that any other family could understand her situation. She thought her daughter was a "bad seed" and would probably never change. That night, Ms. M. called her mother and reported that her therapist had begun to discuss discharge. Mrs. B. didn't sleep well that night, and the next day she called the "head psychiatrist." She complained that Ms. M. needed more time in the hospital and that the staff was making a big mistake by already making day hospital plans just 1 week after admission. Fortunately, the clinical director met daily with the service chiefs and was aware of Mrs. B.'s pessimistic attitude and of the staff's efforts to engage her in treatment. Knowing this, she advised Mrs. B. to discuss the matter with the family therapist.

Families who disagree with staff decisions regarding inpatient treatment, discharge, or aftercare plans may take their opinions either to individual staff members or to higher-level administrators (Harbin 1978). Potentially embarrassing situations can be avoided by working closely with the family and the treatment team: keeping each system informed of decisions being made in the other, respecting the family's opinions, and maintaining a tight, supportive, and well-coordinated administrative hierarchy with an open flow of accurate clinical information.

SPECIFIC FAMILY TREATMENT APPROACHES

The procedures to be described are pragmatic approaches, validated through outcome research, that represent a best guess of what works for families of acutely hospitalized patients with schizophrenic and major affective disorders.

Brief Family Crisis Intervention

Families of female patients with poor premorbid schizophrenia and bipolar disorder respond well to the model of family crisis treatment originally developed by Langsley and Kaplan (1968), applied to acute schizophrenia by Goldstein and colleagues (1978), and adapted to work with acute inpatients with schizophrenic and affective disorders by Glick and colleagues (1985). The Inpatient Family Intervention (IFI) program developed by Clarkin and colleagues (1981) is staged for 6 to 10 problem-focused sessions within the time frame of the inpatient stay. The first goal of treatment is that the family accept the notion that the patient has a genuine illness whose origin is biological but triggered by stress. The therapy then identifies and works to correct stressful family situations or interactive patterns that may have contributed to the patient's acute episode and need for hospitalization. Typical stressors usually involve the expression of criticism and hostility by family members toward the patient for failing to meet responsibilities. The patient's behavior is often interpreted as laziness or disobedience, and the failure to negotiate developmental role transitions may be seen as character weakness.

IFI begins once the patient has responded to psychotropic medication sufficiently to participate in family group sessions. The patient's psychiatrist and primary therapist should attend as many of these meetings as possible, both to lend credibility to the biomedical view of the patient's disorder and to facilitate the transmission of accurate information between the family and the treatment team. Often the first couple of sessions are devoted to helping the family develop an accurate picture of the patient's diagnosis and prognosis.

The four principal objectives of IFI include

1. Identifying typical situations or transactional sequences that were stressful for the patient during the period leading up to the hospitalization;
2. Developing strategies to change these behavioral patterns such that they are less stressful to the patient;

3. Having the family rehearse the new strategies in the session and then practice them at home while the patient is on pass; and
4. Anticipating future situations that could be stressful for the patient and devising solutions for them.

For instance, in Case 3, the family may point out that Robert appears to experience stress when his father reminds him constantly to take his medication, and when his mother yells at him for smoking wherever he pleases and for not doing his chores. Robert's father would agree to stop reminding if Robert would agree to take medication on schedule and to keep an accurate pill diary for a month. Robert's mother would agree to stop criticizing if Robert would agree to confine his smoking to certain rooms and to assume an acceptable schedule of chores. The therapy team would suggest that the family hold daily discussions devoted to the assignment and completion of household chores. In these discussions, more attention would be paid to improvement than to failure.

At least one session should be devoted to making aftercare plans. A functional assessment of the patient will help to determine whether the patient would benefit from placement in a partial hospitalization or psychosocial rehabilitation program (Anthony and Liberman 1986; Linn 1989). Some patients with schizophrenic or schizoaffective disorders may benefit from targeted or dosage-reduction antipsychotic medication strategies that depend on the cooperation of the family to identify early warning signs of impending relapse (Carpenter et al. 1990; Herz et al. 1982; Kane et al. 1983; Schooler 1991). Families wishing to continue treatment after completion of a course of IFI may be referred to an ongoing multifamily support group, a program of supportive family management, or a more intensive course of family therapy. Specific problems requiring continuing family care include persistent noncompliance or refusal to participate in rehabilitation programs, as well as ongoing, severe marital distress of the patient's parents or of the patient and spouse.

The Psychoeducational Workshop

The holding of periodic diagnosis-specific, daylong psychoeducational workshops for relatives or spouses can help to accomplish several objectives.

1. The workshop provides important scientific information in a more cost-effective format than working with individual families or spouses.
2. The workshop serves as a forum in which relatives can share their experiences with professionals and with other families.
3. Otherwise resistant families or spouses may follow the lead of more enthusiastic participants and become more willing to search for effective strategies to manage the patient's disorder.

In protocols developed by Anderson and colleagues (1986a) for schizophrenia and by Holder and Anderson (1990) for depression and bipolar disorder, the morning session provides a description of the scientific basis of the disorders and their medical management, whereas the afternoon session involves a discussion of the psychosocial aspects of symptom development and management, behavior control, recovery, and rehabilitation.

In psychoeducational workshops, an effort is made to present an accurate description of patients' and families' experiences in coping with the disorder. First-person accounts are read aloud (these are published regularly in *Schizophrenia Bulletin* under "First Person Accounts," and occasionally as special articles in *Hospital and Community Psychiatry*). Families are encouraged to set realistic expectations by comparing the patient with his or her own level of functioning in the previous 6 months, rather than with an idealized, "normal" person. Families are asked to relate to the patient in a calm and logical manner, to set realistic goals and limits, and to give praise and attention for specific patient accomplishments. Families are encouraged to expand their social networks and are told about the benefits of joining consumer support and advocacy groups for relatives of people with mental illness, such as local chapters of NAMI. The relatives' group can serve as a nexus from which families are referred to other modalities of family treatment.

Because participation in psychoeducational workshops often promotes the family's engagement in and the patient's compliance with continuing outpatient care, referral should occur soon after the patient's hospital admission. In situations where third-party payors or in-house utilization reviewers require very brief hospital stays, the family should be engaged through family crisis treatment and referred to a workshop soon after hospital discharge.

Multifamily Treatment

Male patients with bipolar, schizophrenic, or schizoaffective disorders who may be overstimulated by a full course of brief family crisis intervention should be referred with their families to an outpatient multifamily support group (multifamily treatment [MFT]). The professionally led multiple relatives group intervention developed by British investigators (Berkowitz 1984; Kuipers et al. 1989) and the multiple family approaches developed by American researchers (Atwood and Williams 1978; Beels 1975; Laqueur 1981; McFarlane 1983, 1990) provide an opportunity for families to continue to practice the stress reduction and problem-solving strategies introduced in the workshop within the secure and supportive atmosphere of the group.

Patient-absent and patient-included multifamily group formats each have distinct advantages. The absence of patients in relatives-only groups permits relatives to freely unburden themselves and to ally with other group members who share their experiential knowledge of the frustrations of coping with severe and persistent mental disorder. Thus relatives-only groups promote stronger peer group identification and bonding than groups that include patients. However, the presence of patients may foster more tolerant attitudes toward patients, enabling relatives to view psychotic behavior more objectively, as relatives other than their own describe hallucinations and delusions. They learn by "analogy and identification" (Laqueur 1981) and by modeling and spontaneous practice, and they serve as cotherapists to other patients and relatives (Gartner and Riessman 1982; McFarlane 1983).

This learning is enhanced while the group as a whole accumulates a repertoire of effective coping and management strategies that are then passed on as "group wisdom" to succeeding generations of new members (Cole 1983; Cole et al. 1979; Markewich 1986; O'Shea and Phelps 1985; Walsh 1987). Professional group leaders in MFT provide scientific information and facilitate the sharing of experiences and practical advice. Many meetings are devoted to problem-solving discussions in which families enact typical stressful situations and suggest alternative ways to understand and solve their problems.

Families who appear initially hesitant to attend may be engaged through individual family sessions or with one or two home visits that serve to underscore the psychoeducational principles of the workshop and the benefits of MFT. Families who drop out after attending several MFT meetings may be referred to individual family treatment (IFT).

A variant of MFT is the couples group for bipolar patients and their spouses.

Case 4

David W. was escorted in his acute manic state to the emergency room by his wife, Carol, and his outpatient psychiatrist. Ms. W. had endured 5 years of her husband's unpredictable mood swings. This had severely strained their marriage until he was correctly diagnosed and placed on lithium. Now Mr. W. had "broken through" lithium for the second time in 2 years. With the failure of lithium to contain her husband's disorder, Ms. W. was desperate. She was skeptical when the emergency room psychiatrist suggested that Mr. W. might respond to one of the new antiseizure drugs and that she should join a support group for manic-depressive couples. Ms. W. met the next day with the ward social worker, who mentioned that several patients in the group had complicated mood disorders.

That night in the group, Ms. W. discovered that there were other people who understood what it was like to live with someone like her husband. Because Mr. W. was still too unstable to join the group, his wife attended the first two meetings alone. By the time Mr. W. had begun to respond to medication, Ms. W. felt quite comfortable in the group and invited him to accompany her to "a place where manic-depressive individuals and their spouses and two therapists all look for ways to cope with mental illness."

In the couples group, close companions or marital partners develop tolerance, set reasonable limits to manic behavior, and identify early warning signs of relapse (Davenport and Adland 1988; Davenport et al. 1977; Mayo et al. 1979).

Combined Individual and Family Treatment

Although patients with uncomplicated primary depression and a benign family environment respond well to medication and individual psychotherapy, those with coexisting medical diagnoses, personality disorders, and family distress present more formidable therapeutic challenges that often require family intervention (Keitner et al. 1989). Because there are no controlled studies that evaluate specific inpatient family treatment approaches to unipolar depressive disorder, the following guidelines are based on what works for outpatients (e.g., O'Leary and Beach 1990) and on sound clinical judgment. Several investigators have recommended the combination of antidepressant medication or electroconvulsive therapy (ECT) with individual psychotherapy and marital or family therapy (Falloon et al. 1988; Haas et al. 1985, 1988; Keitner and Miller 1990; Weissman et al. 1987).

Case 5

Doris H. became severely depressed for the first time after the birth of her third child and second daughter. She was placed in the intensive care unit after taking an overdose of tricyclic antidepressants shortly after starting the medication. Following transfer to the psychiatry service, Mrs. H. was evaluated and a new trial of antidepressant medication begun.

Psychological testing indicated that Mrs. H. had borderline and dependent personality traits. A family interview with her husband, Jim, and two latency-age children revealed a longstanding pattern of family distress. Mr. H. reported that his wife had become "gloomy" since giving up her writing career to become a full-time housewife and mother; during this last pregnancy she had forsaken her household duties, charging that Mr. H. was a "workaholic." Mr. H. admitted staying late at the office to avoid facing a "negative atmosphere" at home. The behavior of the children reflected the distress of their parents: the older daughter's grades had fallen, and the son had been reported several times for truancy.

The treatment plan included medication and interpersonal and cognitive therapy for Mrs. H., in combination with family therapy. Her primary therapist would do the following:

1. Help Mrs. H. to recognize and correct negative "automatic thoughts" and underlying assumptions that helped to maintain her in a subservient family role;

2. Show that Mrs. H.'s chronic dysthymia had arisen with the loss of her identity as a writer; and
3. Coach Mrs. H. to be more assertive with her husband and to negotiate a more equitable distribution of parenting duties so that she could resume writing.

The family therapist would try to convince Mr. H. that the whole family would benefit from his assuming a more active role as father and homemaker. Mrs. H. would be given progressively more demanding responsibilities when visiting her family on weekend passes. The parents were coached to give each other praise rather than criticism, and the children were told to keep track of their parents' efforts. The H. family was taught to make requests, to make "corrective comments," and to listen in a way that conveyed an active interest in each other, and they were given several sessions on how to solve problems. All this required eight twice-weekly meetings, begun while Mrs. H. was an inpatient and continued after discharge, when the family was referred for continuing family therapy.

Thus, brief inpatient hospitalization may serve to engage the family in a more extended course of family treatment in the community. Marital or family therapy will help the patient to cope with distress in the intimate social field that might otherwise interfere with recovery (Keitner et al. 1987; Rounsaville et al. 1979). Because a person with unipolar depression has a tendency to express hostility toward his or her partner when in the acute phase, Friedman (1975) has suggested that family or marital therapy be postponed until the patient has begun to respond to medication or ECT and expresses a more positive attitude toward others. The course of combined family and individual treatment may vary. Coffman and Jacobson (1990) recommend 20 sessions of combined cognitive (12 sessions) and behavioral marital therapy (8 sessions). Falloon's team (1988) suggests beginning with hospital-based treatment and then holding further sessions in the patient's home. Curran and colleagues (1988) specify 12 sessions: 2 for education, 5 for communication training, and 5 for problem solving. Keitner and colleagues (1990) propose a package offering medication and individual treatment to patients while their families are treated with psychoeducation and family therapy and then referred to multifamily support groups.

If the therapist deems that the family situation requires more than crisis intervention or psychoeducational management, family therapy may be undertaken at any time during the acute inpatient stay. It is important to keep in mind that family therapy approaches that explore the past may be upsetting to relatives, whereas those that involve confrontation and the escalation of stress may be overstimulating to patients. In contrast, approaches effective for patients requiring brief hospitalization avoid the attribution of blame, recognize the legitimacy of medical diagnosis, and encourage patients and families to build on strengths through positive connotation and a behavioral program of communication training, problem solving, modeling, enactment, and rehearsal (Anderson et al. 1986a; Coffman and Jacobson 1990; Cole 1982; Cole and Jacobs 1989; Coyne 1984; Epstein and Bishop 1981; Falloon 1981; Falloon et al. 1988; Jacobson and Margolin 1979).

CONCLUSIONS

In this chapter, I have presented a family intervention model suitable for brief inpatient psychiatric hospitalization of patients with schizophrenic and affective disorders.

The strategies and techniques discussed here derive from 20 years of family interaction studies and outcome research that have made us aware of the burdens families bear and of how changes in family transactional patterns can help to reduce patient relapse. The model recognizes the importance of treating the patient's acute symptoms with appropriate drug or ECT intervention. The family treatment model emphasizes the importance of engaging the family as soon as possible and places the family therapist in the role of family advocate and mediator between the family and inpatient service systems.

The psychoeducational approach begins with a course of brief family crisis intervention and referral to a psychoeducational workshop, followed by referral to family treatment tracks organized according to the patient's sex, diagnosis, and level of premorbid functioning. Families of women with bipolar or poor premorbid schizophrenic disorders are given a full course of 6 to 8 sessions of family crisis treatment. Families of men with bipolar or poor premorbid schizophrenic disorders are encouraged to join ongoing, professionally led multiple family groups. Unipolar depressive patients are offered a course of individual psychotherapy, followed by involvement in marital or family therapy.

For most of these families, it is crucial that family treatment be continued after the patient leaves the hospital. Ongoing family treatment helps to improve family problem solving, to ease the burden on the family, and to assure patient compliance with medication and rehabilitation. This program of family treatment will improve the patient's chances of remaining relapse-free and will thereby promote a more complete recovery from acute psychosis.

We can hope that outcome studies over the next 20 years will provide information that will not only strengthen our confidence in the suitability of the brief inpatient family treatment model for patients with schizophrenic and affective disorders, but will also expand our knowledge to include approaches for patients with other psychiatric diagnoses.

REFERENCES

Anderson CM: Family intervention with severely disturbed inpatients. Arch Gen Psychiatry 34:697–702, 1977

Anderson CM, Reiss DJ: Family treatment of patients with chronic schizophrenia: the inpatient phase, in The Psychiatric Hospital and the Family. Edited by Harbin HT. New York, SP Medical & Scientific Books, 1982, pp 79–101

Anderson CM, Reiss DJ, Hogarty GE: Schizophrenia and the Family. New York, Guilford, 1986a

Anderson CM, Griffin S, Rossi A, et al: A comparative study of the impact of education vs process groups for families of patients with affective disorders. Fam Process 25(2):185–206, 1986b

Anthony WA, Liberman RP: The practice of psychiatric rehabilitation: historical and research base. Schizophr Bull 12(4):542–559, 1986

Appleton WS: Mistreatment of patients' families by psychiatrists. Am J Psychiatry 131(6):655–657, 1974

Atwood N, Williams MED: Group support for the families of the mentally ill. Schizophr Bull 4(3):415–425, 1978

Beels CC: Family and social management of schizophrenia. Schizophr Bull 1(13):97–118, 1975

Beels CC, Gutwirth L, Berkeley J, et al: Measurements of social support in schizophrenia. Schizophr Bull 10(3):399–411, 1984

Berkowitz R: Therapeutic interventions with schizophrenic patients and their families: a description of a clinical research project. Journal of Family Therapy 6(3):211–233, 1984

Bernheim KF, Lehman AF: Working With Families of the Mentally Ill. New York, WW Norton, 1985

Biddle JR: Working with families within inpatient settings. Journal of Marriage and Family Counseling 4:43–51, 1978

Birtchnell J: Dependence and its relationship to depression. Br J Med Psychol 57:215–225, 1984

Boyd JH: The interaction of family therapy and psychodynamic individual therapy in an inpatient setting. Psychiatry 42:99–111, 1979

Brown GW, Harris T: Social Origins of Depression: A Study of Psychiatric Disorders in Women. New York, Free Press, 1978

Brown GW, Monck EM, Carstairs GM, et al: Influence of family life on the course of schizophrenic illness. British Journal of Preventive Social Medicine 16:55–68, 1962

Brown GW, Birley JLT, Wing JK: Influence of family life on the course of schizophrenic disorders: a replication. Br J Psychiatry 121:241–258, 1972

Carpenter WT, Hanlon TE, Heinrichs DW, et al: Continuous versus targeted medication in schizophrenic outpatients: outcome results. Am J Psychiatry 147(9):1138–1148, 1990

Clarkin JF, Spencer JH, Peyser J, et al: Training Manual for Inpatient Family Intervention for Affective Disorders. New York, Payne Whitney Clinic, Cornell University Medical Center, 1981

Clarkin JF, Haas GL, Glick ID: Inpatient family intervention, in Affective Disorders and the Family: Assessment and Treatment. Edited by Clarkin JF, Haas GL, Glick ID. New York, Guilford, 1988, pp 134–152

Clarkin JF, Glick ID, Haas GL, et al: A randomized clinical trial of inpatient family intervention. J Affect Disord 18:17–28, 1990

Coffman SJ, Jacobson NS: Social learning-based marital therapy and cognitive therapy as a combined treatment for depression, in Depression and Families: Impact and Treatment. Edited by Keitner GI. Washington, DC, American Psychiatric Press, 1990, pp 3–29

Cole SA: Problem-focused family therapy: principles and practical applications, in Psychopathology in Childhood. Edited by Lachenmeyer JR, Gibbs MS. New York, Gardner Press, 1982, pp 341–374

Cole SA: Self-help groups, in Comprehensive Group Psychotherapy, Vol II. Edited by Kaplan HI, Sadock BJ. Baltimore, MD, Williams & Wilkins, 1983, pp 144–150

Cole SA, Cole DS: Professionals who work with families of the chronic mentally ill: current status and suggestions for clinical training, in Families of the Mentally III: Coping and Adaptation. Edited by Hatfield A, Lefley H. New York, Guilford, 1987, pp 278–306

Cole SA, Jacobs J: Family treatment of schizophrenia, in Treatments of Psychiatric Disorders. Edited by Karasu TB. Washington, DC, American Psychiatric Press, 1989, pp 1543–1567

Cole SA, O'Connor SO, Bennett L: Self-help groups for clinic patients with chronic illness. Prim Care 6(2):325–340, 1979

Coyne JC: Depression and the response of others. J Abnorm Psychol 85(2):186–193, 1976

Coyne JC: Strategic therapy with depressed married persons: initial agenda, themes and interventions. Journal of Marital and Family Therapy 10(1):53–62, 1984

Coyne JC: Depression, biology, marriage and marital therapy. Journal of Marital and Family Therapy 13(4):393–407, 1987

Creer C, Wing JK: Living with a schizophrenic patient. Br J Hosp Med, July 1975, pp 73–82

Curran JP, Faraone SV, Graves DJ: Acute inpatient settings, in Handbook of Behavioral Family Therapy. Edited by Falloon IRH. New York, Guilford, 1988, pp 285–315

Davenport YB, Adland ML: Management of manic episodes, in Affective Disorders and the Family: Assessment and Treatment. Edited by Clarkin J, Haas G, Glick I. New York, Guilford, 1988, pp 173–195

Davenport YB, Ebert MH, Adland ML, et al: Couples group therapy as an adjunct to lithium maintenance of the manic patient. Am J Orthopsychiatry 47(3):495–502, 1977

Doll W: Family coping with the mentally ill: an unanticipated problem of deinstitutionalization. Hosp Community Psychiatry 27(3):183–185, 1976

Drake RE, Sederer LI: Inpatient psychosocial treatment of chronic schizophrenia: negative effects and current guidelines. Hosp Community Psychiatry 37(9):897–901, 1986

Epstein NB, Bishop DS: Problem-centered systems therapy of the family. Journal of Marriage and Family Therapy 7(1):23–32, 1981

Fadden G, Bebbington P, Kuipers L: The burden of care: the impact of functional psychiatric illness on the patient's family. Br J Psychiatry 150:285–292, 1987

Falloon IRH: Communication and problem.solving skills training with relapsing schizophrenics and their families, in Family Therapy and Major Psychopathology. Edited by Lansky MR. New York, Grune & Stratton, 1981, pp 35–56

Falloon IRH, Hole V, Mudray L, et al: Behavioral family therapy, in Affective Disorders and the Family: Assessment and Treatment. Edited by Clarkin JF, Haas GL, Glick ID. New York, Guilford, 1988, pp 117–133

Friedman AS: Interaction of drug therapy with marital therapy in depressive patients. Arch Gen Psychiatry 32:619–637, 1975

Gartner AJ, Riessman F: Self-help and mental health. Hosp Community Psychiatry 33(8):631–635, 1982

Glick ID, Clarkin JF: The effects of family presence and brief family intervention for hospitalized schizophrenic patients: a review, in The Psychiatric Hospital and the Family. Edited by Harbin HT. New York, SP Medical & Scientific Books, 1982, pp 157–171

Glick ID, Clarkin JF, Spencer JH, et al: A controlled evaluation of inpatient family interaction, I: preliminary results of the six-month follow-up. Arch Gen Psychiatry 42:882–886, 1985

Glick ID, Clarkin JF, Haas GL, et al: A randomized clinical trial of inpatient family intervention, VI: mediating variables and outcome. Fam Process 30(1):85–99, 1991

Goldstein MJ, Rodnick E, Evans JR, et al: Drug and family therapy in the aftercare of acute schizophrenics. Arch Gen Psychiatry 35:1169–1177, 1978

Gotlib IH, Whiffen VE: Depression and marital functioning: an examination of specificity and gender differences. J Abnorm Psychol 98(1):23–30, 1989

Gould E, Glick ID: The effects of family presence and brief family intervention on global outcome for hospitalized schizophrenic patients. Fam Process 16(4):503–510, 1977

Greenley JR: The patient's family and length of psychiatric hospitalization, in The Psychiatric Hospital and the Family. Edited by Harbin HT. New York, SP Medical & Scientific Books, 1982, pp 213–237

Greenman DA, Gunderson JG, Canning D: Parents' attitudes and patients' behavior: a prospective study. Am J Psychiatry 146:226–230, 1989

Group for the Advancement of Psychiatry, Committee on the Family: The Family, the Patient, and the Psychiatric Hospital. New York, Brunner/Mazel, 1985

Haas GL, Clarkin JF, Glick ID: Marital and family treatment of depression, in Handbook of Depression: Treatment, Assessment and Research. Edited by Beckham EE, Leber WR. Homewood, IL, Dorsey Press, 1985, pp 151–183

Haas GL, Glick ID, Clarkin JF, et al: Inpatient family intervention: a randomized clinical trial, II: results of hospital discharge. Arch Gen Psychiatry 45:217–224, 1988

Haas GL, Glick ID, Clarkin JF, et al: Gender and schizophrenia outcome: a clinical trial of an inpatient family intervention. Schizophr Bull 16(2):277–292, 1990

Hahlweg K, Nuechterlein KH, Goldstein MJ, et al: Parental expressed emotion: attitudes and intrafamilial communication behavior, in Understanding Mental Disorder: The Contribution of Family Interaction Research. Edited by Hahlweg K, Goldstein MJ. New York, Family Process Press, 1987, pp 156–175

Harbin HT: Families and hospitals: collusion or cooperation? Am J Psychiatry 135(12):1496–1499, 1978

Harbin HT: A family-oriented psychiatric inpatient unit. Fam Process 18:281–291, 1979

Harbin HT: The family treatment of the psychiatric patient, in The Psychiatric Hospital and the Family. Edited by Harbin HT. New York, SP Medical & Scientific Books, 1982, pp 3–25

Hatfield AB: Coping and adaptation: a conceptual framework for understanding families, in Families of the Mentally Ill: Coping and Adaptation. Edited by Hatfield AB, Lefley HP. New York, Guilford, 1987, pp 30–59

Herz MI, Szymanski HV, Simon JC: Intermittent medication for stable schizophrenic outpatients: a alternative to maintenance medication. Am J Psychiatry 139(7):918–922, 1982

Hill R: Generic features of families under stress, in Crisis Intervention. Edited by Parad HJ. New York, Family Service Association, 1965, pp 32–52

Holden DF, Levine RRJ: How families evaluate mental health professionals, resources and effects of illness. Schizophr Bull 8(4):626–633, 1982

Holder ID, Anderson C: Psychoeducational family intervention for depressed patients and their families, in Depression and Families: Impact and Treatment. Edited by Keitner GI. Washington, DC, American Psychiatric Press, 1990, pp 159–184

Hooley JM: Expressed emotion and depression: interaction between patients and high versus low expressed emotion spouses. J Abnorm Psychol 95:237–246, 1986

Hooley JM, Teasdale JD: Predictors of relapse in unipolar depression: expressed emotion, marital distress and perceived criticism. J Abnorm Psychol 98(3):229–235, 1989

Hooley JM, Orley J, Teasdale JD: Levels of expressed emotion and relapse in depressed patients. Br J Psychiatry 148:642–647, 1986

Hooley JM, Richters JE, Weintraub S, et al: Psychopathology and marital distress: the positive side of positive symptoms. J Abnorm Psychol 96(1):27–33, 1987

Hoover CF, Fitzgerald PG: Dominance in the marriages of affective patients. J Nerv Ment Dis 169(10):624–628, 1981

Jacobson NS, Margolin G: Marital Therapy: Strategies Based on Social Learning and Behavior Exchange Principles. New York, Brunner/Mazel, 1979

Janowsky ID, Leff M, Epstein R: The manic game. Arch Gen Psychiatry 22:252–261, 1970

Janowsky ID, Kraft A, Clopton P, et al: Relationships of mood and interpersonal perceptions. Compr Psychiatry 25(6):546–551, 1984

Johnson DL: The family's experience of living with mental illness, in Families as Allies in Treatment of the Mentally Ill. Edited by Lefley HP, Johnson DL. Washington, DC, American Psychiatric Press, 1990, pp 31–63

Kane JM, Rifkin A, Woerner M: Low-dose neuroleptic treatment of outpatient schizophrenics, I: preliminary results for relapse rates. Arch Gen Psychiatry 40:893–896, 1983

Kaplan De-Nour A: Psychosocial aspects of the management of mania, in Mania: An Evolving Concept. Edited by Belmaker RH, van Praag HM. New York, SP Medical & Scientific Books, 1980, pp 349–364

Keitner GI, Miller IW: Family functioning and major depression: an overview. Am J Psychiatry 147(9):1128–1137, 1990

Keitner GI, Miller IW, Epstein NB, et al: Family functioning and the course of major depression. Compr Psychiatry 28(1):54–64, 1987

Keitner GI, Miller IW, Ryan CE, et al: Compounded depression and family functioning during the acute episode and at six-month follow-up. Compr Psychiatry 30(6):512–521, 1989

Keitner GI, Miller IW, Epstein NB, et al: Family processes and the course of depressive illness, in Depression and Families: Impact and Treatment. Edited by Keitner GI. Washington, DC, American Psychiatric Press, 1990, pp 3–29

Krajewski T, Harbin HT: The family changes the hospital? in The Psychiatric Hospital and the Family. Edited by Harbin HT. New York, SP Medical & Scientific Books, 1982, pp 143–154

Kreisman DE, Joy VD: The family as reactor to the mental illness of a relative, in Handbook of Evaluation Research, Vol 2. Edited by Struening E, Guttentag M. Beverly Hills, CA, Sage, 1975, pp 483–518

Kuipers L, Bebbington PE: Expressed emotion research in schizophrenia: theoretical and clinical implications. Psychol Med 18:593–609, 1988

Kuipers L, Sturgeon ID, Berkowitz R, et al: Characteristics of expressed emotion: its relationship to speech and looking in schizophrenic patients and their relatives. Br J Clin Psychol 22:257–264, 1983

Kuipers L, MacCarthy B, Hurry J, et al: Counseling the relatives of the long-term adult mentally ill, II: a low-cost supportive model. Br J Psychiatry 154:775–782, 1989

Langsley DG, Kaplan DM: The Treatment of Families in Crisis. New York, Grune & Stratton, 1968

Laqueur HP: Multiple family therapy, in Family Therapy and Major Psychopathology. Edited by Lansky MR. New York, Grune & Stratton, 1981, pp 57–69

Lefley HP, Johnson DL (eds): Families as Allies in the Treatment of the Mentally Ill. Washington, DC, American Psychiatric Press, 1990

Linn MW: Partial hospitalization, in A Clinical Guide for the Treatment of Schizophrenia. Edited by Bellack AS. New York, Plenum, 1989, pp 163–185

MacCarthy B, Hemsley DR: Unpredictability as a correlate of expressed emotion in the relatives of schizophrenics. Br J Psychiatry 148:727–731, 1986

MacCarthy B, Kuipers L, Hurry J, et al: Counseling the relatives of the long-term mentally ill, I: evaluation of the impact on relatives and patients. Br J Psychiatry 154:768–775, 1989

Markewich I: Multiple family group therapy for schizophrenic patients in a day treatment program: a comparison of patient-included and patient-excluded groups for families with different levels of expressed emotion. New York, New York University School of Education, Health, Nursing and Arts Professions, 1986

Matussek P, Wiegand M: Partnership problems as causes of endogenous and neurotic depression. Acta Psychiatr Scand 71:95–104, 1985

Mayo JA, O'Connell RA, O'Brien JD: Families of manic-depressive patients: effect of treatment. Am J Psychiatry 136(12):1535–1539, 1979

McFarlane WR: Multiple family therapy in schizophrenia, in Family Therapy in Schizophrenia. Edited by McFarlane WR. New York, Guilford, 1983, pp 141–172

McFarlane WR: Multiple family groups and the treatment of schizophrenia, in Psychosocial Treatment of Schizophrenia. Edited by Herz MI, Keith SJ, Docherty JP. New York, Elsevier, 1990, pp 167–189

McGill CW, Falloon IRH, Boyd JL, et al: Family educational interventions in the treatment of schizophrenia. Hosp Community Psychiatry 34(10):934–938, 1983

Miklowitz DJ, Goldstein MJ, Falloon IRH: Premorbid and symptomatic characteristics of schizophrenics from families with high and low levels of expressed emotion. J Abnorm Psychol 92(3):359–367, 1983

Miklowitz DJ, Goldstein MJ, Falloon IRH, et al: Interactional correlates of expressed emotion in families of schizophrenics. Br J Psychiatry 144:482–487, 1984

Miklowitz DJ, Strachan AM, Goldstein MJ, et al: Expressed emotion and communication deviance in the families of schizophrenics. J Abnorm Psychol 95(1):60–66, 1986

Miklowitz DJ, Goldstein MJ, Nuechterlein KH, et al: Family factors and the course of bipolar affective disorder. Arch Gen Psychiatry 45:225–231, 1988

Miklowitz DJ, Goldstein MJ, Doane JA, et al: Is expressed emotion an index of a transactional process? I. parents' affective style. Fam Process 28:153–167, 1989

Miller IW, Kabacoff RI, Keitner GI, et al: Family functioning in the families of psychiatric patients. Compr Psychiatry 27(4):302–312, 1986

O'Connell RA, Mayo JA, Eng LK, et al: Social support and long-term lithium outcome. Br J Psychiatry 147:272–275, 1985

O'Leary KD, Beach SRH: Marital therapy: a viable treatment for depression and marital discord. Am J Psychiatry 147(2):183–186, 1990

O'Shea MD, Phelps R: Multiple family therapy: current status and critical appraisal. Fam Process 24(4):555–582, 1985

Parad HJ, Caplan G: A framework for studying families in crisis, in Crisis Intervention. Edited by Parad HJ. New York, Family Service Association, 1965, pp 53–72

Priebe S, Wildgrube C, Muller-Oerlinghausen B: Lithium prophylaxis and expressed emotion. Br J Psychiatry 154:396–399, 1989

Rabkin R: Crisis intervention, in The Book of Family Therapy. Edited by Ferber A, Mendelsohn M. New York, Science House, 1972, pp 582–596

Reiss ID, Costell R, Jones C, et al: The family meets the hospital. Arch Gen Psychiatry 37:141–154, 1980

Rounsaville BJ, Weismann MM, Prusoff BA, et al: Marital disputes and treatment outcome in depressed women. Compr Psychiatry 20(5):483–490, 1979

Scharfstein B, Libbey M: Family orientation: initiating patients and their families to psychiatric hospitalization. Hosp Community Psychiatry 33(7):560–563, 1982

Schmaling KB, Jacobson NS: Marital interaction and depression. J Abnorm Psychol 99(1):229–236, 1990

Schooler NR: Maintenance medication for schizophrenics: strategies for dose reduction. Schizophr Bull 17(2):311–324, 1991

Spencer JH, Glick ID, Haas GL, et al: A randomized clinical trial of inpatient family intervention, III: effects at 6-month and 18-month follow-up. Am J Psychiatry 145(9):1115–1121, 1988

Steinglass P: Psychoeducational family therapy for schizophrenia: a review essay. Psychiatry 50:14–23, 1987

Stewart RP: Building an alliance between the families of patients and the hospital: model and process. NAPPH Journal 12:63–68, 1982

Strachan AM, Leff JP, Goldstein MJ, et al: Emotional attitudes and direct communication in the families of schizophrenics: a cross-national replication. Br J Psychiatry 149:279–287, 1986

Strachan AM, Feingold ID, Goldstein MJ, et al: Is expressed emotion an index of a transactional process? II: patient's coping style. Fam Process 28:169–181, 1989

Strauss JS, Hafez H, Lieberman P, et al: The course of psychiatric disorder, III: longitudinal principles. Am J Psychiatry 142(3):289–296, 1985

Terkelsen KG: Schizophrenia and the family, II: adverse effects of family therapy. Fam Process 22(2):191–200, 1983

Vaughn CE: Patterns of emotional response in the families of schizophrenic patients, in Treatment of Schizophrenia: Family Assessment and Intervention. Edited by Goldstein MJ, Hand I, Hahlweg K. New York, Springer-Verlag New York, 1986, pp 97–106

Vaughn CE, Leff JP: The influence of family life and social factors on the course of psychiatric illness: a comparison of schizophrenic and depressed neurotic patients. Br J Psychiatry 129:125–137, 1976

Vine P, Beels CC: Support and advocacy groups for the mentally ill, in Psychosocial Treatment of Schizophrenia. Edited by Herz MI, Keith SJ, Docherty JP. New York, Elsevier, 1990, pp 387–405

Walsh J: The family education and support group: a psychoeducational aftercare program. Psychosocial Rehabilitation Journal 10(3):51–61, 1987

Weissman MM, Jarrett RB, Rush JA: Psychotherapy and its relevance to the pharmacotherapy of major depression: a decade later (1976–1985), in Psychopharmacology: The Third Generation of Progress. Edited by Meltzer HY. New York, Raven, 1987, pp 1059–1069

Withersty DJ: Family involvement on a psychiatric inpatient service. Am J Psychiatry 134(1):93–94, 1977

Wynne LC, McDaniel S, Weber TT (eds): Systems Consultation: A New Perspective for Family Therapy. New York, Guilford, 1986

Wynne LC, McDaniel SH, Weber TT: Professional politics and the concepts of family therapy, family consultation and systems consultation. Fam Process 26(2):153–166, 1987

Youngren MA, Lewinsohn PM: The functional relation between depression and problematic interpersonal behavior. J Abnorm Psychol 89(3):333–341, 1980

CHAPTER 5

Group Psychotherapy

Howard D. Kibel, M.D.

Inpatient treatment is multimodal. On the modern, short-term psychiatric unit, patients receive a variety of somatic treatments, usually have individual psychotherapy and group psychotherapy, attend family sessions, may attend a community meeting, and participate in therapeutic activities. Cutting across these separate modalities are the nonspecific effects of the milieu, which are difficult to specify and harder to control. Each of these modalities has its own purpose and role in the treatment system; yet they must be related to one another in a rational way for the overall structure of inpatient treatment to be coherent. This principle applies no less to group psychotherapy. Patients on these units are part of a tightly organized social structure in which they are continually subjected to helpful or noxious influences from treatment personnel and from each other. It is important to integrate the psychotherapy group into this social structure and the treatment program of the hospital rather than to insert it as a foreign body.

Inpatient group psychotherapy is widely used (Yalom 1983). Its practice is quite varied. Each approach has its defined purpose, identifies specific goals, and employs distinctive methodology. In most, the thrust of intervention is pragmatic. Rarely do practitioners consider the relationship of the group to the overall treatment system; the two usually remain unintegrated. In this chapter, after a brief review of the current scope of practice, I define an approach that aims to be integrated with and facilitative to the milieu. I then outline its method, particularly in terms of goals for a short-term unit.

CURRENT PRACTICES

The history of inpatient group psychotherapy is almost as old as group psychotherapy itself, dating back to the end of World War I. However, it was not until the mid-1970s that therapists had to adapt to the clinical realities of shortened lengths of stay and rapid patient turnover with heterogeneous populations on the same unit (Marcovitz and Smith 1986). Clinicians once had the luxury of time, which allowed them to transpose techniques developed with outpatients to the hospital setting. The realities of short-term treatment have necessitated the development of newer group methods. These have been largely structured, directive, and focused on symptom removal rather than addressing underlying processes.

Practice has been diverse. Some have used role-playing, a "hot seat" technique, and videotape feedback (Waxer 1977). Others have employed nonverbal exercises (Cory and Page 1978) or used psychodrama and related experiential techniques (Farrell 1976), whereas still others have used confrontational approaches (Rabiner et al. 1973), didactic methods (Druck 1978), or educational techniques (Maxmen 1978). In an effort to fit the method to the patient, certain workers have advocated the use of a graded group program that is geared to the patient's level of functioning (Betcher et al. 1982; Griffin-Shelley and Trachtenberg 1985). In some programs (Leopold 1976), patients progress from a highly structured and supportive group for regressed psychotic patients, to one in which directive techniques are used to promote interpersonal skills, and finally to one composed of both outpatients and inpatients who are nearing discharge. Kanas (1985) has designed a method for homogeneous groups of schizophrenic patients that can be applied to both inpatients and outpatients. Most practitioners exclude patients who are actively psychotic and disorganized (Marcovitz and Smith 1983; Maxmen 1984), whereas many only use methods that are suited to patients who are motivated and better functioning (Brabender 1985).

Common to most inpatient methods are the use of support and structure, active facilitation by the therapist, problem spotting, and problem solving. This is typified by Yalom's method (1983), to be described below, and those of Rabiner and colleagues (1973) and Maxmen (1978). All of these methods aim to rapidly reduce the problematic behavior that led to hospitalization. Patients are encouraged to identify maladaptive behavior, control it, and detect and avert those situations that could lead to a recurrence of symptoms. The leader's role in Maxmen's method is to literally train the patients to work therapeutically with each other (Marcovitz and Smith 1986). Through this experience, it is hoped that the patients will be more accepting of professional help in the future.

Some practitioners design treatment to take into account the various cognitive deficits displayed by many chronic patients (Erickson 1989). Limited attention and concentration necessitate shorter and more frequent sessions. Deficits in learning and memory may be minimized when repetition and behavioral practice are incorporated into technique. Consequently, various methods are used that aim to develop social skills (Rubin and Locascio 1985) and improve problem solving (Powell et al. 1988). These cognitive therapies are instructional in nature and use techniques ranging from semistructured exercises to fairly didactic ones.

Yalom (1983) developed a structured method for here-and-now interpersonal learning. He describes two separate approaches, one for patients functioning on a higher level and another for those functioning on a lower level. The former approach is better known and more widely used. The latter, used with more impaired patients, employs verbal tasks in a systematic way. These consist of a series of prescribed, graded sentence-completion exercises. In contrast, the higher-level group works with an agenda created by the patients to modify behavior. This method is focused and pragmatic, like many others in current use. Yalom's treatment philosophy is typified by the following:

> Although group therapy is not the most effective format to reduce anxiety, relieve profound depression or ameliorate psychotic thinking or behavioral disturbances, it is the therapy setting nonpareil to help individuals learn about maladaptive interpersonal behavior. (p. 56)

With this method, patients are encouraged to play out their self-identified, interpersonal problems within the here and now of the group session. Given the rapid turnover in a modern hospital, all issues raised in one session are resolved at that time. There is no room for carryover from session to session. Unlike other practitioners who allow discussion of behavior that occurs on the unit but outside the group, Yalom (1983) restricts the focus to the small therapy group itself. He eschews any consideration of genetic, current life, or milieu issues. The therapist assists each member in formulating a personal agenda for that meeting. Typical agendas include reluctance to share personal information, annoyance with others, feelings of rejection, fear of confronting others, difficulty with anger or sexual feelings, and erroneous beliefs about social aspects of personality.

> At one session, a patient stated that she was unable to provide an agenda item because she had nothing of value to contribute. A second patient reported that his wife repeatedly complained that he ignored her. During the ensuing discussion, the therapist directed the man to draw this woman out and tell her what she said that he found interesting.

This method has several characteristics. It is structured and stylized, it is leader directed, and it is behaviorally oriented. Although it is adynamic, it is pragmatic and easily teachable. In contrast, there are few approaches that claim to be psychodynamic. Rice and Rutan (1987) have advocated the consideration of group transferences, resistances, and genetic factors. They have elaborated general principles of treatment but have not developed a specific methodology.

In general, evidence for the effectiveness of one method over another is lacking. Models that encourage the expression of affect have not been shown to be of value (Pattison et al. 1967), and those that uncritically transpose outpatient expressive techniques can be frankly detrimental (Beutler et al. 1984). The earlier reviews of controlled studies were pessimistic as to the benefits of group psychotherapy for inpatients (Stotsky and Zolik 1965; Parloff and Dies 1977). Although another review was more sanguine (Kanas 1986), its conclusions were called into question (Parloff 1986). With shortened lengths of stay, it has become more difficult to isolate the effects of group psychotherapy in a multimodal treatment system. It has therefore become harder for researchers to prove that group helps, much less to discern which method is best.

THE MILIEU AND THE PSYCHOTHERAPY GROUP

People change, learn, and mature as a result of their interpersonal and social relationships and experiences. Knowledge of this has been applied in the treatment of mental illness, notably with the psychotherapies—individual, group, and family. A logical extension of this notion is to use the total environment in a deliberate attempt to shape behavior. This is the principle that underlies milieu treatment.

Klein (1977) reviewed a series of studies on inpatient psychotherapy groups that "provided evidence that the social system of the ward, with its norms, expectations, and values, plays a particularly important role in determining patient behavior in group meetings and has a significant impact on the therapeutic process" (p. 201). Earlier in my career, I had an opportunity to work on two wards at the same time. Both had heterogeneous populations, but with a preponderance of patients with schizophrenic disorders. Admissions were assigned to each at random. Yet patients on one ward were socialized in their behavior, whereas those on the other acted in bizarre ways. In groups on the first ward, patients engaged in orderly discussion; but on the second, the conversations were disorganized and content was often incoherent. This experience was consistent with the studies of psychiatric units as social systems (Astrachan et al. 1968), which showed that each community has its preferred way of thinking, feeling, and behaving. Its values are communicated to new arrivals through various formal and informal structures on the unit.

From a general systems perspective, any organization, such as the psychiatric unit, can be conceived of as an overall system, with dynamically interrelated component subsystems (Kernberg 1978). For practical purposes, the psychiatric unit functions like a large group, with its own norms and internal tensions. The small psychotherapy group, which is convened intermittently, should be viewed as sort of a subgroup of the larger unit as a whole. For this reason, its dynamics symbolically reflect those of the milieu within which it resides (Klein and Kugel 1981). In other words, diagnosis of a group session is like a biopsy of the milieu (Levine 1980) in that it reveals the overall regressive dynamic forces of the unit as these are expressed in the patient subculture. From this perspective, the small psychotherapy group can be designed to function at the interface between the intrapsychic world of each member and shared conflicts that are generated within the milieu at large (Kibel 1987a). It will be shown that the purpose of the group is to bring these two levels of experience together so that the milieu is functional.

The psychiatric unit is a complex social system in which patients must learn with whom to communicate about their problems and how to behave to get what they want (usually unit privileges and a preferred disposition). Tensions within the unit enhance regression in already troubled patients. These tensions encourage the reenactment of conflicted, internal object relations within the interpersonal field of the hospital milieu. Patients play out their inner views of relationships, which contain distortions about others linked with defended notions about themselves. These distortions might cause the patients to view the staff as overly controlling, or even oppressive and punitive. In response, patients can act in ways that make their withdrawal and distrust seem responsive. The milieu thus affords opportunities for the identification of these paradigms; but more importantly, it serves as an arena in which primitive object relations can be gradually influenced and, one hopes, modified (Kernberg 1976; Kibel 1987a).

The group is therapeutic when it operates in one of two ways. First, regressive behaviors (i.e., group processes) can be clarified by explaining to the patients that they are reactions to environmental events. For example, in one group, patients voiced fears that passive behavior could be dangerous. This occurred after a weekend during which a manic patient lashed out at his roommate, who had expressed fears of homosexual assault. In another group, patients protested needlessly some minor procedures that they considered to be restrictive. Yet simultaneously, they complained that the sickest patients were given too much freedom. This occurred at a time when the hours for which the unit's main door was unlocked had been increased.

In the second therapeutic use of the group, milieu issues are introduced directly for discussion and resolution. Whereas the first could be said to be "deductive," because it involves decoding metaphor, the second is "inductive." More will be said about this later.

Patients are dependent on the staff both for psychological sustenance (namely, dependency gratification) and for concrete help in terms of advice and recommendations. They are required to partially surrender autonomy, conform to the unit's regulations, and submit to the decisions of the clinic staff regarding their treatment and discharge planning. In a very real way, they depend on these clinicians to prescribe for their future. Patients are often ambivalent about complying with treatment. They want to have their needs met but resent having to accommodate others.

Patients tend to view others, particularly those invested with authority, in highly ambivalent and fantastic ways. Their yearnings and distrust, their dependency and paranoia, infect all relationships with the unit staff, existing alongside adaptive, realistic, and therapeutic attitudes. In a dynamic sense, ambivalence and resistance are inherent in the treatment process; they are intrinsic to the hospital treatment alliance. This is why everything on the unit, from medication compliance to disposition planning, becomes an issue.

Attention to the hospital treatment alliance has become more important as lengths of stay have been shortened. Longer inpatient stays had been associated with compliance with aftercare, thereby maintaining continuity in the treatment (Axelrod and Wetzler 1989). But relapse and recidivism have become commonplace in recent years on short-term units. Readmission aggravates the experience of these patients with failure. Although recidivism is part and parcel of chronic mental illness, it is often not blamed on the illness but on the patient (Craig and Hyatt 1978). This sets the stage for untoward interactions between patients and staff on the psychiatric unit. Research has shown that rehospitalized patients tend to feel more alienated from professionals compared with their counterparts who are successfully maintained in aftercare (Axelrod and Wetzler 1989). Treatment of the patient-team alliance can facilitate the development of trust that then, one hopes, mitigates the estrangement.

The small therapy group, by virtue of its social nature, dramatizes conflicts between patients and staff. The group therapist becomes the object of projection, because he or she is identified with the treatment team. Therefore, working out the relationship of the therapist to the group will greatly benefit the hospital treatment alliance. In this way, the psychotherapy group can be seen to lie at the center of milieu therapy.

In the following clinical example, the patients' conflicts with the treatment team were prominent, which is not always the case. The focus was on the staff's use of power to control behavior, grant privileges, and plan the patients' future.

A newly admitted patient, Anna L., had yet to join the group because her behavior had been too disorganized. She spent much time in the quiet room, yelling and screaming without apparent reason. Several patients were soon to be discharged, one of whom was to be transferred to a state hospital for custodial care. (The session described here was from a twice-weekly group on a unit with an average length of stay of 4 weeks; the group was led by a staff nurse and a psychiatric resident.)

The nurse began the session by introducing a new member. She then announced that for two patients, this would be their last session, because they would be discharged before the next one. A third patient would probably be transferred to a longer-term unit by then. This man quipped, sarcastically, "What do you mean, 'probably'?," to which he was given a factual answer. One patient reported that she might also leave by then, but this was dependent on arrangements to be worked out by the social worker; this could take longer. The psychiatric resident reported that Ms. L. was improving but was still not ready to join the group.

One of the more disorganized patients began to ramble and claimed that his problems have increased by being in the hospital. He implied that the staff was overcontrolling and needlessly limited the privileges of patients. A more organized patient disagreed and stated that hospital procedures were protective of patients. The resident asked if the patients viewed the restrictions on Ms. L. to be beneficial or detrimental to her and them. Several patients said that they were relieved, because her behavior frightened them and made them anxious.

Next, complaints emerged that some of the nursing staff treated the patients like children. The disorganized patient resumed his ramble, and then the man who was to be transferred to a state hospital requested increased unit privileges. Others complained that the unit's policies were inflexible and that this caused them to feel helpless. One woman reported that she found so-called team decisions about her care to be confusing. She claimed that no one took responsibility for these decisions so that the patients did not know to whom they could address their questions. Another member advised her to talk to her therapist.

Throughout this discussion, the therapists tried to be receptive to the patients' concerns, showed interest in their complaints, and expressed empathy for their frustration and confusion. Finally, the psychiatric resident restated what had been said. He noted that the patients had a great deal of mixed reactions to Ms. L.'s behavior, that they found the unit's restrictions to be oppressive, that they sometimes experienced the staff as needlessly controlling, and that both the treatment system and team decisions often seemed mysterious to them. The other therapist noted that, although patients could address questions to their therapists, the unit's decision-making process must seem mysterious to them, because decisions were often made on the basis of information available only to the staff.

The disorganized patient asked the nurse why his blood pressure was taken several times a day. She explained the medical reason. A few patients had other questions to which factual answers were given. By this point, the group members seemed calmer than they had been, and several talked spontaneously about their disposition plans. However, the man who was to go to the state hospital and the one who was to be transferred to a longer-term unit remained silent.

The discussion inevitably returned to the atmosphere on the unit, which several patients acknowledged was tense. As one stated, "We sit around all day long waiting for the white light to blow." (This was a reference to the emergency buzzer, which was sounded whenever help was needed on another unit to restrain a patient who had gotten out of control.) Again, the disorganized man began to ramble. This time he implored patients to "try to beat the rap" and stated that the staff sits idly by, apparently to watch patients "go off." He reported that the quiet room seemed a mysterious place to him, because patients went there when they were upset and came out later, seemingly improved. Another patient reported that the other night seemed strange and was filled with ironies: it was Halloween; Ms. L. was screaming in the quiet room, while others were watching a horror movie on TV. Recognizing the movie, the resident said that he had seen it too and was disturbed by one element of the story. He objected to the portrayal of an escaped mental patient as a killer. Such a depiction, he said, encourages stereotyping and feeds prejudice.

Following this intervention, the disorganized man calmed down and initiated a long, productive discussion of disposition problems that affect discharge. Others joined in. This time the members addressed both the man who was to be transferred to a state hospital and the one who was to go to a longer-term unit. They were sympathetic and encouraging to both.

Here, the hospital treatment alliance was bought into focus by statements clarifying the staff's realistic use of power. The staff had to control Ms. L. for the benefit of all, and they were instrumental in effecting discharges and dispositions. Throughout the session, the most disorganized patient served as a barometer of the group members' anxieties about loss of self-control and autonomy. He exemplified the paranoid position of the patients. In addition, reactions to Ms. L. were central in that session. On the one hand, the patients identified with her. After all, many of them had shown similarly regressed behavior and, at the very least, all had the potential to lose control. On the other hand, the group therapists—a physician and a nurse—were part of the team that had to control her behavior. Thus, the relationship between Ms. L. and the staff paralleled the transference in the group.

The therapists helped the patients by showing interest in what they said, being concerned for them, and providing clarification. However, more was needed. First, the patients were told that some of their confusion about decision making was justified, because they did not have access to all the facts. Second, the resident, in a crucial maneuver, made use of the metaphor of the TV movie. His intervention showed that he empathized with the patients and refused to accept the view that their aggressive potential is nefarious. He thereby diminished their anticipation of countervailing distrust, fear, and retaliation by the staff. Once all this was done, the patients were able to attend to a realistic task of milieu treatment—namely, to be supportive of one another.

THE PARAMETERS OF PRACTICE

To be successful, group psychotherapy programs need to have solid administrative and staff support. Group programs that fail or flounder have goals at odds with those of the treatment team. When key members of the medical and nursing hierarchies appreciate how the therapy benefits them (i.e., by helping patients to be more receptive to milieu treatment), they are more likely to cooperate with the program. Sometimes it is advantageous to involve various multidisciplinary staff in the group program by having them rotate as cotherapists or observe sessions on a regular basis.

It is the responsibility of both the group psychotherapists and the medical leadership to remind the staff how the therapy group complements the overall treatment. For their part, the staff should expect the patients to participate in the group as they do with other modalities. The group should not be subordinate or have second-class status. In this regard, the boundaries of the group—its membership, time, and location—must all be respected. When scheduling conflicts are unavoidable, the group therapist should be included in the planning, and he or she should then explain to the members what is to happen and why. Scheduling conflicts may be minor (e.g., when one patient cannot attend a session because of a concurrent meeting) or major (e.g., when the group session must be canceled or rescheduled to suit changes in the unit's schedule).

The therapist should be fully informed of significant events in the milieu. These events will affect the group, and patients' reactions need to be worked out there. As a corollary, the therapist should share information from the sessions with the staff, preferably on a regular basis. This prevents divisions in the staff, which patients quickly sense and respond to by withdrawing or fostering dissension.

The overall composition of the group varies from setting to setting. As I have noted previously, some programs have a series of hierarchical groups in which each is designed for a particular level of patient functioning. In other programs, patients are placed in group according to team assignment. Assignment by team has certain advantages: Communication within the staff occurs more readily, and the entire arrangement conveys a clear message that group is an integral part of the treatment system. In other words, team groups are more easily integrated into the social structure of the milieu.

Patient Selection

The patients who populate hospital groups are the very ones who would ordinarily be excluded from outpatient group psychotherapy. They lack the motivation and ego controls that are prerequisites for outpatient treatment. Yet it is possible for them to participate and benefit from group in the hospital for two reasons. First, inpatient group psychotherapy is integrated into the overall milieu treatment. Second, the experience of hospitalization causes patients to have a natural affinity for one another. The latter is the basis for group cohesion.

Inclusion criteria for inpatient groups are quite broad. Virtually every kind of patient (with a few exceptions) can benefit. Thus it is only relevant to consider exclusion criteria. These are limited to those patients who are unable to appreciate what is happening in the group and those who threaten its integrity. Specifically, it is advisable to exclude the following (Rutchick 1986):

1. Patients who are cognitively impaired, such as those with marked organic brain syndromes;

2. Patients who are so severely regressed that they cannot communicate even the simplest of needs;
3. Patients who are unable to tolerate modest external stimulation;
4. Patients with tenuous impulse control who threaten the safety of the group; and
5. Patients who are so self-injurious as to require close, constant observation lest they harm themselves.

The group should be a safe place where patients can say what they wish without worrying that it will precipitate aggressive or self-destructive behavior in their peers. Although patients whose uncontrolled behavior poses serious management problems should be excluded, those with psychotic thinking and nonintrusive, bizarre behavior should be accepted. Inclusion of such patients lets the others know that the therapist can tolerate their psychotic potential too.

Preparation and Structural Elements

Unlike outpatient treatment, there is usually no formal process of evaluating patients for the inpatient group. Staff can usually spot those who need to be excluded. Some units allow newly admitted patients to attend the next scheduled session, but it is often preferable to have them wait one out and join the group thereafter. This short delay allows the new patient time to adjust to the unit and for the other patients to acclimate to the new patient.

Frequently, patients are told little about the group prior to entry—perhaps just its time and place. Because of limited time, it is often impossible to prepare patients individually for the group. Yet they must somehow be oriented to their role, the group's function, and its ground rules. This can sometimes be done through written information. Usually, the therapist begins each session with an orientation statement that includes the specifics of time and place, the group's purpose, and other key elements of the treatment contract. However, certain elements (e.g., items 3 and 4 below) may remain implicit in the treatment culture. In any case, the therapist should keep in mind this treatment's contract components. They include 1) the structural boundaries of the group (i.e., the time of the meeting, its length and frequency of sessions, and its location) and

2) the flow of information (i.e., the informational boundaries) between the rest of the unit and the group. This latter component means that

1. Members (both patients and therapists) bring for discussion outstanding events on the unit, and the patients discuss significant information regarding their treatment.
2. Members do not discuss information revealed by other group members with patients who are not in the group.
3. Members bring outside, group-related discussions back to the sessions.
4. Therapists share information as needed with other members of the treatment team.

The statement of purpose at the start of the session should help the group members define their role. It is usually broad and encourages patients to talk about and share concerns regarding their problems, treatment, or experience on the unit. A round of introductions may also be useful when there are new members. It is inadvisable to ask patients to reveal why they came into the hospital. This (common) procedure is embarrassing at best and usually deteriorates into a repetition of standard platitudes. In contrast, an invitation for newcomers to comment on their experience since admission can be less threatening.

In practice, the size of groups varies from 5 to 12; however, 7 to 9 is optimal. Although outpatient groups are usually 90 minutes long, inpatient groups are generally shorter, because inpatients have a much shorter attention span (Erickson 1989). Most inpatient groups are 45–60 minutes long. Less than 45 minutes does not allow sufficient time for orientation, introductions, discussion, and closure. The frequency of the sessions varies from two to five per week. As a rule of thumb, the more rapid the patient turnover, the more frequent sessions need to be, because acute patients create a bustling and tumultuous environment. The shorter the length of stay, the more often destabilizing factors need to be discussed and worked on.

Cotherapy is a common practice. Although it is costly, its use speaks to the stress therapists feel conducting inpatient groups. Inpatients are difficult to engage and tax therapists by attributing noxious, oppressive qualities to them and then inducing them to fulfill the corresponding role.

METHOD AND TECHNIQUE

Although the literature reflects considerable variations in practice, there is a fair degree of consensus as to the group leader's role. A passive, reflective stance and a laissez-faire approach to treatment can have deleterious effects and are contraindicated (Beutler et al. 1984). Specifically, patients can decompensate unless the therapist takes a vigorous role in structuring the sessions. A leader who figures prominently in the process provides the members with an anchoring point against which they can better define themselves. The leader needs to be active and moderately directive and to facilitate interaction. He or she should be accepting, noncritical, gentle with confrontations, and generally highly supportive. Clinicians would agree that getting patients to talk and interact with one another is the first task of treatment. Beyond this, there is little consensus as to the technique of treatment. Goals must first be clarified, because they dictate technique.

Goals for Treatment

The goals of treatment are many and range from the most basic and apparent to the more complex and sophisticated. They are listed here in progressive order:

1. *Engaging patients in conversation and promoting verbal interchange among them.*
   Because inpatients tend to be withdrawn and resistive, the therapist should take an active role in fostering discussion and interaction. Given patients' pervasively fearful and paranoid attitudes, the therapist must work diligently, yet tactfully, to engage them.
2. *Making the group interactive so that it can serve as an instrument for peer support and assistance.* It is well known that patients can be helpful to one another and that self-esteem is enhanced by giving help. This group goal is similar to that of any support group.
3. *Using the group to cultivate an atmosphere of open communication on the unit.*
   The therapist must share with the patients information from the milieu that is relevant to their concerns. Often this relates to events on the unit, treatment plans, administrative decisions, and staff issues. Of

course, this must be done with respect for rights of privacy, particularly for the staff.

4. *Bringing for discussion and clarifying milieu issues so as to make the social system of the unit comprehensible to the patients.*
The therapist needs to be sensitive to issues that concern, confuse, and mystify patients. The unit's structures and procedures should be explained in the group. More importantly, disruptive milieu events are common on short-term units and readily become a source of distortions. These disruptive events can quickly convert a salutary environment into a noxious one. Clarifying that patients' behavior in group is a response to these environmental influences serves to demystify their experience on the unit (Levenson 1981). It is important for patients to learn that their reactions to these upsetting events are comprehensible and similar to those of nonpatients. This process improves reality testing and is ego supportive.

5. *Relieving and correcting negative transference reactions to the group leader, which function as a paradigm for all patient-staff relationships.*
These patients generally operate by using projective mechanisms, which in effect creates a persecutory system that usually incorporates all of the unit staff. Addressing the transference can rectify paranoid distortions that affect the hospital treatment alliance (Kibel 1987b). Positive results here reap benefits for all treatments on the unit.

On short-term units, the milieu is most often unstable and sometimes volatile. This curtails the consolidation of working alliances within the small therapy group itself. Under these circumstances, it is best to view intragroup processes as reflecting milieu dynamics. The goals for treatment listed above are in accord with this perspective. On longer-term units, the situation is different and, in some respects, more complex. Because the patient population is more stable and less acute, the milieu develops a more organized culture. This in turn permits relationships within the small group to consolidate in a way that allows some degree of group cohesion to develop. Then, intragroup experiences have greater emotional import. Work on the resulting transferences within the small psychotherapy group develop more potential to be mutative. Goals for treatment on longer-term units can therefore be more elaborate and be based on the interdependence and concurrence of both milieu and small group dynamics. However, discussion of such goals is beyond the scope of this chapter (Kibel 1986).

Techniques for Intervention

Prior to each session, the therapist should prioritize in his or her own mind recent events on the unit in terms of their overall impact on the patients. For example, fire and assaultive behavior are more emotionally charged than suicidal or psychotic behavior. Relapses and treatment failures have a moderately high level of priority. Staff issues are always important. Secrets about the staff have enormous impact, because the "unspoken" is threatening. It is rare that a staff issue does not filter down to the patients in some way. With this in mind, the decision to be explicit about staff problems will have to be made on a case-by-case basis, often with administrative input.

Although the therapist should enter each session with a mental list of events that might affect patients, he or she should not introduce them for discussion in a vacuum. First, the therapist should listen to the material for relevant unconscious content. When that is present, he or she can suggest the relationship of the material to recent unit events. When patients are withdrawn or avoidant, the therapist can suggest a topic to see if they respond to it. Thus, the therapist should always mention relevant milieu issues. At the very least, this puts the subject "on the table" for patients to pick up at some point. Sometimes, the therapist may insist that a matter not be ignored because it is ripe for discussion or urgent. However, more often than not, items that are avoided one day become less threatening with time; distance serves as a buffer for anxiety.

It is important to ask questions in a manner that allows for a concrete focus rather than an abstract response. Thus, patients respond better when discussing an incident to being asked "what happened?" rather than "how did you react?" Because paranoid patients often have difficulty "owning" their responses, unit events often are discussed first in terms of how others were affected. Externalization relieves anxiety by permitting the fiction that others are more upset. Providing an outside focus enables members to unite in opposition. This serves group cohesion and can organize experience for the moment, albeit in a somewhat paranoid way (Feilbert-Willis et al. 1986).

It is important for the therapist to set a supportive tone for the group. He or she can do this in both subtle and overt ways. Examples of the former include offering one patient a chair or another a tissue, inviting some to join the circle, attending to each one's physical comfort, and sitting next to a disturbed patient who needs additional attention. The therapist should show interest in what patients say, no matter how negativistic or bizarre it may seem. Patients' comments, questions, or complaints should never be labeled "inappropriate," for this word conveys denigration. Interest in one patient's jumbled verbiage shows respect for the psychotic potential in others. When members need to be interrupted or topics deferred, this should be done tactfully.

The therapist also should attend to his or her own behavior. He or she should apologize for mistakes (e.g., lateness) and then make up the lost time. Patients should be told well in advance of any structural or schedule changes, even to be reminded of missed sessions because of holidays, vacations, and the like.

Overall, support is provided when the therapist structures the treatment. This includes starting each session on time, ending each without cutting patients off, welcoming new members, orienting them, and carrying out the provisions of the treatment contract as previously outlined. The therapist is the administrator of the group who convenes it, managing its external boundaries and its internal components. It is the therapist's job to engage the retiring members (e.g., by asking silent ones for their observations or merely checking in with them by asking how they are managing). Silences should not last too long. The active therapist quietly orchestrates the flow of the session without imposing his or her preconceived ideas or will on the patients.

Patients frequently compare themselves to one another, but also to some idealized image of recovery. They envy those who appear to be favored by the staff with early discharge. Yet they become anxious when an obviously disturbed individual is permitted to sign out against medical advice. They repeatedly seek feedback on the staff's evaluation of their clinical progress. But they worry that self-exposure will yield negative assessments and prolong their stay. The therapist must show that he or she understands their envy and recognizes their distrust and worry, but then needs to demonstrate that talking about their inner experiences is valued.

The inexperienced clinician often asks how the therapist should deal with a group of patients who refuse to talk, are disorganized, or are overly hostile. This is the wrong question to ask. More relevant is why the patients are resistive. What on the unit is making them anxious and/or impeding communication?

When impasses occur, the therapist can ask the group members for help. This shows respect. Yet it is the therapist who must manage inter-member conflict and diminish scapegoating. A useful device here is to interpret the process. Interpretations can curtail actions by telling patients that they are contentious for inadvertent reasons and by clarifying that the source of the behavior is beyond conscious design. Ironically, interpretations also serve as gentle admonition and help to make dysfunctional behavior ego-dystonic.

The most fascinating part of group psychotherapy is discerning meaning from metaphor. With inpatient work, the task of making interpretations is more complicated than with other kinds of groups. When the content reflects a concern of the membership, the therapist needs to do more than translate its meaning. He or she must relate it to the event to which the patients are reacting. In fact, discussion of the event is often more important than exploration of the affect. After all, the aim is to improve the hospital treatment alliance, not to gain insight. Thus, the therapist may draw analogies between the discussion and the precipitating event, or even raise the latter as a parallel issue.

> In one group, the therapist returned from vacation and was greeted by complaints about the nursing staff, who seemed to have little time for the patients in the group because they had to provide additional attention to a few regressed patients. The therapist first acknowledged that the patients' frustration was realistic and then remarked how the patients must have felt similarly when he was away. Thus, a milieu issue was introduced and discussed in a fashion that was both timely and acceptable to the patients.

CONCLUSION

Inpatient group psychotherapy is an arduous craft. The small group itself has many dynamic components, including the transference to the leader, as well as group-as-a-whole, subgroup, dyadic, and individual processes. Its levels of meaning are multitudinous. Although many uses can be made of the group, one useful approach treats the small therapy group as a subgroup of the larger unit. Reflections of environmental events allow the clinician to use the group to facilitate milieu treatment. The therapeutic work in the group (and with the transference in particular) bears heavily on the hospital treatment alliance. This viewpoint integrates group psychotherapy into the overall treatment.

Because the group therapist, like the patients, is part of the larger unit, his or her perspective may be limited by the same dynamics that affect group members. For this reason, supervision of junior therapists is imperative and, for more experienced therapists, peer supervision or regular, outside consultation is needed.

REFERENCES

Astrachan BM, Harrow M, Flynn HR: Influence of the value system of a psychiatric setting on behavior in group therapy meetings. Social Psychiatry 3:165–172, 1968

Axelrod S, Wetzler S: Factors associated with better compliance with psychiatric aftercare. Hosp Community Psychiatry 40(4):397–401, 1989

Betcher RW, Rice CA, Weir DM: The regressed inpatient group in a graded group treatment program. Am J Psychother 36:229–239, 1982

Beutler LE, Frank M, Schieber SC, et al: Comparative effects of group psychotherapies in a short-term inpatient setting: an experience with deteriorating effects. Psychiatry 47:66–76, 1984

Brabender VM: Time-limited inpatient group therapy: a developmental model. Int J Group Psychother 35:373–390, 1985

Cory TL, Page D: Group techniques for effecting change in the more disturbed patient. Group 2:149–155, 1978

Craig AE, Hyatt BA: Chronicity in mental illness: a theory on the role of change. Perspect Psychiatr Care 16:139–153, 1978

Druck AB: The role of didactic group psychotherapy in short-term psychiatric settings. Group 2:98–109, 1978

Erickson RC: Applications of cognitive testing to group therapies with the chronic mentally ill. Int J Group Psychother 39:223–235, 1989

Farrell D: The use of active experiential group techniques with hospitalized patients, in Group Therapy 1976. Edited by Wolberg LR, Aronson ML. New York, Stratton Intercontinental Medical Book Corp, 1976, pp 44–51

Feilbert-Willis R, Kibel HD, Wikstrom T: Techniques for handling resistances in group psychotherapy with severely disturbed patients. Group 10:228–238, 1986

Griffin-Shelley E, Trachtenberg J: Group psychotherapy with short-term in-patients. Small Group Behavior 13:97–104, 1985

Kanas N: Inpatient and outpatient group therapy for schizophrenic patients. Am J Psychother 39:431–439, 1985

Kanas N: Group therapy with schizophrenics: a review of controlled studies. Int J Group Psychother 36:339–351, 1986

Kernberg OF: Toward an integrative theory of hospital treatment, in Object Relations Theory and Clinical Psychoanalysis. New York, Jason Aronson, 1976, pp 241–275

Kernberg OF: Leadership and organizational functioning: organizational regression. Int J Group Psychother 28:3–25, 1978

Kibel HD: From acute to long-term inpatient group psychotherapy. Psychiatric Journal of the University of Ottawa 11:58–61, 1986

Kibel HD: Inpatient group psychotherapy: where treatment philosophies converge, in The Yearbook of Psychoanalysis and Psychotherapy, Vol 2. Edited by Langs R. New York, Gardner Press, 1987a, pp 94–116

Kibel HD: Contributions of the group psychotherapist to education on the psychiatric unit: teaching through group dynamics. Int J Group Psychother 37:3–29, 1987b

Klein RH: Inpatient group psychotherapy: practical considerations and special problems. Int J Group Psychother 27:201–214, 1977

Klein RH, Kugel B: Inpatient group psychotherapy: reflections through a glass darkly. Int J Group Psychother 31:311–328, 1981

Leopold HS: Selective group approaches with psychotic patients in hospital settings. Am J Psychother 30:95–102, 1976

Levenson EA: The rhetoric of intimacy. Group 5(4):3–11, 1981

Levine HB: Milieu biopsy: the place of the therapy group on the inpatient ward. Int J Group Psychother 30:77–93, 1980

Marcovitz RJ, Smith JE: An approach to time-limited dynamic inpatient group therapy. Small Group Behavior 14:369–376, 1983

Marcovitz RJ, Smith JE: Short-term group therapy: a review of the literature. International Journal of Short-Term Psychotherapy 1:49–57, 1986

Maxmen JS: An educative model for inpatient group therapy. Int J Group Psychother 28:321–338, 1978

Maxmen JS: Helping patients survive theories: the practice of an educative model. Int J Group Psychother 34:355–368, 1984

Parloff MB: Discussion of "Group therapy with schizophrenics." Int J Group Psychother 36:353–360, 1986

Parloff MB, Dies RR: Group psychotherapy outcome research: 1966–1975. Int J Group Psychother 27:281–319, 1977

Pattison EM, Brissenden E, Wohl T: Assessing special effects of inpatient group psychotherapy. Int J Group Psychother 17:283–297, 1967

Powell M, Illovsky M, O'Leary W, et al: Life-skills training with hospitalized psychiatric patients. Int J Group Psychother 38:109–117, 1988

Rabiner EL, Wells CF, Yager J: A model for the brief hospital treatment of the disadvantaged psychiatrically ill. Am J Orthopsychiatry 43:774–782, 1973

Rice CA, Rutan JS: Inpatient Group Psychotherapy: A Psychodynamic Perspective. New York, Macmillan, 1987

Rubin JH, Locascio K: A model for communication skills group using structured exercises and audiovisual equipment. Int J Group Psychother 35:569–584, 1985

Rutchick IE: Group Psychotherapy, in Inpatient Psychiatry, 2nd Edition. Edited by Sederer LI. Baltimore, MD, Williams & Wilkins, 1986, pp 263–279

Stotsky BA, Zolik ES: Group psychotherapy with psychotics: 1921–1963—a review. Int J Group Psychother 15:321–344, 1965

Waxer PH: Short-term group psychotherapy: some principles and techniques. Int J Group Psychother 27:33–42, 1977

Yalom ID: Inpatient Group Psychotherapy. New York, Basic Books, 1983

Inpatient Cognitive-Behavioral Therapy of Depression

Michael E. Thase, M.D.

INTRODUCTION

There has been a dramatic increase in the application of cognitive and behavioral approaches to psychotherapy over the past decade (e.g., Arkowitz and Hannah 1989; Norcross 1986; Simons and Thase 1990). In this chapter, the basic principles of Beck's model of the cognitive-behavioral treatment of depression (Beck 1976; Beck et al. 1979) are reviewed as they pertain to the inpatient psychiatric setting.

There are a number of strengths that point to the applicability of cognitive-behavioral therapy (CBT) as an inpatient treatment paradigm:

1. The psychoeducational aspects of CBT provide a structure and framework of treatment that are well suited for use with hospitalized patients.
2. The standard outpatient protocol of Beck and colleagues (1979) has already been condensed for use in the hospital (Thase and Wright 1991).

Completion of this chapter was supported in part by grants MH-41884, MH-40023, and MH-30915 (MHCRC) from the National Institute of Mental Health. The author thanks Ms. Lisa Stupar for her assistance in the preparation of this chapter.

3. CBT can be adapted for treatment of even the most severely depressed inpatients, because a wide range of behavioral interventions are applicable for patients who are relatively inactive or virtually incapacitated (Beck et al. 1979).

4. The cognitive focus of treatment is particularly relevant for use with patients with suicidal ideation (Freeman and White 1989). For example, Beck and colleagues (1979) specify the importance of rapid identification of exaggerated pessimistic and/or hopeless beliefs that are likely to underlie suicidal thoughts and a wide range of intervention methods are available for addressing such symptoms.

5. CBT is compatible with other models of treatment, most notably the somatic therapies (Wright and Schrodt 1989; Wright et al. 1992a). In fact, both the cognitive-behavioral and biomedical models of depression emphasize the importance of objective evaluation of outcomes and empirical verification of the utility of interventions (Wright and Schrodt 1989).

6. CBT is viewed as an ongoing process, with a detailed emphasis on importance of learning new skills for coping in vivo. This is particularly important with respect to preparing for discharge while on passes from the hospital (Thase and Wright 1991). Moreover, specific attention to relapse prevention is routinely provided in the latter phase of a course of CBT (Beck et al. 1979; Thase 1992).

Following an overview of the various types of cognitive and behavioral disturbances that have been documented in depression, the fundamental principles of inpatient application of CBT are described. This discussion includes consideration of the basic psychotherapeutic skills, methods, and techniques utilized in CBT. Finally, relevant research from outpatient studies of clinical depression is extrapolated to the inpatient setting, and more recent research pertaining to the use of CBT with hospitalized depressed patients is reviewed.

COGNITIVE DISTURBANCES IN DEPRESSION

The depressed person is usually plagued by two major types of cognitive dysfunction: 1) difficulties in learning, concentration, and memory, and

2) negatively biased thoughts, information processing, attitudes, and assumptions. Learning and memory deficits, which are principally manifest on cognitive tasks that are complex or require considerable effort, necessitate the use of straightforward and stepwise psychotherapeutic strategies (Wright and Salmon 1990). Severely depressed inpatients also may show subtle impairments of abstract thought (Braff and Beck 1974; Rubinow et al. 1984), further compromising their ability to engage in psychotherapy. These difficulties must be taken into account as the therapist "calibrates" the pacing and depth of therapy sessions; patients whose depression is greater typically benefit more from interventions that are more structured and focused on specific problems or symptoms.

Automatic thoughts represent a special type of cognition, which have been shown to be of particular significance to the depressive disorders (e.g., Beck 1976; Clark 1988). Automatic thoughts typically accompany emotional reactions and occur spontaneously (i.e., without deliberation). Some illustrative examples of automatic negative thoughts are described in Table 6–1. Automatic negative thoughts tend to be repetitive and personalized, and they often have unquestioned believability when ini-

Table 6–1. A three-column summary sheet of automatic thoughts in relation to situations and feelings

Situation	Feeling	Automatic thoughts
1. Awoke early; unable to go back to sleep	Depressed, anxious	Why can't I even get a decent night's sleep? I'll never get better. I can't stand this much longer!
2. Spilled coffee in cafeteria	Embarrassed, depressed	I'm such a klutz. I can't do anything right.
3. Not able to speak up in group therapy	Depressed	How can treatment help if I can't do my part? People will think I'm stuck-up. Why can't I relate?
4. Husband 1 hour late for visit	Depressed, anxious, angry	He's mad at me. I'm driving him away. Why can't he be more supportive? I don't deserve him.
5. Playing volleyball in gym	Depressed	I'm so out of shape. I used to be athletic. I'm just going through the motions. This fatigue is unbearable.

tially explicated. Thus, while the statement may seem to be grossly exaggerated or distorted to a more objective person, the individual experiencing the thought may swear to its veracity. The constellation of automatic thoughts specifically linked to the depressed person's appraisals about self, world, and future have been called the cognitive triad (Beck 1976).

The themes revealed in a patient's automatic thoughts may be further sorted into patterns that, in turn, can be used to infer more complex cognitive processes (Beck 1976). Such processes include a person's beliefs or attitudes, as well as "deeper" cognitive structures known as schemas. In more traditional approaches to psychopathology, beliefs and attitudes would be considered "preconscious" processes, whereas schemas are "unconscious." Dysfunctional attitudes generally set rigid, unrealistically demanding, or unobtainable standards, such as perfectionism or the belief that one must always be loved. Beliefs and attitudes thus often may be surmised from a patient's use of "should" or "must" statements or repeated patterns of problematic behavior. As I describe later, it is the CBT therapist's task to help the patient begin to recognize and collate examples of such dysfunctional attitudes and beliefs so that their validity, utility, and changeability can be addressed (Beck et al. 1979; Persons 1989). Examples of common dysfunctional attitudes in depression and anxiety are provided in Table 6–2.

In the cognitive model of psychopathology, schemas are hypothetical constructs that serve as unspoken rules or basic principles. They are presumed to have been shaped by developmental experiences and, by adulthood, their more fundamental and enduring nature serves to provide a source of consistency (i.e., to help bring order to the complexities

---

Table 6–2.   Common dysfunctional attitudes in depression

---

1. To be happy, I have to be successful in whatever I undertake.

2. To be happy, I must be accepted by all people at all times.

3. If I make a mistake, it means that I am inept.

4. I can't live without you.

5. If somebody disagrees with me, it means that person doesn't like me.

6. My value as a person depends on what others think of me.

Source.   Adapted from Beck 1976.

of life [Beck 1976]). Nevertheless, some investigators propose that schemas may be continually evolving (e.g., Guidano and Liotti 1983). An individual's set of schemas runs the range from simpler, perceptional-organizational phenomena (e.g., object constancy or conversation of volume) to more complex and highly specific problem-solving strategies. Maladaptive schemas in psychopathological states typically concern more fundamental components of psychological well-being, such as trust, safety, lovableness, self-worth, and competence (Persons 1989; Thase and Beck 1992). Three research groups have reported that ratings of vulnerability within the schematic area of connectedness (i.e., interpersonal dependence) are predictive of depressive relapse following the occurrence of specific types of environmental stress (Hammen et al. 1989; Robins and Block 1989; Segal et al. 1989).

As noted previously, schemas (even ultimately maladaptive ones) benefit the individual by organizing and simplifying a vast and ongoing universe of perceptual experience. Schemas thus have been described as serving the individual as a "mental filter" (Beck et al. 1979). This filtration function can be indirectly observed through recognition of mental processes subserving information processing (e.g., selective abstraction or selective recall). For example, personally relevant memories are stored or retrieved, whereas extraneous material is disregarded. At times of intense affect or arousal, the presumed filtration function appears to perform such that information processing and decision making are consistent with the overarching view dictated by this schema. As a result, a number of examples of faulty or erroneous information processing can be observed in emotionally distressed persons that may reinforce or prolong the affective response (see Table 6–3). Unfortunately, although such strong mood states may only transiently affect the information processing of a relatively invulnerable person (i.e., the relevant schema is not pathogenic), more pronounced and protracted changes are seen in clinical samples (Beck 1976; Shaw and Segal 1988).

BASIC PRINCIPLES OF INPATIENT CBT

CBT is typically a short-term treatment in which the therapist helps the patient to learn more effective methods for coping with problematic thoughts, feelings, and behavior. It is thus a pragmatic or problem-oriented psychotherapy that was developed to address the patient's psychopathological reactions to both situational problems and more episodic long-standing underlying difficulties. In inpatient settings, CBT may be provided as an individual therapy or in groups of 4 to 8 patients. The relatively short length of stay and "turnover" of patients on most psychiatric inpatient units is now such that the closed group model of CBT

Table 6–3.   Patterns of faulty information processing in depression

---

1. *Emotional reasoning:* A conclusion or inference that is based on an emotional state (i.e., "I *feel* this way, therefore I *am* this way).

2. *Overgeneralization:* Evidence that is drawn from one experience or a small set of experiences to reach an unwarranted conclusion with far-reaching implications.

3. *Catastrophic thinking:* An extreme example of overgeneralization, in which the impact of a clearly negative event or experience is amplified to extreme proportions.

4. *All-or-none (black-or-white) thinking:* An unnecessary division of complex or continuous outcomes into polarized extremes (e.g., "either I am a success at this, or I'm a total failure").

5. *Shoulds and musts:* Imperative statements about self that convey rigid standards or, when about others, reflect an unrealistic degree of presumed control over external events.

6. *Negative predictions:* Use of pessimism or earlier experiences of failure to prematurely or inappropriately predict failure in a new situation. Also known as "fortune-telling."

7. *Mind reading:* Negatively toned inferences about the thoughts, intentions, or motives of another person.

8. *Labeling:* An undesirable characteristic of a person or event that is made definitive of that person or event.

9. *Personalization:* Interpretation of an event, situation, or behavior as salient or personally indicative of a negative aspect of self.

10. *Selective negative focus:* Undesirable or negative events, memories, or implications focused on at the expense of recalling or identifying other, more neutral (or positive) information. In fact, positive information may be ignored *or* disqualified as irrelevant, atypical, or trivial.

Source.   Adapted from Beck et al. 1979.

typically utilized for outpatients is generally not feasible. Instead, inpatient CBT groups generally operate with an open enrollment policy and a rotating curriculum. The open enrollment approach is an efficient way to utilize staff, although it is more difficult to tailor to an optimal pace for each patient. As a result, it is harder to build progressively toward discharge and probably should be viewed as a secondary or adjunctive therapy with a primary psychoeducational focus. Individual therapy, which is significantly less time-efficient from an economic standpoint, may be reserved for patients who cannot or will not take antidepressant medications.

Although a majority of practicing cognitive therapists are clinical psychologists, psychiatrists, social workers, and nurse-clinicians with advanced degrees, when selecting candidates for training as CBT therapists, it is important to select individuals who have sufficient clinical experience so that the cognitive model of treatment can be adapted for use with patients of diverse backgrounds and clinical presentations (Rush 1982). Therapists must be able to be relatively active within sessions (i.e., so that they can help the patient learn to apply the therapeutic methods and strategies prescribed in the CBT model). They also need to learn to maintain high levels of empathy, genuineness, and understanding while following the CBT protocol (Beck et al. 1979; Persons and Burns 1985). Typically, it takes a year or more of supervised training to become an effective cognitive therapist.

The high level of therapeutic intensity also pertains to the patient, who will be asked to collaborate actively within sessions and complete homework assignments between sessions (Beck et al. 1979). Such self-help assignments play an integral role in broadening or generalizing the impact of the therapy (Persons 1989). As a general rule, homework assignments are most effective when they are relevant to the material addressed in sessions. Moreover, compliance with homework assignments appears to be maximized when the therapist remembers to attend to these assignments at the beginning of each subsequent session. Conversely, vague or overlooked assignments tend to lead to noncompliance and may weaken the treatment alliance (Persons 1989).

The actual style or nature of the therapeutic relationship in CBT has been referred to as collaborative empiricism (Beck et al. 1979). In the cognitive model of treatment, it is the therapist's task to establish this type of working alliance, which helps to ensure development of compatible goals, reduction of potential points of resistance, and enhancement of communication. Like other core therapeutic qualities (e.g., genuineness or accurate empathy), an effective therapeutic alliance is considered to be a necessary, but not sufficient, ingredient of CBT (Beck et al. 1979). The therapist must draw upon his or her experience to guide each session, in a manner analogous to the methods used by a skilled coach or teacher. Moreover, like many effective teachers, CBT therapists often use Socratic questioning to help patients to explore and identify relationships between thoughts, feelings, and behavior (Beck et al. 1979; Persons 1989). The therapist also provides and elicits a liberal amount of feedback, both within and across sessions, to explicate and strengthen the collaboration between therapist and patient. The timely provision and receipt of such feedback also provides an explicit method by which the therapist can help the patient to cope with the concentration difficulties, distortion of new information, and pessimism so characteristic of severe depression (Wright and Salmon 1990).

The empirical tone of CBT is introduced early in the course of therapy. Therapeutic interventions thus may be described as ways to collect data and test hypotheses concerning aspects of a patient's condition (Beck et al. 1979; Thase and Beck 1992). Thus, the therapist and patient often jointly develop experiments to address a problem, either within a session or as a homework assignment. Once the experiment is performed and the pertinent evidence is collected, the results are reviewed so that the patient can decide whether to accept or reject the hypothesis. Based on the stage of the therapy, these experiments may range from relatively straightforward behavioral tasks (e.g., increasing a particular type of activity as a way of counteracting fatigue or procrastination) to more complex cognitive-emotional interactions (e.g., an assignment to test the relationship between feelings of loneliness and thoughts about reactivating an ungratifying relationship). One of the therapist's most important tasks is to help the patient to design experiments that (while not too demanding) help to illuminate the cognitive case formulation, challenge maladaptive beliefs and assumptions, or increase "antidepressant" behavior.

A typical course of outpatient treatment usually involves once- or twice-weekly sessions for a total of 12 to 20 weeks of therapy (Beck et al. 1979; Persons 1989). As I explain later, the frequency of inpatient group or individual sessions is recommended to range from 3 to 5 times a week (Bowers 1990; Scott 1988; Shaw 1981; Thase and Wright 1991). Patients may thus receive a course of therapy ranging from as few as 6 to as many as 20 sessions during an inpatient hospitalization.

INDICATIONS FOR INPATIENT CBT

The medical model that often guides care on psychiatric inpatient units, as well as practical constraints imposed by utilization review policies and cost-containment efforts, provide strong conceptual and pragmatic disincentives against the routine use of CBT as a single or primary treatment of hospitalized patients. Further, the efficacy of CBT as a principal inpatient treatment has not yet been demonstrated. However, there are several special circumstances in which individual CBT may be useful as a primary treatment for nonpsychotic, nonbipolar depression. These clinical indications include

1. When patients are adamantly opposed to treatment with medication (i.e., inpatient CBT is preferable to discharge against medical advice);
2. When patients have not been able to tolerate a number of standard antidepressants from different classes;
3. When patients have not responded to adequate therapy with antidepressants and refuse to receive electroconvulsive therapy (ECT); or
4. When there are strong contraindications to antidepressant medication (Thase and Wright 1991; Wright and Schrodt 1989).

The fourth category may include patients with serious cardiovascular or hepatic disease, women in their first trimester of pregnancy, or nursing mothers who are opposed to discontinuation of breast-feeding.

Other clinical criteria for use of individual CBT as a primary treatment modality (in lieu of pharmacotherapy) have not yet been fully developed (Bowers 1989; Shaw 1981; Thase and Wright 1991). Although considerable research remains to be done, primary treatment with CBT may be most clearly indicated for dysphoric patients admitted in an intense crisis situation (i.e., a severe adjustment disorder according to DSM-III-R terminology [American Psychiatric Association 1987] or milder, acute nonpsychotic major depression). Inpatient CBT also may prove to have a valuable, additional role as a nonsomatic treatment for research purposes (Thase et al. 1991a). This is particularly true with respect to provision of an ethically acceptable nonsomatic treatment during an antidepressant washout period (Thase and Simons 1992). Indeed, when CBT is effective in this scenario, it has the added research benefit of eliminating the potentially confounding effects of somatic antidepressant treatments on brain functions during longitudinal studies of the recovery process.

There are few contraindications for use of CBT as an adjunctive treatment in combination with pharmacotherapy. In our program at the Western Psychiatric Institute and Clinic (WPIC) of the University of Pittsburgh School of Medicine, we have not had much success treating patients with severe Cluster B-type personality disorders (e.g., borderline or antisocial disorders) with individual CBT, which has reinforced the assumption that such patients have a low likelihood of benefit from a short-term psychotherapeutic intervention. We do include severely characterologically disturbed patients in more psychoeducationally oriented therapy groups if their behavior within group is not too disruptive.

With respect to other proposed contraindications, concurrent provision of CBT during a course of bilateral ECT may prove to be an inefficient use of therapy, given the amnestic effects of this treatment. Similarly, depressed patients with a mild or early stage of dementia may have a more difficult time learning to use the concepts of this therapy; but again, CBT would not be specifically contraindicated. Even delusionally depressed patients may benefit from the structure and behavioral techniques of CBT while pharmacologic treatment is ongoing (Bishop et al. 1986; Wright et al. 1992a). Finally, although the utility of CBT as an adjunctive treatment for inpatients with bipolar affective disorder has not yet been studied, evidence is available to suggest that, even in this most "biological" form of affective disorder, CBT may enhance treatment adherence and improve overall outcome (Cochran 1984). The remaining conditions in which inpatient CBT would be relatively contraindicated are few. Attempting to tailor therapy for use with moderately to severely mentally retarded patients would represent one extreme circumstance, as would trying to identify interventions for patients who are essentially stuporous or catatonic.

The nature of contemporary hospital practice necessitates certain modifications in the delivery of individual CBT. Nevertheless, the outpatient treatment manual of Beck and colleagues (1979) is suitable for inpatient use with appropriate condensation (Thase and Wright 1991). Many of the adaptations reflect the type of patients seen on inpatient units. For example, the average inpatient will be more severely depressed than the average outpatient, which dictates that the early stages of therapy need to be modified to include a greater initial emphasis on behavioral strategies (Scott 1988; Thase and Wright 1991). Moreover, sessions sometimes need to be shortened to about 30 minutes to prevent overburdening a severely depressed patient with too much new information (Scott 1988). And as I noted previously, despite the slower pace within sessions, a greater frequency of sessions is recommended for more severely ill individuals. Wright (1986) utilized inpatient CBT (in combination with pharmacotherapy) on a thrice-weekly basis, whereas other researchers provided four or five sessions per week (Bowers 1990; Miller et al. 1989a; Scott 1988; Thase et al. 1991a).

Inpatient CBT also must take into account the greater likelihood that patients will have made a suicide attempt or will have active suicidal ideation. Suicidality is the most common reason for hospitalization of a depressed person (Mezzich et al. 1984). The initial emphasis on recognition of hopelessness, with attention given to both the historical and situational factors that may maintain such a negative view of future, is an important component of CBT (Beck et al. 1979). It is incumbent upon the therapist to identify specific strategies that are likely to lead to a lessening of hopelessness, beginning with the initial session of therapy.

Yet other modifications are related to the ward's milieu and the overall team approach to treatment (see Thase and Wright 1991). As a result, inpatient CBT must fit well within an integrated treatment plan. In our setting, this works best when the therapist develops a written addendum to the treatment plan. The CBT "addendum" may thus serve to facilitate communication with the patient, the treatment team, and other affiliated inpatient staff. A well-specified CBT addendum to the treatment plan also may reduce some of the mystery that traditionally surrounds psychotherapy. Further, it is important that the CBT therapist function as a well-integrated member of the treatment team. This requires regular attendance at treatment team meetings, at which time the progress and problems in the course of therapy are incorporated into the assessment of the patient's overall progress. Finally, the support of each member of the treatment team is vital to prevent undercutting of the therapy.

In an ideal circumstance, one might wish that all team members would be trained in CBT (Thase and Wright 1991; Wright and Schrodt 1989). However, such uniform training is quite unlikely in most inpatient settings and many not even be justifiable. Therefore, the onus of coordinating communication, as well as the delivery of CBT, will continue to fall on the therapist. To simplify this process, two steps are recommended: the explicit training of nursing staff as cotherapists, and conjoint meetings with the patient's family and the treatment team's social worker. In our program at WPIC, we accomplish the former through regular in-service training of nurses (Bowler et al. 1992), whereas the latter is addressed (whenever feasible) in weekly meetings involving the patient, the patient's spouse or significant other, the CBT therapist, and the social worker (Thase and Wright 1991).

THE STRUCTURE OF INPATIENT THERAPY SESSIONS

During the patient's initial or introductory session the therapist has several major goals. These initial goals include 1) developing rapport, 2) establishing a specific problem list and initial case formulation, and 3) educating the patient about the cognitive model of therapy. The therapist often begins to achieve these goals while obtaining a comprehensive history of the patient's current situation, past difficulties, and syndromal presentation (Beck et al. 1979; Persons 1989). As I noted previously, the therapist also has a fourth goal: to learn about the patient's feelings of pessimism, hopelessness, and, specifically, suicidality (Beck et al. 1979). Moreover, whenever possible, the therapist needs to initiate an intervention that will lessen these symptoms.

After the initial session, CBT sessions typically follow a semi-standardized sequence (Beck et al. 1979; Thase and Wright 1991). First, an agenda is set for the work that will be accomplished within that session. The agenda always includes a symptomatic check-in, an update of new developments, and a review of homework assigned at the previous session. The problem list next may be used to set priorities regarding what difficulties will be dealt with first. Normally, the decision is made to focus initially on the life problems, affective symptoms, or thought patterns that are both central to the patient's difficulties *and* potentially amenable to change. Therapist and patient thus select several items from the problem list to work on within the session. Generally, it is possible to make progress on only one or two problem areas in a particular session.

In addressing a typical problem, the therapist usually begins by asking a series of questions to clarify the nature of the patient's difficulty. Is the patient misinterpreting events, or is the perception of the problem accurate? Are the patient's assumptions and attributions about the problem realistic, and has the patient thought of alternative possible explanations? When problems are symptomatic or behavioral in nature (e.g., insomnia, appetite disturbance, decreased activity, or anhedonia), obtaining a more detailed history of the antecedent, concomitant, and consequent factors associated with the problem is helpful. At the end of this data-collecting process, the therapist typically summarizes the evidence and suggests a framework for understanding the problem in psychoeducational terms. This in turn leads to the therapist's recommendation for an intervention designed to address the thoughts, assumptions, or behaviors related to the problem.

After an intervention is complete, the therapist elicits feedback from the patient. To facilitate this process, the therapist may ask the patient to summarize the major points of the session. It is helpful to identify and, if necessary, gently correct any distortions revealed in the patient's understanding of the formulation of the problem or the rationale for the intervention before moving on. Therapist and patient may then move on to address another problem or item from the agenda, if time permits, or they may proceed to develop relevant homework assignments. As I have noted, homework assignments are then crafted to help the patient to begin to apply and expand on the material covered during the session.

Although the structure of a CBT session as illustrated here may not change as treatment progresses, the content typically does. In general, the initial sessions are devoted to learning to cope with thoughts of hopelessness, applying behavioral methods to reduce distressing symptoms, and confirming the relationship between thoughts and feelings (see below). During the second and third weeks of intensive inpatient therapy, the focus is likely to shift to problems that require more focused cognitive interventions so as to first test and subsequently modify dysfunctional attitudes and attributions (Thase and Wright 1991). This middle phase of individual therapy (typically between sessions 5 and 15) thus is spent helping the patient to apply in vivo the cognitive component of CBT. As I describe later, such work is enhanced by use of homework assignments emphasizing a systematic approach to thought recording and application of specific rational responses to counter specific automatic negative thoughts (Beck et al. 1979; Thase and Wright 1991).

In the later phase of therapy (e.g., during the third or fourth week of inpatient treatment, if appropriate), the patient is usually less symptomatic, and targets for therapeutic intervention may shift again to address schemas or long-standing patterns of dysfunctional behavior (Thase and Wright 1991). An example of a schematic issue addressed in this phase of therapy would be found in the interventions that follow recognition of the unspoken assumption that "Unless I perform perfectly, I am a failure." Patients also are encouraged to take an increasing amount of responsibility in the later phase of therapy, including generating their own homework assignments and applying therapy techniques while on predischarge passes. As discharge approaches, the therapist may serve more as a consultant, and the patient is encouraged to apply CBT techniques without such a high level of constant feedback or support (Thase 1992). For many patients who must be discharged earlier, schema-focused treatment will need to be continued after discharge from the inpatient unit.

SPECIFIC THERAPEUTIC TECHNIQUES

Behavioral Techniques

Behavioral techniques are particularly useful in the early stages of therapy. Their principal use is to help patients cope with symptoms and address interpersonal skills deficits. This is especially true in the treatment of more severely depressed patients who are less active, socially withdrawn, and/or have marked difficulties with concentration. Although behavioral techniques thus tend to be more focused and concrete, they also may be used as the vehicle to help patients begin to identify, test, and modify dysfunctional cognitions. For example, a patient who complains of marked anhedonia often can use the results of a behavioral assignment intended to increase pleasurable activity to also test the accuracy of the catastrophic thought "I don't enjoy anything!" The most commonly used behavioral methods are described in the following subsections.

Activity scheduling. The activity schedule specifically helps the patient learn to monitor and modify behavior and to increase productivity (Beck and Greenberg 1974; Thase and Beck 1992). Patients are given a rating form and instructed how to keep a record of their activities on an hour-by-hour basis. Ratings of mood may then be added so as to help to establish functional relationships between the scheduled activity or changes in behavior and mood. Scheduling new activities is usually one of the first techniques used with a depressed patient and may be targeted to counteract hopelessness, inactivity, anhedonia, or loss of motivation. The inpatient therapist helps the patient to identify unscheduled blocks of time that are empty and to consider alternative, potentially rewarding activities that may be scheduled into these time slots. Such activities would include those already on the ward's "menu" (e.g., occupational therapy, recreation, or exercise groups) or may be developed de novo to fit the needs of a given patient (e.g., blocking out 1 hour to complete laundry or 2 hours to watch a videotape of a favorite movie or sporting event on TV). Indeed, a regularly scheduled period of exercise may exert a modest antidepressant effect (Simons et al. 1985). In an optimally functioning inpatient CBT program, the plan for a scheduled activity is passed on to ward staff from shift to shift to ensure that the patient has the necessary supervision and support to complete the task successfully. An example of an experiment devised around an activity schedule would be for the patient to monitor his or her mood and thoughts during an unstructured time period in comparison to a similar time period spent engaged in a preferred, formerly rewarding activity.

It is important to help the patient understand that his or her inactivity and loss of enjoyment are *symptoms* of depression and therefore likely to be transient (rather than enduring) and potentially amenable to change. Conversely, an informed therapist appreciates that the patient's anhedonia may actually be the result of dysfunction in the pleasure-reward centers of the brain (Thase et al. 1985) and, as a result, the reinforcing aspects of many formerly desirable activities have a reduced salience. In cases of an apparently diminished capacity to enjoy, therapeutic expectations are temporarily set lower (i.e., to complete a task rather than to enjoy it), and an illustration such as "priming a pump" or "establishing a foundation" to lessen dysphoria and build on is often helpful.

Mastery and pleasure ratings.   Activity scheduling is often necessary, because patients may feel too anergic and/or dysphoric to spontaneously seek out pleasurable activities. Moreover, many patients minimize or devalue their remaining intellectual and interpersonal assets and areas of competence. The process of gaining greater objectivity is facilitated by having patients begin to rate scheduled activities according to their experiences of mastery (M) or pleasure (P). Although most patients can readily identify with the concept of pleasure, the term "mastery" often requires a brief psychoeducational lesson. Mastery is used to refer to any feelings associated with accomplishment or performance of tasks that require skill or competence. For example, completion of an overdue tax form is not likely to elicit pleasure, but it does require a certain measure of competence.

Once patients understand the concepts underlying M and P ratings, they are asked to begin to use a scale from 0 to 10 to rate M and P experiences. These ratings are then used to identify areas of deficit in the experience of pleasure or mastery. Such deficits can then be addressed with new homework assignments emphasizing increased access to reinforcement or esteem-enhancing activities. Persistently low M and/or P ratings also often provide a helpful clue that the patient's perceptions about the assignments (i.e., negative predictions, ruminations, and automatic negative thoughts) may be interfering with their intended effect. Identification of such a process would readily lead to the therapist's use of cognitive interventions, as I describe later.

Diversion techniques.   These techniques are used to help patients cope with the most painful or overwhelming affects, including dysphoria, anxiety, and anger. The rationale for the use of diversion techniques (rather than methods intended to have more fundamental or enduring effects on cognitions or behaviors) is that strong affects may be too overwhelming to overcome early in the course of therapy. The use of diversion thus enables the patient to cope more effectively at times of intense distress and/or to "dampen" an otherwise escalating emotional reaction. Patients thus obtain the added benefit of being able to regain a sense of control. Diversion may be accomplished through the use of physical activity (e.g., riding an exercise bike), a distracting social contact, or visual imagery. Thought stopping, a specific elaboration of a diversion technique, may be particularly useful in coping with more intrusive ruminations or images. The therapist teaches the patient to use a distressing rumination as the cue to visualize an alternate image, such as a stop sign or a mountain brook. By focusing intently on the visual image, the patient typically achieves some respite from the emotionally charged rumination.

Patients sometimes disparage diversion techniques as a superficial or "trivial" approach. It is important for the therapist to elicit negative cognitions at such times (e.g., "My problems are overwhelming and the only help you can offer is to ride an exercise bike!"). The therapist also must make sure that the rationale and time-limited nature of the use of diversion techniques are understood explicitly. Moreover, when the patient uses a negative image to describe the technique (e.g., "This is just a Band-Aid."), it is helpful to use reattributions of that image to address the problem. For example, the therapist might ask, "What is it about the idea of our using a Band-Aid technique that is so upsetting for you?" and "Can you think of any real-life circumstances in which you would find a Band-Aid helpful?"

Graded task assignments.   To help severely depressed patients initiate more complex activities, the therapist often needs to break down an activity into a series of steps, beginning with the simplest part of the task and progressing to the most demanding (Beck et al. 1979). This step-by-step approach permits the patient to eventually complete assignments that at first seem impossible or overwhelming. Graded task assignments thus serve as a key behavioral method of addressing problems associated with procrastination and inertia. In the early phases of treatment, graded task assignments also may help a markedly depressed patient realize that some accommodations need to be made to cope with impairments caused by the disorder. Such graded tasks also teach the utility of a stepwise approach to problem solving and thus may be generalized and applied to more complicated life problems following discharge (Thase 1992).

Behavioral rehearsal and role-playing. Rehearsal strategies help patients to prepare for and ultimately accomplish difficult tasks or responses. Role-playing usually includes the therapist's use of modeling and coaching of the patient's approximations of the target behaviors. For example, the patient may be asked to play the role of a significant other, while the therapist "models" an appropriately assertive or confrontational response in the patient's role.

Monitoring of automatic thoughts during the use of rehearsal methods also may help the patient identify cognitive distortions that may exacerbate an emotionally charged situation. Imagery also may be used to help a patient to covertly rehearse for specific tasks that cannot be explicitly practiced (Beck et al. 1979). These methods may be modified or expanded to enable the patient to develop new patterns of behavior, such as enhanced social skills (Hersen et al. 1984), assertiveness, or improved management of anger.

Relaxation training. The technique of progressive deep muscle relaxation introduced by Jacobson (1964) is a useful adjunctive method for managing generalized anxiety, psychomotor agitation, and initial insomnia. Relaxation training has been shown to have a modest additive effect when used along with antidepressant therapy (Bowers 1990), and we have found it to be a particularly helpful adjunct to CBT when medications are not utilized (Thase and Wright 1991).

Cognitive Techniques

Four general steps are involved in a cognitive intervention:

1. Eliciting automatic thoughts and understanding their personal significance in terms of the cognitive triad (i.e., the meaning of the perception with respect to thoughts about self, world, or future);
2. Testing the accuracy of the automatic thoughts;
3. Identifying logical errors, distortions, maladaptive underlying assumptions, and schema; and
4. Analyzing the validity of maladaptive assumptions and schema.

These methods are discussed in the following subsections.

Identification of dysfunctional automatic thoughts.   The patient is taught to identity automatic negative thoughts as the first step of cognitive intervention. Automatic thoughts are described to patients in a didactic manner, and relevant reading material is provided early in the course of therapy (see, e.g., Beck and Greenberg 1974; Burns 1981; Howell and Thase 1991). The therapist and patient next work collaboratively to identify examples of such thoughts in vivo. Through repetition of this process, the patient learns to become more aware of his or her internal dialogue and patterns of thinking. The central hypothesis of CBT—namely, that feelings of depression or anxiety are related to the patient's tendency to think in a distorted or unrealistically negative manner—is thus introduced. However, the therapist does not explicitly try to "correct" the accuracy of a patient's thoughts until the process for identifying and evaluating negative automatic thoughts is established.

Several techniques are used to help the patient to identify automatic negative thoughts. The therapist may ask about what "passed through" the patient's mind during an emotional state. Mood shifts that occur during the session provide a particularly timely opportunity for the therapist to ask about the patient's thoughts. Similarly, upsetting events from the patient's past can be examined by asking him or her to recall specific thoughts and feelings while imagining that the troubling event is taking place. Role-playing also may be used to facilitate recall of thoughts and feelings associated with an unpleasant circumstance.

Homework assignments are similarly used to improve the patient's recognition of automatic negative thoughts and their relation to emotional reactions. The Daily Record of Dysfunctional Thoughts ([DRDT] Young and Beck 1982; see Table 6–4) is an especially helpful form for patients to use as they begin to record variations in mood in relation to both the situations or events associated with dysphoric mood or, conversely, the automatic thoughts that accompany a change in emotions. Thought counting may be used as an homework assignment when a patient is skeptical about the occurrence of a certain type of automatic thought. Patients may use a wrist counter or a golf scorer to count the "targeted" thoughts.

Testing the accuracy of automatic negative thoughts.   After the patient's pattern of automatic negative thoughts has been demonstrated to covary

Table 6-4. Daily record of dysfunctional thoughts

Situation	Emotion(s)	Automatic thought(s)	Rational response	Outcome
Describe: 1. Actual event leading to unpleasant emotion, or 2. Stream of thoughts, daydreams, or recollection, leading to unpleasant emotion.	1. Specify sad/ anxious/angry, etc. 2. Rate degree of emotion, 1–100.	1. Write automatic thought(s) that preceded emotion(s). 2. Rate beliefs in automatic thought(s), 0–100%.	1. Write rational response to automatic thought(s). 2. Rate belief in rational response, 0–100%.	1. Rerate belief in automatic thought(s), 0–100%. 2. Specify and rate subsequent emotions, 0–100.
DATE:				
6/25 Husband 1 hour late for visit	Sad (80%)	He's mad at me. (80%) I don't deserve him. (80%)	Maybe he just got tied up and is running late. Even if he is mad, it is not my fault. We've been married 8 years, and up to recently, I've pulled my weight. He tells me he still love me.	50%
	Anxious (50%)	I'm driving him away. (25%)	Ditto. I have no evidence that he's planning to leave. My hospitalization is stressful but, all-in-all, he doesn't run away from stress.	0%
	Angry (20%)	Why can't he be more supportive? (50%)	No one's perfect. When I'm not depressed, he's better. Maybe the social worker can help us with this.	40%
				30%

Explanation: When you experience an unpleasant emotion, note the situation that seemed to stimulate the emotion. (If the emotion occurred while you were thinking, daydreaming, etc., please note this.) Then note the automatic thought associated with the emotion. Record the degree to which you believe this thought: 0% = not at all; 100% = completely. In rating degree of emotion, 1 = a trace; 100 = the most intense possible.

with disturbances of mood (i.e., a process that typically takes one to three sessions to establish), therapy shifts to testing the accuracy of the patient's thoughts. The goal of this step is to help the patient learn to think more objectively (i.e., like a scientist or judge). As a result, the patient learns through guided discovery that his or her thoughts and conclusions are hypotheses rather than facts and, because these hypotheses often have ominous implications, they require verification against all available evidence. A majority of therapist-patient interactions during the midphase of therapy (i.e., inpatient sessions 5 to 15) utilize this method (Thase and Wright 1991). The novice CBT therapist must learn that this method differs from simple persuasion, in which an expert (i.e., the therapist) attempts to persuade or convince the patient that the automatic thoughts are wrong or irrational. This step represents a fundamental element of Beck's approach to CBT (Beck 1976; Thase and Beck 1992).

The patient next is asked to record emotionally charged situations and the corresponding automatic negative thoughts on an hour-by-hour basis. Material elicited during doctor's rounds or group therapy may be particular useful, as are the patient's thoughts and afterthoughts about family therapy sessions or visits. These recordings are examined in the subsequent session to evaluate their accuracy. At the most pragmatic level, patients need to learn to ask themselves four basic questions regarding their automatic negative thoughts (Thase and Beck 1992):

1. "What is the evidence to support these thoughts?"
2. "Are there any alternative interpretations?"
3. [If a negative event has happened] "What is my role/responsibility, and can I do anything about it?"
4. "So what if my interpretation is true (or partly true), what does it really say about me (or the world, or my future)?"

Development of rational alternatives for automatic negative thoughts.
Learning to identify more rational responses to dysfunctional automatic thoughts accompanies the process described above. At first, patients are encouraged to write down their alternative explanations or more rational counterresponses to automatic negative thoughts within the session, followed shortly thereafter by written homework. The therapist often needs to help the patient flesh out or expand upon these rational alternatives.

The written approach to coping with affectively laden situations is viewed as an important aid for learning these skills. Later, patients are encouraged to begin to answer their dysfunctional automatic thoughts in vivo (i.e., first by writing them down and, once successful, through covert verbalizations).

Many patients find that their initial efforts to construct rational responses trigger a new "wave" of automatic negative thoughts. Often, these thoughts undercut the mood-altering goal of the rational response intervention. The skilled CBT therapist learns to perceive when a patient is experiencing unstated thoughts questioning the accuracy of his or her rational responses (Persons 1989). Such reservations usually can be recognized by changes in the patient's posture or facial expression. These derivative or "second-order" automatic thoughts need to be recognized, tested, and countered within therapy sessions if the patient is to reach maximum benefit from the rational response technique (Thase and Beck 1992).

Identification of schemas and dysfunctional silent assumptions. In later stages of treatment, explicit identification of basic schemas becomes a high priority. An assignment to review past homework assignments to collate themes or patterns of rigid, harsh, or maladaptive attitudes is often a useful way to begin to identify schemas. An autobiography also may be assigned as a way to collect historical data to document the development of pertinent schemas (Thase and Wright 1991).

A number of strategies are available to modify schemas and silent assumptions (see, e.g., Beck et al. 1979; Persons 1989). For example, patients may be asked to list the advantages and disadvantages of retaining the attitudes and beliefs that are derived from a schema. Drawing upon a technique used in the behavioral treatment of obsessive-compulsive disorder, a modified form of response prevention also may be effectively used (Thase and Beck 1992). This technique involves encouraging the patient to conduct experiments in which he or she behaves opposite to his or her normal tendency (i.e., the stereotypic response typically dictated by the attitude or silent assumption in question). For example, patients with perfectionistic attitudes may be encouraged to develop and perform an experiment in which they must complete a task in an "only satisfactory" manner. In the hospital setting, participation in occupational or recreational therapies provides ample opportunity for such homework assignments (Wright et al. 1992b). While performing this experiment, a patient typically encounters automatic negative thoughts that trigger anxiety or dysphoria, which in turn may interfere with performance or trigger ruminations. The patient may then apply methods learned in therapy to cope with the symptoms in vivo. Parallels then can be drawn to circumstances from the past or anticipated situations in which the standard of perfection would be impossible to achieve.

Continuity of Care

By the end of psychiatric hospitalization, most patients have improved but have not yet achieved a complete or full remission. Moreover, the first several months following an inpatient admission are times of high risk for relapse (Thase 1992). Therefore, careful attention to continuity of outpatient care and discharge planning are essential ingredients of a high-quality inpatient service (Thase 1992). As noted earlier, CBT is conceptually well suited for this need. One approach is to provide a period of outpatient continuation CBT treatment for patients who have been treated as inpatients (Thase 1992). Such continuation therapy ordinarily consists of up to 20 weekly sessions provided over a 4- to 6-month period (Miller et al. 1989a; Thase et al. 1991a). Continuation treatment provides additional support during the transition from inpatient to outpatient status and allows for the consolidation of new skills learned during hospital-based treatment. Moreover, outpatient therapy may permit more extensive work on underlying cognitive vulnerabilities to relapse (e.g., depressogenic schemas), as well as promote more pragmatic changes in stressful life circumstances (Thase 1992).

It is not clear if the value of inpatient CBT is compromised by an aftercare plan that does not include further cognitive therapy. In our preliminary experience utilizing CBT as the principal treatment of unmedicated depressed patients (Thase et al. 1991a), patients who receive continuation therapy are significantly less likely to relapse during the first 4 months after discharge than patients who decline such further treatment. These findings may not generalize to patients receiving concomitant pharmacotherapy; however, the question of an enduring benefit following inpatient CBT warrants further study.

Studies of Effectiveness of CBT

CBT is the best-studied psychotherapeutic treatment of depression in the outpatient setting. Several comprehensive reviews document the utility of this approach in a variety of samples and settings (see, e.g., Dobson 1989; Hollon and Najavitis 1988). Follow-up studies also suggest more enduring prophylactic benefits when patients treated with CBT are compared with patients withdrawn from tricyclic antidepressants (TCAs; Blackburn et al. 1987; Kovacs et al. 1981; Shea et al. 1992; Simons et al. 1986). In one study, the TCA imipramine was more effective than CBT in a subgroup of patients with higher initial depression severity scores (Elkin et al. 1989). We similarly found CBT to be somewhat less effective in more severely depressed outpatients when compared with less severely depressed patients, although our study did not include a TCA-treatment comparison group (Thase et al. 1991b).

The finding of poorer response to CBT in more severely depressed patients may "activate" the common assumption in the mental health field that more severe depressions are likely to have a stronger biological basis and, hence, require concomitant pharmacotherapy (Rush 1982; Thase 1983; Williams 1984). Although few data are as yet available to test this important hypothesis, it is quite relevant to determinations of the ultimate role of CBT as a treatment for hospitalized patients. With respect to treatment of depressed outpatients, several groups have failed to find any relationship between the presence of so-called endogenous features and responsivity to CBT (Blackburn et al. 1981; Kovacs et al. 1981; Simons and Thase 1992; Teasdale et al. 1984; Thase et al. 1991a). Moreover, neither of two research groups (Jarrett et al. 1990; Thase and Simons 1992) found that the reduced rapid eye movement (REM) sleep latency, an objective biological correlate of endogenous depression (Thase et al. 1985), was associated with a poor response to individual CBT. However, two groups reported small but essentially negative outpatient trials of CBT in patients resistant to antidepressant treatment (Fennell and Teasdale 1982; Harpin et al. 1982).

There are as yet no controlled studies of inpatient CBT as a primary treatment modality. Preliminary reports (de Jong et al. 1986; Scott 1988; Shaw 1981; Thase et al. 1991a) suggest that some depressed inpatients can be treated with CBT instead of pharmacotherapy. However, examination of the first 30 unmedicated inpatients treated in our CBT program revealed that marked severity, diagnostic comorbidity, and hypercortisolemia were associated with significantly poorer response (Thase, in press).

Inpatient CBT may have broader application when used in combination with pharmacotherapy. Two reports (Bowers 1990; Miller et al. 1989a) document that patients receiving CBT in addition to standardized pharmacotherapy responded better than those receiving pharmacotherapy alone. In one study, the addition of CBT resulted in more sustained remissions (Miller et al. 1989b) and greater improvements on measures of cognitive dysfunction (Whisman et al. 1991).

SUMMARY

Beck's model of CBT is well suited for adaption as an inpatient therapy for major depression and related disorders. Programmatic options range from development of ideologically "pure" inpatient units (specifically devoted to the delivery of an intensive CBT-centered milieu) to the addition of a trained cognitive therapist to provide group and individual therapy as part of a more eclectic inpatient treatment team. Review of available research suggests that an adjunctive course of inpatient CBT (i.e., provided in addition to standard treatment) may enhance the response of hospitalized depressed patients, particularly those who have failed to respond to outpatient pharmacological treatment and/or who manifest a high level of dysfunctional attitudes. Some patients who decline pharmacotherapy benefit from an intensive course of CBT as the primary treatment modality. In either case, the prognosis following discharge appears to be enhanced by provision of additional sessions of outpatient CBT. When taken together, these factors and findings illustrate the potential utility of inpatient CBT and point to the need for both broader application and further scientific study.

REFERENCES

American Psychiatric Association: Diagnostic and Statistical Manual of Mental Disorders, 3rd Edition, Revised. Washington, DC, American Psychiatric Association, 1987

Arkowitz H, Hannah MT: Cognitive, behavioral, and psychodynamic therapies, in Comprehensive Handbook of Cognitive Therapy. Edited by Freeman A, Simon KM, Beutler LE, et al. New York, Plenum, 1989, pp 143–167

Beck AT: Cognitive Therapy and the Emotional Disorders. New York, International Universities Press, 1976

Beck AT, Greenberg RL: Coping with Depression [booklet]. New York, Institute for Rational Living, 1974

Beck AT, Rush AJ, Shaw BF, et al: Cognitive Therapy of Depression. New York, Guilford, 1979

Bishop S, Miller IV, Norman W, et al: Cognitive therapy of psychotic depression: a case report. Psychotherapy 23:167–173, 1986

Blackburn IM, Bishop S, Glen AIM, et al: The efficacy of cognitive therapy in depression: a treatment trial using cognitive therapy and pharmacotherapy, each alone and in combination. Br J Psychiatry 139:181–189, 1981

Blackburn IM, Eunson KM, Bishop S: A two-year naturalistic follow-up of depressed patients treated with cognitive therapy, pharmacotherapy, and a combination of both. J Affect Disord 10:67–75, 1987

Bowers WA: Cognitive therapy with inpatients, in Comprehensive Handbook of Cognitive Therapy. Edited by Freeman A, Simon KM, Beutler LE, et al. New York, Plenum, 1989, pp 583–596

Bowers WA: Treatment of depressed inpatients: cognitive therapy plus medication, relaxation plus medication, and medication alone. Br J Psychiatry 156:73–78, 1990

Bowler KA, Moonis LJ, Thase ME: The role of the nurse in the cognitive milieu, in Cognitive Therapy With Inpatients: Developing a Cognitive Milieu. Edited by Wright JH, Thase ME, Beck AT, et al. New York, Guilford, 1992, pp 247–270

Braff DL, Beck AT: Thinking disorder in depression. Arch Gen Psychiatry 31:456–459, 1974

Burns D: Feeling Good: The New Mood Therapy. New York, Morrow, 1981

Clark DA: The validity of measures of cognition: a review of the literature. Cognitive Therapy and Research 12:1–2, 1988

Cochran SD: Preventing medical noncompliance in the outpatient treatment of bipolar affective disorders. J Consult Clin Psychol 52:873–878, 1984

de Jong R, Treiber R, Henrich G: Effectiveness of two psychological treatments for inpatients with severe and chronic depressions. Cognitive Therapy and Research 10:645–663, 1986

Dobson K: A meta-analysis of the efficacy of cognitive therapy of depression. J Consult Clin Psychol 57:414–419, 1989

Elkin I, Shea MT, Watkins JT, et al: National Institute of Mental Health Treatment of Depression Collaborative Research Program: general effectiveness of treatments. Arch Gen Psychiatry 46:971–982, 1989

Fennell MJV, Teasdale JD: Cognitive therapy with chronic, drug-refractory depressed outpatients: a note of caution. Cognitive Therapy and Research 6:455–460, 1982

Freeman A, White DM: The treatment of suicidal behavior, in Comprehensive Handbook of Cognitive Therapy. Edited by Freeman A, Simon KM, Beutler LE, et al. New York, Plenum, 1989, pp 321–346

Guidano VF, Liotti G: Cognitive Processes and Emotional Disorders. New York, Guilford, 1983

Hammen C, Ellicott A, Gitlin M, et al: Sociotropy/autonomy and vulnerability to specific life events in patients with unipolar depression and bipolar disorders. J Abnorm Psychol 98:154–160, 1989

Harpin RE, Liberman RP, Marks I, et al: Cognitive-behavior therapy for chronically depressed patients: a controlled pilot study. J Nerv Ment Dis 170:295–301, 1982

Hersen M, Bellack AS, Himmelhoch JM, et al: Effects of social skill training, amitriptyline, and psychotherapy in unipolar depressed woman. Behavioral Therapy 15:21–40, 1984

Hollon SD, Najavitis L: Review of empirical studies on cognitive therapy, in American Psychiatric Press Review of Psychiatry, Vol 7. Edited by Frances AJ, Hales RE. Washington, DC, American Psychiatric Press, 1988, pp 643–666

Howell JR, Thase ME: Beating the blues: recovery from depression, in Insights to Recovery Series. Edited by Daley DC. Skokie, IL, GT Rogers Productions, 1991, pp 1–27

Jacobson E: Anxiety and Tension Control. Philadelphia, PA, JB Lippincott, 1964

Jarrett RB, Rush AJ, Khatami M, et al: Does the pretreatment polysomnogram predict response to cognitive therapy in depression outpatients? a preliminary report. Psychiatry Res 33:285–299, 1990

Kovacs M, Rush AJ, Beck AT, et al: Depressed outpatients treated with cognitive therapy or pharmacotherapy. Arch Gen Psychiatry 38:33–39, 1981

Mezzich JE, Evanczuk KJ, Mathias RJ, et al: Symptoms and hospitalization decisions. Am J Psychiatry 141:764–769, 1984

Miller IW, Norman WH, Keitner GI, et al: Cognitive behavioral treatment of depressed inpatients. Behavioral Therapy 20:25–47, 1989a

Miller IW, Norman WH, Keitner GI: Cognitive-behavioral treatment of depressed inpatients: Six- and twelve-month follow-ups. Am J Psychiatry 146:1274–1279, 1989b

Norcross JC: Handbook of Eclectic Psychotherapy. New York, Brunner/Mazel, 1986

Persons JB: Cognitive Therapy in Practice: A Case Formulation Approach. New York, WW Norton, 1989

Persons JB, Burns DD: Mechanisms of action of cognitive therapy: the relative contributions of technical and interpersonal interventions. Cognitive Therapy and Research 9:539–551, 1985

Robins CJ, Block P: Cognitive theories of depression viewed from a diathesis-stress perspective: evaluations of the models of Beck and of Abramson, Seligman, and Teasdale. Cognitive Therapy and Research 13:297–313, 1989

Rubinow DR, Post RM, Savard R, et al: Cortisol hypersecretion and cognitive impairment in depression. Arch Gen Psychiatry 41:279–283, 1984

Rush AJ: Diagnosing depressions, in Short-Term Psychotherapies for Depression. Edited by Rush AJ. New York, Guilford, 1982, pp 1–18

Scott J: Cognitive therapy with depressed inpatients, in Developments in Cognitive Psychotherapy. Edited by Dryden W, Trower P. London, Sage, 1988, pp 177–189

Segal ZV, Vella DD, Shaw BF: Life stress and depression: a test of the congruency hypothesis for life event content and depressive subtype. Canadian Journal of Behavioral Science 21:389–400, 1989

Shaw BF: Cognitive therapy with an inpatient population, in New Directions in Cognitive Therapy. Edited by Emery G, Hollon SD, Bedrosian RC. New York, Guilford, 1981, pp 29–49

Shaw BF, Segal ZV: Introduction to cognitive theory and therapy, in American Psychiatric Press Review of Psychiatry, Vol 7. Edited by Frances AJ, Hales RE. Washington, DC, American Psychiatric Press, 1988, pp 538–553

Shea MT, Elkin I, Imber SD, et al: Course of depressive symptoms over follow-up: findings from the National Institute of Mental Health Treatment of Depression Collaborative Research Program. Arch Gen Psychiatry 49:782–787, 1992

Simons AD, Thase ME: Mood Disorders, in Handbook of Outpatient Treatment of Adults. Edited by Thase ME, Hersen M, Edelstein BA. New York, Plenum, 1990, pp 91–138

Simons AD, Thase ME: Biological markers, treatment outcome, and 1-year follow-up of endogenous depression: electroencephalographic sleep studies and response to cognitive therapy. J Consult Clin Psychol 60:392–401, 1992

Simons AD, Epstein LH, McGowan CR, et al: Exercise as a treatment for depression: an update. Clin Psychol Rev 5:553–568, 1985

Simons AD, Murphy GE, Levine JL, et al: Cognitive therapy and pharmacotherapy of depression: sustained improvement over one year. Arch Gen Psychiatry 43:43–48, 1986

Teasdale JD, Fennell MJV, Hibbert GA, et al: Cognitive therapy for major depressive disorder in primary care. Br J Psychiatry 144:400–406, 1984

Thase ME: Cognitive and behavioral treatments for depression: a review of recent developments, in Affective Disorders Reassessed. Edited by Ayd FJ, Taylor IJ, Taylor BT. Baltimore, MD, Ayd Medical Communications, 1983, pp 234–243

Thase ME: Transition and aftercare, in Cognitive Therapy With Inpatients: Developing a Cognitive Milieu. Edited by Wright JH, Thase ME, Beck AT, et al. New York, Guilford, 1992, pp 414–435

Thase ME: Cognitive behavior therapy of severe unipolar depression, in Severe Depressive Disorders. Edited by Grunhaus L, Greden J. Washington, DC, American Psychiatric Press (in press)

Thase ME, Beck AT: Overview of cognitive therapy, in Cognitive Therapy With Inpatients: Developing a Cognitive Milieu. Edited by Wright JH, Thase ME, Beck AT, et al. New York, Guilford, 1992, pp 3–34

Thase ME, Simons AD: The applied use of psychotherapy to study the psychobiology of depression. Journal of Psychotherapy Practice and Research 1:72–80, 1992

Thase ME, Wright JH: Cognitive behavior therapy with depressed inpatients: an abridged treatment manual. Behavioral Therapy 22:579–595, 1991

Thase ME, Frank E, Kupfer DJ: Biological processes of major depression, in Depression: Basic Mechanisms, Diagnosis, and Treatment. Edited by Beckham EE, Leber WR. New York, Plenum, 1985, pp 816–913

Thase ME, Bowler K, Harden T: Cognitive behavior therapy of endogenous depression, part 2: preliminary findings in 16 unmedicated patients. Behavioral Therapy 22:469–477, 1991a

Thase ME, Simons AD, Cahalane J, et al: Severity of depression and response to cognitive behavior therapy. Am J Psychiatry 148:784–789, 1991b

Whisman MA, Miller IW, Norman WH, et al: Cognitive therapy with depressed inpatients: specific effects on dysfunctional cognitions. J Consult Clin Psychol 59:282–288, 1991

Williams JMG: Cognitive-behavior therapy for depression: problems and perspectives. Br J Psychiatry 145:254–262, 1984

Wright JH: Nortriptyline effects on cognition in depression. Dissertation Abstracts International 47 (Section B):2667, 1986

Wright JH, Salmon PG: Learning and memory in process, in Depression: New Directions in Theory, Research, and Practice. Edited by McCann CD, Endler NS. Toronto, Canada, Wall and Emerson, 1990, pp 211–236

Wright JH, Schrodt GR: Combined cognitive therapy and pharmacotherapy, in Comprehensive Handbook of Cognitive Therapy. Edited by Freeman A, Simon KM, Beutler LE, et al. New York, Plenum, 1989, pp 267–282

Wright JH, Thase ME, Sensky T: Cognitive and biological therapies: a combined approach, in Cognitive Therapy With Inpatients: Developing a Cognitive Milieu. Edited by Wright JH, Thase ME, Beck AT, et al. New York, Guilford, 1992a, pp 193–218

Wright JH, Thase ME, Beck AT, et al (eds): Cognitive Therapy With Inpatients: Developing a Cognitive Milieu. New York, Guilford, 1992b

Young JE, Beck AT: Cognitive therapy: clinical applications, in Short-Term Psychotherapies for Depression. Edited by Rush AJ. New York, Guilford, 1982, pp 182–214

II

SPECIAL POPULATIONS

Inpatient Psychotherapy With Chronically Mentally Ill Patients

Francine Cournos, M.D.
Ewald Horwath, M.D.

INTRODUCTION

Psychotherapy for chronically mentally ill patients on short-term inpatient units bears little resemblance to the open-ended explorations of most office-based psychotherapies. Patients on these units have multiple problems and extensive treatment histories, but the goal of the therapy is to resolve the immediate problems that brought the patient to the hospital. Any verbal interaction that enhances the patient's understanding of the situation, promotes better adaptation, or improves the quality of the patient's life constitutes the psychotherapy needed to achieve this goal.

The use of brief hospitalization in the management of chronic illness requires accepting that patients may be repeatedly hospitalized during certain phases of the illness. This can be discouraging, but the team approach helps by providing needed support to both patient and staff. For the patient, each member of the team is a resource and has something unique to contribute. For the staff, the team approach allows shared

The authors acknowledge Pelligrino Sarti, M.D., without whose clinical insights this chapter could not have been written.

responsibility and collegial support when dealing with patients whose treatment is difficult and often only partially successful.

The literature on expressed emotion (EE; see Chapter 4) is also relevant to the milieu of an inpatient unit treating chronically mentally ill individuals. The approach in this chapter is grounded in evidence suggesting that overzealous therapies and high-expectation environments may be harmful to patients with schizophrenia (Cournos 1987; Drake and Sederer 1986; Kuipers 1979; Linn et al. 1980; Linstrom 1988; Wing 1978). Moreover, there is no place for blame in this approach. Staff convey the message that neither the patient nor the family has caused the patient's illness, but they nevertheless can be immensely helpful by sharing responsibility with the staff for managing it.

REASONS FOR HOSPITALIZATION

Generally, patients with chronic mental illness are hospitalized because a problem with some aspect of their care outside of the hospital has interfered with their ability to live in the community. Even though the patient is now in the hospital, the center of his or her treatment in the long run is still outside of it. Undoubtedly, the patient has significant psychiatric symptoms, but focusing only on how to improve them is almost never sufficient. Symptoms are only one aspect of the problem and may correlate modestly with social functioning, which is often more directly responsible for hospitalization (Dohrenwend et al. 1983). Thus, a broader view of the patient's problem is required. Table 7–1 lists some common reasons for the admission of severely and persistently ill patients.

It is essential for the entire treatment team to use the first few days of hospitalization to identify which of the factors listed in Table 7–1 were involved in the patient's current admission and to begin immediate and aggressive work to resolve them.

For example, if a young man was admitted to the hospital after he threatened his mother with a knife, convinced his outpatient therapist that he was no longer manageable outside the hospital, and provoked his landlord to begin eviction proceedings because he was harassing other tenants, staff must contact the mother, the therapist, and the landlord as quickly as possible if they expect to return the patient to the setting he came from. It is not possible to wait until the time of discharge and expect the patient to get a good reception because he is now much better. By then, the system may well have solidified in a way that excludes the patient, and the possibility of successful reentry into his previous situation may be forever closed (Drake and Sederer 1986).

Table 7–1.   Reasons for hospitalization

Patient factors

1. Exacerbation of symptoms caused by noncompliance with prescribed regimen and/or use of nonprescribed or illicit drugs

2. Exacerbation of symptoms caused by patient fragility to minor stresses outside the hospital (e.g., a call from a bill collector, the therapist's vacations)

3. Exacerbation of symptoms caused by serious stresses (e.g., failure to achieve an important goal, loss of a significant relationship)

4. Unremitting psychopathology, especially disorganized and/or dangerous behavior that occurs because the patient is refractory to standard treatment

5. Complicating medical problems, including those caused by prescribed psychotropic medication

Disruption of personal social supports

1. Inability of caretakers to cope with the patient

2. Illness or death of the primary caretaker

3. Severe family disturbances (e.g., psychiatric illness in more than one family member, significant separation difficulties between the patient and the family)

Societal pressure to compel the mental health system to control undesirable social behavior

1. Decisions by law enforcement authorities to triage disturbed dangerous people into the mental health system

2. Community pressure to exert control over people who engage in recurrent nuisance behavior

Systems deficiencies

1. Lack of affordable housing

2. Insufficient support from social welfare programs

3. Deficiencies in the mental health system itself (e.g., fragmentation of services, limited long-term hospitalization, program cutbacks)

4. Poor matches between patients and their therapists or programs

---

STABILIZATION AND ESTABLISHMENT OF THE THERAPEUTIC ALLIANCE

For most patients, the first phase of hospitalization follows a medical model in which somatic interventions are used to ameliorate psychopathology. During this period, many patients are limited in their capacity to observe their own problems. Dangerous or agitated behavior is often a prominent issue (Leibenluft and Goldberg 1987). Although medication is usually essential to restoring a patient's control, the therapist's verbal interventions to set limits and contain regression can be very helpful.

For example, the sense of self of psychotic patients may be threatened by delusions of control, thought withdrawal, thought broadcasting, or formal thought disorder. These symptoms contribute to a sense of bewilderment, fragmentation, and lack of ego boundaries. The sense of invasion experienced by such patients can be mitigated by supportive statements, such as reassuring patients that others cannot read their minds or control their thoughts.

Angry, threatening patients can be asked in a straightforward way if they feel they can stop what they are doing or need time in a quiet room or some other form of restraint. The fears of paranoid patients are often reduced when therapists offer straightforward descriptions of the diagnosis and treatment plan, even if the patients totally disagree with what they are told. While waiting for medication to take effect, it is possible to talk to patients in ways that make them feel safer and encourage their own efforts to stay in control.

However, even after cognitive functioning and reality testing have improved to the extent possible using somatic treatments, chronically ill patients will often still be far from having the insight they need into their situations. The psychological defenses that most commonly interfere with insight in this patient population are projection and denial (Sarti and Cournos 1990).

Chronically ill patients often view the goal of hospitalization as discharge from the hospital rather than treatment for their illnesses. Those who have been admitted involuntarily or under pressure often experience genuine fear, anger, and confusion about the reasons for admission. Denial is often accompanied by patients' projection of their problems onto others, which may take the form of persecutory or grandiose delusions that persist despite adequate doses of antipsychotic medication. Paranoid defenses preserve a patient's sense that he or she is all right by externalizing the blame for the predicament onto the hostile outside world (Meissner 1978). Direct confrontation of these defenses often makes such patients feel frightened, misunderstood, and unfairly treated. Addressing these attitudes presents one of the most common and frustrating problems for therapists who work with severely mentally ill people.

The job of the therapist is to encourage the patient to accept an alternative view by empathizing with his or her feelings without agreeing with unrealistic ideas. The perception of a patient that the therapist is sympathetic and interested is the beginning of the successful therapeutic alliance. Through the daily intensive contact that characterizes short-term hospitalization, the therapist searches with the patient for realistic and shared goals. For example, the therapist may align him- or herself with a patient's interest in remaining out of the hospital and suggest they discuss ways to avoid conflicts with neighbors or the police.

In doing this, the experienced therapist moves at a pace the patient can tolerate and avoids minimization of the problem, anger in response to resistance, and futile attempts to confront entrenched denial or delusional convictions. Patients use psychological defenses for the purpose of protecting self-esteem and warding off fears of invasion and disintegration. Yet most patients have some awareness that something is wrong. The therapist knows that regardless of how patients characterize their problems, he or she must help them understand how their behavior brought them to the hospital and what they can do to change it.

PSYCHOTHERAPY TECHNIQUES WITH CHRONICALLY MENTALLY ILL INPATIENTS

Most patients need a combination of individual, group, and family therapy to maximize the chances of successful discharge and follow-up care.

Supportive Versus Exploratory Approaches

Studies of individual and group psychotherapy for schizophrenic patients have often had serious design flaws or inconsistent and unimpressive outcomes (Gunderson et al. 1984; Mosher and Keith 1979; Stanton et al. 1984). Sometimes the studies were targeted to carefully selected patients (Gunderson et al. 1984). Given this general lack of guidance, clinicians must rely on their own impressions. In our experience with this population, supportive, structured approaches are much more successful than open-ended exploratory therapies, which is probably one reason clinicians gravitate toward the former (Zahniser et al. 1991).

Open-ended exploration is often not well tolerated (Drake and Sederer 1986; Gunderson et al. 1984; Stanton et al. 1984). Usually it produces little useful information. For a variety of reasons, it may also lead to increased anxiety and further regression.

Open-ended approaches can inadvertently delay dealing with the crises that have precipitated the patient's hospitalization, and such delays can result in harm to the patient. In addition, attempting to help a psychotic patient by uncovering repressed sexual and aggressive desires may lead to deterioration in a fragile patient with limitations in reality testing. Such a patient may not be able to distinguish between the forbidden sexual or aggressive wish on the one hand and the act on the other. For example, a frightening dream may provide an important avenue of access to unconscious material in a well-functioning psychotherapy patient, but a chaotic primitive dream in a hospitalized psychotic patient is often best handled by assuring the patient that it was just a dream.

> Katherine M. was a 33-year-old woman with bipolar disorder and many prior psychiatric hospitalizations. On this occasion, she was admitted with increasingly severe symptoms, revolving around a belief that the priest in her church had developed strong sexual feelings for her. Once in the hospital, Ms. M.'s inpatient therapist helped her to recognize the connection between her preoccupation with the priest and sexual feelings toward other important men in her life, in particular her outpatient therapist and her father. Although the therapist's statements were probably accurate, Ms. M. became progressively worse. Whereas her multiple previous admissions had lasted on average only 1 month, this time Ms. M. remained in the hospital for 6 months before she improved enough to be discharged.

Although cause and effect cannot be proven here, it appears that the therapist's interpretation frightened the patient without producing any resolution of the problem. Moreover, even if it is sometimes useful to encourage regression, explore certain conflicts, and arrive at a new understanding and level of integration, this is not a realistic strategy for the brief hospitalization of a psychotic patient.

Psychodynamic insight works best when the therapist uses it to understand the patient's experiences and conflicts with others. However, the therapist is not attempting to help the patient get in touch with his or her unconscious inner life, which is already overwhelming. Rather, to the extent the therapist reveals a psychodynamic understanding to the patient, it is to discourage regression and help the patient make contact with day-to-day reality. This manner of encouraging higher-level functioning can be very useful.

> William B. was a 25-year-old chronically ill schizophrenic man who had trouble recognizing his difficulties in controlling his anger. Instead, he was preoccupied with the idea that World War III was about to occur. The therapist witnessed an interaction in which Linda K., another patient, accidentally poked Mr. B. with a pool cue, and Mr. B. began shouting about the coming of World War III. "Don't get so upset," the therapist said, "Ms. K. hit you by accident." Following this comment, Mr. B. calmed down. The therapist presented Mr. B. with the link between his abstract and externalized worries about World War III and his own angry feelings in response to the ordinary event of being poked by another patient. He did so to help Mr. B. regain control.

In fact, much of the psychotherapy with this population involves providing patients with tools to differentiate between frightening internal ideas and ordinary external reality. The therapist tries to encourage adaptive rather than infantile responses to stressful situations.

> This was the sixth hospitalization for Barbara F., a 42-year-old woman with chronic schizophrenia who always came into the hospital in a disorganized state. On this admission, her symptoms improved rapidly on medication, but she habitually disrobed in public, which thwarted any attempts to discharge her. The therapist surmised that Ms. F. was using this childlike behavior to express her anxiety about going home. He told Ms. F. that she didn't have to take her clothes off to show him how frightened she was to leave the hospital. He understood her fear, and he

would be meeting with her and her family to help her handle the problems she had been having at home. Ms. F. listened without acknowledging the comment, but she did not disrobe in public again for the remainder of her hospital stay.

The therapists' interventions with Mr. B. and Ms. F. were brief. However, they were highly effective because they contained accurate perceptions of the patients' immediate distress and because the therapists modeled more direct and effective ways of dealing with frightening feelings. Psychotherapy with this population requires a more flexible model than adhering to a rigid schedule of planned 45-minute sessions. Brief, focused daily contact with a psychotic patient is often more effective and better tolerated than extended sessions several times a week (Sarti and Cournos 1990).

Psychoeducation

All successful psychotherapies with severely mentally ill patients use psychoeducation as a component of the approach. In an individual treatment, this involves attaching names and descriptions to the patient's illness and symptoms, a process that is essential if the patient is to have any control over his or her problem.

In the next exchange, a psychiatrist is encouraging a young woman admitted for her third episode of mania to monitor her own progress:

> Patient: "Do you think I'm ready to go home?"
> Psychiatrist: "What's your impression?"
> Patient: "I'm still talking too fast."
> Psychiatrist: "Then I guess you're not quite ready yet."

In a similar manner, patient and therapist need to develop successful management strategies, especially for those symptoms that do not remit with somatic treatment. Many patients with psychotic illnesses develop their own techniques for reducing symptoms or distracting themselves from them, such as lying quietly, exercising, changing activities, and so on. In addition, the therapist can work with the patient on techniques for ignoring symptoms.

Patient: "The voices I hear are telling me to hurt myself."
Therapist: "You know when you hear those voices, the part of your mind that is ill is playing tricks on you."
Patient: "Yes, we've talked about that before. I know they're not real, and I don't need to listen to what they tell me to do."

Although not every patient is capable of self-observation at the beginning of treatment, many can develop these techniques over time.

Groups

In addition to individual sessions, psychoeducational groups on inpatient units can play an important adjunctive role. In a group setting, the therapist can explain the signs and symptoms of psychotic illnesses without directly confronting any individual patient's need to deny being ill. Patients are familiarized with the medical explanation for their symptoms. Often, even acutely psychotic patients can attend a series of educational sessions that describe the stages of psychosis, its early warning signs and later manifestations, the problem of violent impulses, and the impact of prescribed and illicit drugs. Patients who may otherwise seem out of touch with reality can nonetheless ask relevant questions or coherently share their own experiences. Those who are further along in treatment and less invested in denial serve as a model for expressing curiosity about their symptoms and acknowledging the impact of their illnesses. In any case, patients have the option of either participating or sitting quietly and absorbing the information. In our experience, these groups increase patient involvement with their treatment, and many patients will discuss with their individual therapists issues that first arose in the group.

Psychoeducational groups are a suitable forum for discussing the problem of stigma and how to handle negative attitudes toward mentally ill people. Educational groups for family members are also extremely helpful (see Chapter 4). They offer support and reduce distress among family members while promoting management techniques that will assist the staff in carrying out the treatment plan.

Other groups also augment individual work with severely ill patients. The most effective groups focus on specific tasks, such as improving social and daily living skills and preparing for discharge (Cournos 1987; Drake and Sederer 1986). Helpful group techniques include the presentation of information followed by discussion, the completion of tasks, role-playing and other skill-training techniques, and the development of peer norms and support. Open-ended verbal groups are usually not as helpful for seriously ill patients (Drake and Sederer 1986; Linn et al. 1979).

Groups are sometimes the best way to perform certain evaluative functions, such as assessing a patient's concentration or ability to get along with others. They are also an efficient way to provide counseling on topics such as health care and safer sexual practices.

Integrating Family and Systems Work

Effective family approaches to the treatment of severe mental illness are now well described (see Chapter 4). During brief hospitalization, the first meeting with the family should occur as close to the time of the patient's admission as possible. It is equally important to make early contact with the patient's current outpatient therapist and prescribing psychiatrist. If the patient lives in a supervised living setting, this in effect becomes an extension of his or her family, so staff there should be involved as well. The knowledge other parties have about the patient is essential to every treatment decision, including choice of medication, alterations in the direction of future outpatient treatment, and any modification of living arrangements. When the obvious usefulness of these collaborations is overlooked, the result is often prolongation of the hospital stay or increased recidivism following discharge.

It is usually not helpful to impose a rigid theoretical model on the nature of these contacts. Questions of whom to contact, when, and whether or not to include the patient in a meeting should be considered pragmatically. If the patient feels it is in his or her interest for the therapist to speak with a boss, a landlord, an agency providing benefits, or others, the therapist should consider doing so within the defined limits of confidentiality and sensible therapeutic practice. It is crucial to preserve the patient's existing support network, which is often irreplaceable.

One particularly common pitfall is to accept at face value a patient's stated desire to separate from his or her family. Such attempts, as any therapist who works with this population can attest, frequently fail. Most commonly, patients with severe mental illness are discharged to live with family members (New York State Office of Mental Health 1985) and, however conflicted, the bonds are intense. When separation is desirable, the occasion of a particular brief hospital stay may be neither the practical nor the therapeutically appropriate moment to achieve it. Separation from the family is thus too complex to be accomplished under pressure and should be viewed as a long-term goal.

NONCOMPLIANCE

Noncompliance is an important issue not just in psychiatry but in all of medicine. Patients are concerned about autonomy; they may have difficulty grasping information about the proposed treatment; often, their deeply held beliefs about health and illness conflict with medical advice; and strong emotional reactions, including fear and denial, can interfere with rational decision making. Health care professionals may also contribute to patient noncompliance when they fail to offer persuasive reasons for their recommendations, or when they respond with abruptness or anger to patient resistance.

Studies of medical patients show comparable rates of noncompliance to those of psychiatric patients (Conrad 1985; Zisook and Gammon 1981). But because of the nature of mental illness, noncompliance has received special attention in psychiatric treatment. Factors associated with noncompliance among psychiatric patients vary from psychotic ideas to rational responses and include thought disturbance, grandiosity, hostility, denial of illness, chronicity, paranoia, side effects, lack of drug efficacy, and a desire to be in control (Appelbaum and Hoge 1986, 1988; Marder et al. 1983, 1984; Van Putten et al. 1974, 1976).

The therapist's approach to the noncompliant chronically mentally ill patient must begin with this realistic expectation: gaining patient cooperation is a long-term process. Although it is common to assume that with healthier patients it may take years of psychotherapy to change repetitive patterns of behavior, therapists often get frustrated with severely mentally ill patients who don't immediately give up their denial and their unrealistic ideas about their own illnesses. But why should severely ill patients be expected to change more rapidly than those who are less ill, or behave in a more reasonable manner than the general population?

Perhaps the temptation to be impatient grows out of the severity and urgency of a patient's problem, the seeming unreasonableness of refusing help for symptoms that are so clearly incapacitating or even dangerous, and the time pressures of brief hospitalization. In spite of these facts, the therapist's impatience is not a helpful contribution. The therapist needs to view noncompliance as a problem that, over a period of months or years, is amenable to change. Brief hospitalization is one of the many events in the course of a patient's illness that affords an opportunity to shift the patient's view.

When 28-year-old Mark P. insisted on his being released from the hospital, his psychiatrist took him to court to retain him against his will. Despite 10 years of recurrent psychotic episodes and multiple hospital-izations caused by his refusal to accept outpatient treatment, Mr. P. insisted that there was nothing wrong with him. At the court hearing, the psychiatrist described Mr. P.'s problems in a manner that was con-siderably more detailed and explicit than any Mr. P. had heard before, including a description of his symptoms, his diagnosis, and the course of his illness. The judge granted the order of retention and told Mr. P. that continuing treatment when he left the hospital would be in his best interest.

On return to the hospital, Mr. P. declared for the first time that he was willing to go to a clinic and take medication after discharge. He announced to a group of staff members, "If I knew you felt that way about me, I would have done it sooner." Mr. P. had heard himself discussed in an austere courtroom setting in a tone that was consider-ably more blunt than a tactful clinician would normally use with a patient. For Mr. P., this experience was a turning point in his ability to accept his illness, and in fact he did follow through with aftercare for the first time.

It is important to maintain hope that even chronically resistant patients will eventually be able to accept some responsibility for managing their illnesses.

Compliance with medication is often the issue over which the greatest struggles occur. It is important for the therapist to listen to what the patient has to say about the medicine, to ensure that he or she under-stands the recommended regimen, and to take seriously any complaints about side effects. Informed patients are better equipped to identify medication problems and find solutions to them rather than discontinue medication.

Some therapists feel reluctant to mention all the various problems that medications can cause, out of concern that patients may perceive them as more harmful than helpful. This is an error for several reasons. First, patients are entitled to be fully informed about the effects of medications prescribed for them, including the possibility of tardive dyskinesia if they are on antipsychotic medications. Such information usually does not lead to drug refusal (Munetz and Roth 1985), and even acutely psychotic patients can understand and benefit from it. Second, the therapist is trying to persuade the patient that medications, despite their risks and the discomfort they cause, are justified by the gravity of the illness. Any other position on the part of the therapist is a form of participation in the patient's denial of the problem. Third, withholding information may undermine trust in the therapist, which can be especially problematic for the paranoid patient.

Patient-Therapist Conflicts

It is helpful to be prepared for the conflicts that often occur between staff and patients with severe mental illness. The most common is the adversarial position between a therapist and a patient who is involuntarily hospitalized or medicated, or who feels pressured into accepting a treatment. Other conflicts may include the pressure staff feel to return a patient to his or her family when the family objects; reporting a patient for suspected child abuse; management of forensic problems, such as threats to others or a crime the patient committed; or differences of opinion over financial matters, such as whether the patient will accept a conservator, should apply for disability, or is willing to spend existing savings to become eligible for a critical government benefit.

These conflicts are painful, awkward, and unavoidable. They should not be viewed as incompatible with preserving the therapeutic alliance. The therapist should help the patient face the painful consequences of his or her illness while balancing encouragement of the patient's autonomy on the one hand and preservation of the patient's health and the public's safety on the other.

COMORBIDITY

The presence of more than one problem among severely mentally ill people is the rule and not the exception. Comorbidity among such patients may refer to the occurrence of more than one Axis I diagnosis, to the presence of a personality disorder on Axis II, to a serious concurrent medical illness, or to the presence of mental retardation or neurological impairment. Even certain social problems, such as homelessness, can reasonably be viewed as a form of comorbidity. The most frequently discussed form of comorbidity in this population is the presence of a psychotic illness and a psychoactive substance abuse disorder. Nonetheless, all forms of comorbidity are common and often lead to confusion about etiology, diagnosis, and effective treatment.

In addition to the standard treatment of the psychotic disorder, specialized techniques for the concurrent problem are usually necessary. For example, a schizophrenic patient with mental retardation may get considerable benefit from behavioral therapy and cognitive training, whereas a manic-depressive patient with borderline personality disorder will be more likely to require confrontational and limit-setting techniques. It is beyond the scope of this chapter to discuss all the possible forms of comorbidity seen in this population, but many of the issues described in the following discussion on comorbid substance abuse apply to other forms of comorbidity.

Comorbid Substance Abuse

A number of studies have shown high rates of comorbidity between substance abuse and other mental disorders. In a comprehensive investigation of community and institutional settings, the Epidemiologic Catchment Area Study (ECA) found that approximately 22% of people surveyed in mental hospitals had a lifetime diagnosis of drug abuse or dependence (Anthony 1991).

Comorbid substance abuse is common among people with severe mental illness, and it complicates diagnosis and management. Surveys of various settings have given clinicians some idea of the scope of the problem. The ECA study found a strong association between schizophrenia and drug or alcohol abuse/dependence (Anthony 1991). Of 15,078 psychiatric inpatients surveyed by the New York State Office of Mental Health (1988), clinicians recorded a 20.5% rate of alcohol or drug abuse in the 30-day period prior to the survey (Way and McCormick 1990). Other studies of psychiatric inpatients have recorded rates of 25% to 50% of comorbid substance abuse (Caton et al. 1989; Sheets et al. 1982).

The issue of comorbidity is complicated by the fact that substance abuse may by itself cause symptoms of psychosis and affective disturbance. However, among chronically mentally ill patients, it is common to see symptoms whose time course, severity, and persistence suggest that two diagnoses are in fact present.

Psychiatric inpatients with substance abuse disorders are more difficult to manage than those without this diagnosis. They tend to be more unkempt, disruptive, uncooperative, suicidal, and homicidal than psychiatric patients without substance abuse disorders (Drake and Wallach 1989; Kay et al. 1989).

The therapist must be aware of possible relationships between substance abuse problems and chronic mental illness. For example, schizophrenic patients, who tend as a group to use amphetamines, cocaine, cannabis, hallucinogens, inhalants, caffeine, and tobacco at rates greater than or equal to control groups consisting of other psychiatric patients or subjects without psychiatric illness (Scheier and Siris 1987), may be doing so to counteract neuroleptic side effects or to self-medicate unpleasant symptoms.

There is uncertainty about the degree to which approaches now used for treating primary substance abuse need to be modified for treatment of chronically mentally ill patients. Mental health professionals have expressed concern that established substance abuse approaches, such as that of Alcoholics Anonymous (AA), depend on a high level of motivation to maintain abstinence, require the ability to tolerate confrontation, express bias against the use of psychotropic medication, and require good interpersonal skills. By contrast, the chronically mentally ill patient may not be prepared to accept abstinence or tolerate confrontation. He or she is likely to require psychotropic medication and may fit poorly into existing groups created for people without chronic mental disease. Of course, these generalizations may not apply to any particular patient or program.

A number of authors have suggested using an integrated treatment approach for comorbid substance abuse that emphasizes engagement, detoxification, education, and relapse prevention (Brown et al. 1989). Minkoff (1989) views patients as having two primary chronic biologically based mental illnesses that require concomitant treatment. He proposes integrating the 12-step model of AA with the biopsychosocial and rehabilitation models for chronic mental illness. Osher and Kofoed (1989) have proposed introducing the initial elements of substance abuse treatment while the patient is still in the psychiatric hospital.

Nonetheless, the literature remains scanty. Debate continues over whether to integrate mental health and substance abuse approaches and if so, how, or whether the two disorders should be treated concurrently in separate systems. In 1987, the National Institute of Mental Health (NIMH) Community Support Program funded 13 demonstration programs for patients with both mental illness and substance abuse problems (Drake et al. 1991). These programs test a variety of ways to combine treatment of these two disorders. Eventually, data will emerge to help clarify which approaches work best for which patients.

In the meantime, brief hospitalization on a general psychiatric inpatient unit can still accomplish the goals outlined in the following subsections.

Diagnostic assessment. History taking and physical assessment should be done with an awareness of substance abuse diagnoses. It is helpful to routinely perform urine toxicology screens on all new admissions. These measures will ordinarily permit the diagnosis of a substance abuse disorder if it is present.

It is also important to establish the relationship between the substance abuse disorder and the chronic psychiatric illness. Some patients use substances only during periods of symptom exacerbation, and once the psychiatric condition is under control, the substance abuse remits. These patients may not need additional treatment.

Detoxification. Detoxification will ordinarily occur in the course of hospitalization and may require medical monitoring or intervention. Enough supervision should be provided to discourage patients from bringing drugs or alcohol onto the ward or arranging for visitors to do so. If this supervision is not provided, length of stay may be prolonged by the patient's continued intoxication.

Confrontation of the substance abuse problem. Confrontation can be used in a supportive and caring way to address the patient's tendency to deny a drug or alcohol problem and minimize its consequences (Fine and Miller, in press). Looked at another way, patient and therapist can work together to confront the patient's denial, contradictions, and pathological defenses. To tacitly ignore an addiction is to encourage its continuation.

Referral. The acute hospitalization can be used as an opportunity to link the patient to an appropriate substance abuse program. This is best done while the patient is still in the hospital and can visit the program prior to discharge. The type of program(s)—inpatient, residential, outpatient, or self-help—will depend on the nature of the patient's problem and the local resources available.

In addition to these individual goals with patients, it is sometimes possible to arrange for groups like AA and Narcotics Anonymous to run meetings inside the hospital. If funds are available, more specialized substance abuse counseling and group programming can be provided.

As with other forms of therapy with this population, it is important for the clinician to be realistic without becoming discouraged. It may take several tries before a patient can accept help for an alcohol or drug problem. Although abstinence is a desirable goal, staff need not demand that the patient achieve it. There is a range of outcomes seen in the treatment of all substance abuse patients, and the degree of abstinence is proportional to the degree of recovery that is accomplished.

Discharge

In the model we have described, discharge planning begins the first day of admission. However, there are some specific tasks as the day of discharge approaches. Most important is to prepare the patient to leave the hospital unit by encouraging passes that are used to clarify the patient's ability to function adequately without the structure of the hospital, and to increase the patient's contact with family and outpatient staff (Leibenluft and Goldberg 1987). These passes are essential, because they test the discharge plan and allow for modifications to make it more realistic. This avoids discharging patients prematurely only to have them quickly return. Manic patients in particular reach a point where they begin to look euthymic in the hospital but become rapidly disorganized or excited when sent out on pass. Only when the manic patient can return from a pass without reporting significant problems does discharge become clinically realistic.

Predischarge visits to the aftercare program improve patient compliance. Techniques for preventing relapse should be reviewed at this time and are similar to those described for other recurrent mental disorders (see Chapter 8).

Satisfactions

In spite of the difficulties, there are many rewards to working with chronically mentally ill patients. Many of these patients show great courage in the face of severe disease and considerable gratitude for the help they receive. Even when symptomatic improvement is limited, it is usually possible to improve the quality of life of both the patient and his or her family. Managing these illnesses requires several simultaneous interventions and allows all members of the treatment team to contribute something important. Even when patients return to the hospital with a relapse, staff often take satisfaction in knowing the patients well and knowing what kinds of treatment have been proven to work. There is immense challenge and satisfaction in treating patients with some of the most severe and complex diseases known to medicine.

REFERENCES

Anthony JC, Helzer JE: Syndromes of drug abuse and dependence, in Psychiatric Disorders in America. Edited by Robins LN, Regier DA. New York, Free Press, 1991, pp 116–154

Appelbaum PS: The right to refuse treatment with antipsychotic medications: retrospect and prospect. Am J Psychiatry 44:413–419, 1988

Appelbaum PS, Hoge SK: The right to refuse treatment: what the research reveals. Behavioral Science and Law 4:279–292, 1986

Brown VB, Ridgely MS, Pepper B, et al: The dual crisis: mental illness and substance abuse. Am Psychol 44:565–569, 1989

Caton C, Gralnick A, Bender S, et al: Young chronic patients and substance abuse. Hosp Community Psychiatry 40:1037–1040, 1989

Conrad P: The meaning of medications: another look at compliance. Soc Sci Med 20:29–37, 1985

Cournos F: The impact of environmental factors on outcome in residential programs. Hosp Community Psychiatry 38:848–852, 1987

Dohrenwend BS, Dohrenwend BP, Link B, et al: Social functioning of psychotic patients in contrast with community cases in the general population. Arch Gen Psychiatry 40:1174–1182, 1983

Drake RE, Sederer LI: Inpatient psychosocial treatment of chronic schizophrenia: negative effects and current guidelines. Hosp Community Psychiatry 37:897–901, 1986

Drake RE, Wallach MA: Substance abuse among the chronically mentally ill. Hosp Community Psychiatry 40:1041–1046, 1989

Drake RE, McLaughlin P, Pepper B, et al: Dual diagnoses of major mental illness and substance disorder: an overview, in Dual Diagnosis of Major Mental Illness and Substance Disorder. Edited by Minkoff K, Drake RE. San Francisco, CA, Jossey-Bass, 1991, pp 3–12

Fine J, Miller NS: Evaluation and acute management of psychotic symptomatology in alcohol and drug addiction. Journal of Addictive Diseases (in press)

Gunderson JC, Frank AF, Katz HM, et al: Effects of psychotherapy in schizophrenia, II: comparative outcome of two forms of treatment. Schizophr Bull 10:564–598, 1984

Kay SR, Kalathara M, Meinzer AE: Diagnostic and behavioral characteristics of psychiatric patients who abuse substances. Hosp Community Psychiatry 40:1062–1064, 1989

Kuipers L: Expressed emotion: a review. British Journal of Social and Clinical Psychology 18:237–243, 1979

Leibenluft E, Goldberg RL: Guidelines for short-term inpatient psychotherapy. Hosp Community Psychiatry 38:38–42, 1987

Linn MW, Caffey EM, Klett CJ: Day treatment and psychotropic drugs in the aftercare of schizophrenic patients. Arch Gen Psychiatry 36:1055–1066, 1979

Linn MW, Klett CH, Caffey EM: Foster home characteristics and psychiatric patient outcome. Arch Gen Psychiatry 37:129–132, 1980

Linstrom LH: The effect of long-term treatment with clozapine in schizophrenia: a retrospective study in 96 patients treated with clozapine for up to 13 years. Acta Psychiatr Scand 77:524–529, 1988

Marder SR, Mebane A, Chien CP, et al: A comparison of patients who refuse and consent to neuroleptic treatment. Am J Psychiatry 140:470–473, 1983

Marder SR, Swann E, Winslade WJ, et al: A study of medication refusal by involuntary psychiatric patients. Hosp Community Psychiatry 35:724–726, 1984

Meissner WW: The Paranoid Process. New York, Jason Aronson, 1978

Minkoff K: An integrated treatment model for dual diagnosis of psychosis and addiction. Hosp Community Psychiatry 40:1031–1036, 1989

Mosher RL, Keith SJ: Research on the psychosocial treatment of schizophrenia: a summary report. Am J Psychiatry 136:623–631, 1979

Munetz MR, Roth LH: Informing patients about tardive dyskinesia. Arch Gen Psychiatry 42:866–871, 1985

New York State Office of Mental Health: Report, Bureau of Statistical Analysis, Office of Planning and Program Evaluation. Albany, NY, New York State Office of Mental Health, 1985

Osher FC, Kofoed LL: Treatment of patients with psychiatric and psychoactive substance abuse disorders. Hosp Community Psychiatry 40:1025–1030, 1989

Sarti P, Cournos F: Medication and psychotherapy in the treatment of chronic schizophrenia. Psychiatr Clin North Am 13:215–228, 1990

Scheier FR, Siris SG: A review of psychoactive substance use and abuse in schizophrenia: patterns of drug choice. J Nerv Ment Dis 175:641–652, 1987

Sheets JL, Prevost JA, Reihman J: Young adult chronic patients: three hypothesized subgroups. Hosp Community Psychiatry 33:197–203, 1982

Stanton AH, Gunderson JG, Knapp PH, et al: Effects of psychotherapy in schizophrenia, I: design and implementation of a controlled study. Schizophr Bull 10:520–563, 1984

Van Putten T: Why do schizophrenic patients refuse to take their drugs? Arch Gen Psychiatry 31:67–72, 1974

Van Putten T, Crumpton E, Yale C: Drug refusal in schizophrenia and the wish to be crazy. Arch Gen Psychiatry 33:1443–1446, 1976

Way BB, McCormick LL: The mentally ill chemical-abusing population: a review of the literature. Albany, NY, Bureau of Evaluation and Services Research, New York State Office of Mental Health, June 1990

Wing JK: The social context of schizophrenia. Am J Psychiatry 135:1333–1339, 1978

Zahniser JH, Coursey RD, Hershberger K: Individual psychotherapy with schizophrenic outpatients in the public mental health system. Hosp Community Psychiatry 42:906–913, 1991

Zisook S, Gammon E: Medical noncompliance. Int J Psychiatry Med 10:291–303, 1981

CHAPTER 8

Inpatient Psychotherapy With Alcoholic Patients

Lisa Borg, M.D.
Richard J. Frances, M.D.

INTRODUCTION

It is estimated that approximately 29% of men and 4% of women will have a lifetime incidence of alcoholism (Helzer and Pryzbeck 1988). In the general population, people who abuse alcohol have a comorbidity rate of 37% for additional mental illness. Conversely, 29% of psychiatric patients have had a problem with substance abuse (Regier et al. 1990). In this chapter, we cover the special psychotherapeutic issues involved in treating alcoholic patients on general psychiatric units. First, the initial phase of inpatient treatment of these patients is described. This discussion includes indications for hospitalization and techniques for facilitating the admission, establishing a therapeutic alliance and treatment contract, setting goals, and establishing a treatment plan. This section is followed by a discussion on modifying standard individual psychotherapy approaches for the alcoholic inpatient and also on integrating the individual work with other modalities. The management issues raised by comorbidity of other psychiatric disorders are covered next; finally, prognostic factors are explored.

THE INITIAL PHASE OF TREATMENT

Indications for Hospitalization and Interventions to Facilitate Admission

A variety of circumstances necessitate inpatient treatment of the alcoholic patient. These include history of medical problems (e.g., complicated alcohol withdrawal), current serious medical conditions (e.g., hypertension or diabetes), acute suicidality or psychosis, outpatient treatment failure, lack of social supports, and polysubstance addiction (Frances and Franklin 1989). The inpatient unit provides a safe, controlled environment for patients who need close monitoring. Many of these patients enter inpatient treatment very unwillingly—not with a primary interest in abstinence, but because of pressures exerted by their employers, their families, the courts, or their physicians. Patients can present as quite uncooperative, with denial of both the seriousness and the consequences of the illness and a consequent denial of the need for help and treatment. The initial resistance to hospital treatment must be addressed from the outset as a critical factor in the development of a therapeutic relationship.

The hospital psychotherapist should begin with a detailed exploration of the patient's life history in relation to the areas in which alcohol has caused problems. The therapist can help the patient begin to see the more direct consequences of the alcoholism. For example, the patient may not realize how he or she has been using alcohol to change mood and may not recognize the full effects of the drinking on work performance. This focused approach guides the patient gradually and inevitably to the diagnosis of alcoholism (Frances et al. 1989). Corroboration from significant others including family members, employers, probation officers, friends, and referring physicians will help the clinician confront the patient's denial. Collateral evidence such as abnormal physical findings and laboratory tests, including toxicology results, can also be very powerful in getting the patient to begin to admit to the severity of his or her problem and the need for help. Questionnaires and screening devices such as CAGE (Ewing 1984) and the Michigan Alcoholism Screening Test (MAST [Selzer 1971]) may be useful adjuncts that help the patient to accept the diagnosis.

If a patient is particularly intransigent, the clinician might want to arrange an intervention. This is a meeting conducted by the clinician where the family, employer, probation officer, and others confront the patient about his or her alcoholism. An intervention may be used to initiate hospitalization or when the crises in the patient's life need to be underlined during hospitalization to aid in compliance. For example, a patient may resist the recommendation to continue treatment in a long-term residential setting after completion of the acute inpatient stay. The key people in the patient's life can come in to support the clinician's recommendation and to describe to the patient how failure to comply will affect relationships with them. This may include the patient's spouse refusing to let the patient come home and perhaps even obtaining a court order of protection, or the employer reporting the patient to a disciplinary board at work.

Discharge planning should begin on admission to the hospital and requires thorough assessment of finances and benefits, social supports, and the availability of aftercare. Careful initial evaluation for comorbid psychiatric disorders and suicide potential is essential, in consultation with the team psychiatrist. The clinician must decide whether to admit the patient to a general psychiatric unit or (if available) to a specialized alcohol rehabilitation unit. Alcoholic patients with severe psychiatric problems such as psychosis or major depression are usually better handled initially on a general psychiatric unit. A necessary consideration in this decision is the nature of the patient's current and lifetime insurance coverage for one type of unit versus the other. When the psychiatric symptoms are under control, the patient can be transferred to a specialized chemical dependency unit with continued psychiatric monitoring.

Some institutions do not have separate facilities for treating substance abuse patients. Treating the alcoholic patient on the general psychiatric unit requires a staff that is informed and trained to treat the disease. A separate team and program can be set up on the unit to deal with the special problems of alcoholic patients. This includes focused groups, psychoeducation lectures, 12-step program participation, and social work services tailored to the treatment and discharge planning needs of alcoholic patients. Given the high prevalence of alcoholism in the general psychiatric inpatient population, a program like this helps meet the needs of many patients.

Establishing a Therapeutic
Alliance and Treatment Contract

With shortening lengths of stay, psychiatric hospitalization has become a period of extended evaluation. This is particularly true for the alcoholic patient. The inpatient stay affords an opportunity to carefully assess the patient and to begin to develop an alliance while protecting the patient in a controlled environment. The therapist must realize that his or her primary function is to lay the groundwork and set up the structure for the patient's ongoing recovery program. At this stage, the patient requires extensive assessment, support, therapeutic intervention, and discharge planning. The patient needs to be educated about the disease model of alcoholism and engaged in Alcoholics Anonymous (AA).

After a comprehensive evaluation, the clinician formulates a treatment plan with a broad-based biopsychosocial perspective (Frances and Franklin 1989). The therapist should approach the patient with a high level of activity and concern. The approach should include medical and psychiatric knowledge of alcoholism, informed optimism, and a capacity for both persistence and patience. These therapist attributes aid in the formation of a treatment alliance that will help the patient begin to accept and attack the problem of his or her alcoholism (Frances 1988). The therapist attempts to work through the patient's initial resistances to treatment so as to establish a treatment alliance and develop a therapeutic contract. The therapeutic contract is the part of the treatment plan that refers to the patient's relationship with the primary therapist and is the agreement between patient and therapist as to the boundaries and expectations of the relationship.

The treatment alliance is best forged with an acknowledgment of both the patient's suffering and his or her need for help. The patient should be supported and also empathically confronted. Implicit in this approach is the notion that the clinician will help the alcoholic patient to come to terms with his or her unhappiness and to do something about it. For example, a patient may be focused on the disintegration of his marriage and his relationship with his wife. The pain of this loss must be addressed, and sobriety discussed with the patient as a fundamental aspect of his recovery from this loss. The patient may begin to feel that the psychotherapist is someone to respect and trust, and the therapy helps to provide the patient with an all-important sense of hope (Frances and Allen 1986).

The therapeutic contract should be explicit. The clinician will need to remind the patient many times of its existence and its terms. It must exist because the newly admitted alcoholic patient requires explicit parameters for abstinence, honesty, self-care, and program attendance. The therapist should explain to the patient what the patient's problems are, what needs to be done about them, and how the therapist can help. The alcoholic patient frequently responds to this discussion with resistance if not anger. The clinician should listen to the patient's objections, be willing to discuss them within reason, and stand firm but not fixed. The explicit contract thus provides a framework within which the alcoholic patient can begin to recover.

A number of basic conditions must be addressed in this contract. First, the patient must accept the necessity for abstinence. This may seem self-evident; yet even hospitalized alcoholic patients do not always accept this premise and may be able to illicitly obtain substances within the hospital. The patient often does not view him- or herself as someone who cannot drink. He or she may appear to agree to the need for abstinence in an effort to comply with the expectations of staff and loved ones, yet in fact may be unable to grasp the concept of life without alcohol. It is essential that the clinician ask the patient direct questions about sobriety. Many alcoholic individuals have trouble understanding or even thinking about whether they really can or want to be sober and what this would mean to them. Raising these questions opens up a meaningful discussion.

Another critical aspect of the therapeutic contract is the issue of honesty. By the time they enter the hospital, most alcoholic patients have developed a complex system of rationalizations and cover-ups for their behavior and predicament. By balancing confrontation and support, the clinician helps the alcoholic patient to recognize these rationalizations and begin to open up. Honesty is fundamental to all of the relationships of the recovering alcoholic patient, including those with the therapist, the rest of the staff, the other patients, and the support system at home. The therapist can help the patient to see that this process of covering up is part of the disease. Confidentiality is another key issue that must be discussed with the patient at the very beginning. The alcoholic patient is understandably fearful that "leaked" information could further damage relationships and exacerbate or even create legal problems. The clinician must raise the issue and talk with the patient about the boundaries and limits of confidentiality. Specifically, the patient should be told that information will be shared among staff members, but he or she must also be reassured that disclosure of information outside the hospital (e.g., to family or employer) will only be with the patient's permission.

The psychotherapist can also explain to the patient that the treatment approach is one of working together on self-care and the reduction of self-harm. Because many alcoholic patients have grown up in chaotic or otherwise difficult families and have continued to perpetuate dysfunctional relationships, the notion of a nonexploitative relationship based on cooperation and trust may be both bewildering and uplifting. Finally, the psychotherapist should explicitly address the issues of both suicidality and violence and explain to the patient how these risks will be handled should they arise.

Setting Goals and Establishing a Treatment Plan

Having developed a therapeutic contract, the patient and the psychotherapist must set goals and establish a treatment plan. Because the alcoholic person who requires psychiatric hospitalization usually presents with an array of difficulties, this plan should be worked out with the treatment team. The psychotherapist works with the treatment team to sort through the confusion and decide which problems can be handled in a simple and direct way, and which ones of greater depth and complexity demand more complicated solutions. Ideally, in addition to individual psychotherapy, the plan should include ongoing medical assessment and treatment, as needed; consideration of pharmacotherapy including disulfiram (Antabuse), antidepressants, and other agents for additional psychiatric disorders; group and family psychotherapy; AA meetings; and individual and family education about alcoholism. Additional important areas include nutritional assessment and counseling, use of Breathalyzer tests and urine drug screens, and recreational, vocational, and social assessment and guidance. A good treatment plan will mesh the skills and approaches of the various disciplines and modalities. The treatment plan is usually worked out and updated in a once- or twice-weekly team meeting.

The specific combination of psychotherapies should be tailored to the patient's needs and the resources of the unit. Most patients do best with a mix of individual, group, and family therapy. The individual therapy develops the therapeutic alliance and in many cases is the pivotal aspect of the hospitalization. The group therapy provides peer support and confrontation and is particularly helpful (as described below) for patients who have problems with authority. Family therapy places the patient's illness in a social context and begins to expose the underlying family psychodynamics. AA provides education, structure, and a strong link to the discharge plan. The patient may have a refused a number of these modalities in prior treatments. The therapist may therefore need to push the patient to try a combined approach in the hospital.

> A self-punitive alcoholic schoolteacher with recurrent depression developed severe difficulties getting along with the school principal and became acutely suicidal. The focused goals of a hospital-based treatment included abstinence from alcohol and compliance with tricyclic antidepressants. The targeted psychotherapeutic approach was cognitive-behavioral and included providing assertiveness training, decreasing dependency and self-blame, learning new coping and social skill techniques to deal with the school situation, and changing school jobs.
>
> At the same time, the psychotherapist addressed the psychodynamic conflicts underpinning the patient's masochism. This involved a harsh, perfectionistic view of herself that was frequently projected onto parental figures. Although these dynamics would only be resolved with long-term work, the inpatient therapist could engage the patient's interest in collaborating to better understand herself and to focus on self-esteem and self-care. Some of her denial regarding major life issues initially was left untouched; however, denial about alcoholism was challenged early on, so that the patient began to constructively wonder about her motivations without overwhelming anxiety.

INDIVIDUAL PSYCHOTHERAPY

General Considerations

As we have described, inpatient treatment of the alcoholic patient on the acute unit is primarily directed toward evaluation and treatment planning. However, at the same time, the therapist needs to begin to engage and prepare the patient for psychotherapy.

The best rule of thumb for psychotherapy with alcoholic patients is for the therapist to work with the patient wherever he or she is at that moment. Otherwise, there is the risk of losing the patient to treatment altogether because of overwhelming unexplored resistances.

> An alcoholic male patient in need of a kidney transplant from his father had difficulty accepting help from his male therapist, who clearly represented his father. A major problem had been getting him to admit to his alcoholism and accept his strong dependence on substances to deal with problems. Interpretation of the transference both helped him to open up in treatment and ultimately helped him to accept his father as a kidney donor.

Time-limited psychodynamic therapy theories such as those that focus on specific conflicts (Malan 1980), Oedipal issues (Sifneos 1972), or separation and loss (Mann 1973) can be modified for this population. The proper focus and approach will come from a careful evaluation of the patient's specific conflicts and needs. Cognitive and behavioral approaches as described by Marlatt and Gordon (1985) and Beck and colleagues (1990) can be applied to a brief focal therapy. As we explain below, the therapist may need to interweave a cognitive-behavioral approach with a psychodynamic understanding. He or she should first focus on the addiction, but gradually expand to other issues. Addressing the alcoholism should be the first priority. In a case such as the schoolteacher described previously, the patient's alcoholism and acute stressors require a pragmatic, behavioral treatment in which the therapist is very directive and structuring. Early childhood issues and resultant personality problems are then approached with a focused psychodynamic model.

Psychodynamic Psychotherapy

The attempt to engage the newly sober alcoholic patient in psychodynamic psychotherapy can be daunting for the clinician. At this stage, the alcoholic patient is often quite unreceptive to the concept of internal, intrapsychic problems that require self-scrutiny and internal change.

Using a strict model, such patients have often been excluded from this type of therapy because of their impulsivity and difficulty tolerating anxiety and other painful affects. When stressed by an insight-oriented approach, they may become dependent, regressed, and passive and employ primitive defenses (Frances et al. 1989). However, some of the principles of brief psychodynamic therapies can still be usefully applied to the newly sober hospitalized alcoholic patient. For example, in the approach described by Malan (1978), the therapist keeps the therapy focused and moving, often making transference interpretations based on past as well as present relationships. The approach can be used with patients who have fairly significant psychopathology if the conflict is highly focused or the motivation reasonably high. In the case example of the schoolteacher, the therapist begins to address the patient's underlying core conflicts while the patient is in the hospital; however, the primary focus remains the patient's alcoholism. Sifneos (1979) confronts the patient's defenses around the Oedipal conflict. Though it is not appropriate for the majority of inpatients who are alcoholic, this approach may be applied to some primarily with Oedipal conflicts.

> An alcoholic physician had succeeded far beyond his pharmacist father's dreams. He felt guilty about surpassing his father in his career and would exhibit his drinking in ways that were self-destructive. This behavior led to his dismissal from a major hospital post. Understanding his need to fail helped him in preventing relapses.

Mann (1973) concentrates on the issues of separation and loss. He identifies and presents the "central issue" to the patient as a statement that captures and reflects back to the patient his or her painful inner experience. The treatment focus here is on the time limit of hospitalization and the need to deal with a variety of losses both past and present including the loss of alcohol. Khantzian and colleagues (1990) emphasized self-care, self-esteem, affect regulation, and exploration of dependency and interpersonal problems as central to the psychotherapy of the addicted patient.

Alcoholic patients often view the therapist in distorted ways. On the one hand, the therapist may be perceived as a cold, judgmental, punitive figure who will ridicule and reject them. At the same time, they may feel overwhelmed and dependent on the therapist, which is frightening and confusing. These patients also often idealize the therapist in their tremendous desire to be taken care of, and then feel crushed when their irrational expectations are inevitably disappointed. Past and present transferential relationships are relevant, and transference must be addressed insofar as it interferes with the treatment. However, it is not the central issue. The therapist must be careful not to be distracted by the patient from the primary problem (Malan 1980).

The treatment plan includes a schedule for individual psychotherapy. A likely arrangement is two or three 45-minute sessions per week. In the sessions, the therapist keeps bringing the patient back to discussing the alcoholism and its consequences. For example, if the patient complains about unit policies or worries about his or her children, the therapist at first can listen and explore the overt issue. The therapist then empathically reminds the patient that the unit is quite restrictive in some ways, because this is particularly necessary for the newly sober alcoholic individual as part of the recovery from out-of-control drinking. At the same time, the therapist can agree that although it is worrisome that the patient's children are having some difficulties, the fact remains that some if not most of the problems are tied to the patient's inability to function as a parent when drinking.

Those patients who have never developed mature ego function need habilitation to reach a more healthy state. Efforts to split staff can be interpreted in the context of patients' previous patterns of getting everyone to fight over them. For patients who have regressed in function, rehabilitation provides an environment to rediscover and practice relatedness. As ego function improves, there is improvement in impulse control, judgment, and reality testing along with the adaptive use of defenses such as reaction formation, intellectualization, and sublimation.

From the beginning of treatment, the psychotherapist helps the patient prepare for discharge from the safety of the hospital. Given the current short length of stay for most inpatient hospitalizations, one of the challenges to the psychotherapist is to engage the patient in the treatment process adequately enough to carry him or her into outpatient treatment without promoting excessive attachment to the therapist and the hospital (Leibenluft and Goldberg 1987). From the outset of the admission, the therapist should focus on discharge planning—the patient and the family need to always keep in mind that the patient is expected to get better and leave the hospital. While in the hospital, the patient should attend AA and outpatient clinic and therapy appointments, which will aid in the transition to discharge.

The patient must deal with a variety of conflicts around loss and separation. By the time of discharge, he or she is expected to leave the relative safety of the inpatient unit and be ready to relinquish an addiction to a substance that is like a best friend. Typically, the patient regresses close to discharge and becomes hostile and dependent. The therapist points out this behavior to the patient and explores the underlying concerns about separation. The therapist also uses a supportive approach to help anchor the patient in reality, pointing out the resources and options available to the patient after discharge, and emphasizing the patient's strengths and abilities.

Unfortunately, alcoholic individuals often receive less psychotherapy as inpatients than other types of patients (McCarrick et al. 1988) even though patients with substance abuse problems have been shown to derive substantial benefit from psychotherapy, particularly if there are coexistent psychiatric problems (Woody et al. 1984).

Cognitive-Behavioral Treatment

The specific objectives of the cognitive-behavioral aspect of the treatment are to reduce negative views of the self and the future and to help the patient anticipate and prepare for "people, places, and things" that may produce relapse. The psychotherapist should help the patient to openly discuss fears about the future and his or her ability to handle stressful situations. Some patients who have been active in AA may have difficulty expressing their fears because that may be considered a form of unacceptable self-pity.

Marlatt and Gordon (1985) and others have written extensively about "relapse prevention." Using this approach, the therapist helps the patient identify problem areas that are likely to lead to drinking, and then to develop new coping skills to avert the slip. For example, a patient may be able to pinpoint problems that produce the urge to drink, such as loneliness, an argument with a friend, work pressure, or sexual inhibition. The patient is encouraged to think of the recovery process and the development of coping skills as a type of journey—a gradual process of learning new strategies to deal with urges and craving, anticipate pitfalls, and recognize early warning signals of relapse. The psychotherapist helps the patient to make changes in life-style and habits. Perhaps most importantly, the therapist teaches the patient to think not so much in terms of absolute sobriety versus total failure, but instead in terms of learning from experience and "studying" setbacks as a means of increasing self-confidence and self-efficacy. The patient's role as "coinvestigator" and objective observer helps to build self-esteem and lessens the sense of humiliation and the tendency to develop power struggles.

From a psychodynamic perspective, a cognitive-behavioral relapse prevention approach helps the patient to use more highly developed ego functions, which then leads to a sense of competence and independence. Instead of rationalizing, denying, and avoiding, the patient begins to take pleasure in self-mastery and personal responsibility. The major limitation of the relapse prevention approach is that it requires a fairly motivated, engagable patient. Other cognitive-behavioral–based approaches such as assertiveness training (Hirsch et al. 1978), social skills training (Intagliata 1978), and contracting can also be used with the alcoholic patient. These can be incorporated into the psychodynamic conceptualization and approach to the patient. For example, the schoolteacher described previously could be taught concrete ways of dealing with her difficult colleagues and negotiating job interviews.

OTHER MODALITIES

Milieu

The staff working with alcoholic patients needs to be able to tolerate pain and anxiety in both themselves and others. These patients benefit from an inpatient unit where the tone is one of warmth and caring, with clear structure and low expressed emotion. There should be a high level of both patient-staff and staff-staff interaction and a nurturing, family feeling on the unit. The unit approach should be to reward health, not sickness. The unit leadership should recognize the various points of view of the staff and invite open discussion but ultimately maintain a medical, hierarchical structure. In general, when things go wrong (e.g., a patient elopes, alcohol is found on the unit, or a suicide occurs), the event should be discussed and processed, and the stabilizing rules and traditions of the unit should be upheld.

On the general psychiatric unit, addicted patients can be quite disruptive—refusing to adhere to ward routine, expecting special treatment, and requiring large amounts of staff time. The psychotherapist (and treatment team) may begin to feel helpless, inadequate, unappreciated, and angry. The staff's sense of alienation from the patient may be heightened by a commonly held prejudice: the alcoholic patient is wreaking havoc because of his or her inherent "badness" and deserves punishment, not compassion. Some staff may feel that the alcoholic patient needs to suffer and atone in order to become abstinent (Musto 1989). Some staff members may have difficulty with a psychotherapeutic, nonpunitive approach to dealing with alcoholic people. These beliefs may supersede health care training and can be very damaging to the patient.

Staff members need to be educated about alcoholism and the disease model. At the same time, the psychotherapist has to recognize and empathize with the staff's frustration and anger toward alcoholic patients so that they in turn are able to work empathically with them. As described by Kernberg (1976) in the treatment of borderline personality disorders, the staff needs to be alert to the problem of splitting. Some members of the team may be devalued and others idealized; some patients may idealize the staff members who are in recovery or those who are medically trained. The team needs to work closely together to avoid fragmentation of the treatment plan.

Family/Couples Treatment

Inpatient family therapy is an important adjunct to individual psychotherapy and may be carried out by the patient's individual psychotherapist or another clinician.

The patient's drinking may be one aspect of a dysfunctional family system that requires treatment for the patient to begin to change. For example, the husband of an alcoholic woman may be uneasy at the prospect of a healthier, independent, and in some ways more demanding spouse. He may be unhappy with their present relationship but afraid of the possible upheaval that may occur with her recovery. In other instances, the patient may initially appear very resistant to treatment and the family may be very eager to work. This imbalance often shifts back and forth during the course of the treatment (Heath and Stanton 1991). Family members may be substance abusers or have other impulse control disorders that can sabotage the patient's recovery and thus require concurrent treatment. Overall, however, most families are quite eager to see their alcoholic family members recover.

The psychotherapist (or another staff member who functions as the family therapist) may elect to see patient and family separately or in some combination. For example, if the patient is driving a wedge between his or her parents, the psychotherapist may decide to see them several times without the patient. If the family is using the patient as a scapegoat for family conflicts, the psychotherapist may choose to keep the patient's treatment more separate from the family. Multiple family groups can be very helpful in breaking up entrenched family patterns.

Inclusion of the employer in family sessions can be very effective. Sometimes an alcoholic patient rationalizes difficulties with spouse or children, blaming their erratic behavior and avoiding responsibility. When the employer confronts the patient with the concrete reality of his or her absenteeism and poor performance at work, the patient may have a much harder time defending a position as the victim of unreasonable people. For some patients, the potential loss of a job is more threatening to self-esteem and a sense of security than the threatened or real loss of family.

Just as the patient needs to continue in treatment to prevent relapse after discharge, so must the family in most instances. This can be in the form of family, individual, and self-help group therapy such as Al-Anon (Kaufman 1986).

Finally, the therapist needs to recognize situations where the patient or the family do not want conjoint treatment and perhaps should not have it at the present time. This includes situations where the family is unusually toxic (e.g., with physically or sexually abusing parents or spouses) or where the patient is trying to extricate him- or herself from a very constricting, destructive family. The clinician should assess the family's capacity to work constructively in treatment and not automatically assume that working with them closely is best for the patient.

Medication

Much has been written regarding the issue of the use of medication in combination with psychotherapy (Miller et al. 1989). In the treatment of alcoholic patients, the issue is complicated by the fact that patients in recovery usually become involved in a 12-step AA program. Although AA officially supports medical authority, some members are opposed to the use of any medication, including disulfiram, and this stance may contribute to noncompliance. The psychotherapist (or treating psychiatrist) should explain to the patient that medication may be necessary if he or she has a psychiatric illness in addition to the alcoholism. Medication can include the use of methadone maintenance treatment for concurrent heroin addiction. Other substances with addictive properties are avoided except in rare instances (e.g., very selected treatment-resistant patients with anxiety disorders or where pain medication is indicated [Frances and Borg, in press]). Disulfiram can be helpful for patients who are highly motivated yet are having difficulty maintaining sobriety because of severe stressors or intense craving.

Alcoholics Anonymous

Although it is difficult to scientifically study treatment outcome with AA, many patients seem to do best early in recovery if they get involved. It may be that the most motivated patients self-select to participate in this program (Bebbington 1976). An important task of the inpatient therapist is to help the patient work through ambivalent feelings about AA. As we have described, the patient needs to be exposed to a 12-step program as early as possible in the hospital stay. If the patient does not view him- or herself as alcoholic, much of the work will be directed at helping the patient to recognize how much the principles of AA do apply to his or her current situation.

In the 12-step program, Step 1 helps the patient to accept the diagnosis of alcoholism. Step 2 helps the patient to accept his or her dependency needs and the importance of getting help. Other steps involve introspection, assessment of character defects, efforts to make amends, and efforts to help others. This approach requires the therapist to have a working knowledge of the program, which is best obtained by reading about the subject, talking with patients about their experience of the program, and attending at least a few meetings. Having the AA experience early in recovery gives a patient a structure and an identity as a recovering person. Instead of feeling isolated and "bad," patients can be proud to be recovering from alcoholism. Participation in AA gives many patients hope and pride, and promotes self-care, self-regard, and self-regulation.

Group Treatment

Group therapy is an important adjunct to the individual psychotherapy of the alcoholic patient and may be led by the psychotherapist or other members of the treatment team. Groups can help the patients to deal with social relationships, feelings of shame, and resistance to treatment. The patient can also increase self-esteem and improve ego function by helping other members of the group. There are a variety of different group therapy approaches used with alcoholic patients, including interactional, behavioral, insight-oriented, supportive, educational, and interpersonal problem-solving therapies (Galanter et al. 1991).

The modality chosen should be determined by the goals of treatment and should reinforce or complement the individual psychotherapy. For example, problems such as difficulty with self-assertion, priority setting, affect regulation, or divulging of feelings can be discussed in the individual therapy and then further explored in an insight-oriented group. If the patient is hospitalized on a general psychiatric unit, the group leader needs to be particularly attentive to the patient's alcoholism as a primary problem from which many of these other problems may originate. Forming a homogeneous group selecting for patients with dual diagnosis is useful. The leader working with alcoholic patients in the group setting often needs to provide limits and focus (Vanicelli 1982). Again, it is helpful if staff have subspecialty training or experience in the field of alcoholism.

Galanter and colleagues (1991) point out certain aspects of group therapy treatment with alcoholic patients that are particularly relevant. For example, many patients are unable to tolerate anxiety. The group leader needs to be sensitive to this limitation and to modulate the affect and level of confrontation in the group accordingly. The optimal style for the group therapy leader working with alcoholic patients is one of encouraging interpersonal process as well as demonstrating knowledge of alcoholism.

COMORBIDITY

Associations have been demonstrated between alcoholism and certain other psychiatric illnesses. In men, drug use, antisocial personality, and phobic disorder are most prevalent, whereas in women, depression, drug use, phobias, and antisocial personality are found. In both sexes, other diagnoses that are found less frequently but more often than in the general population include panic disorder, somatization, and mania (Helzer and Pryzbeck 1988). Inpatients are particularly likely to have psychiatric comorbidity (Hesselbrock et al. 1985).

In discussing comorbidity, it is probably most useful to distinguish between Axis I and Axis II pathology, because the two types raise very different treatment issues. Patients with Axis I problems require a more supportive approach and often need medication. They may do better on a primary psychiatric unit rather than a rehabilitation unit and can require a longer length of stay because of the complexity of their problems. Patients with Axis II pathology require an empathic yet firm stance. These patients often require strong limit setting and confrontation. At the same time, the staff needs to be alert to countertransference issues and avoid overly punitive reactions to these difficult patients.

The psychiatrist on the treatment team makes sure that the comorbid diagnoses are recognized and addressed. In these cases, the psychiatrist also evaluates whether these other illnesses are primary or secondary to the heavy drinking and how the comorbid disorders interact. This may be difficult to ascertain, but it is essential in determining treatment and prognosis. The psychotherapist must help the patient gain perspective and set priorities in this as in all other areas.

A newly admitted 34-year-old male patient met DSM-III-R (American Psychiatric Association 1987) criteria for alcohol dependence, anxiety disorder with severe panic attacks, and antisocial personality disorder. The therapist educated the patient regarding his alcoholism, helped the patient to recognize the damage it had caused in his life, and guided him in a directive way to try to rectify his problems. This included handling his pending court dates for a DWI (driving while intoxicated) offense, working out a contract with his wife and his employer, and planning a structured aftercare treatment program.

At the same time, the patient received a psychiatric assessment of his panic attacks (which in this case were primary) as well as pharmacotherapy with a (nonaddictive) antidepressant and psychiatric follow-up. He also received cognitive-behavioral treatment for the panic from the psychotherapist. The patient's antisocial tendencies dictated firm limit setting and external controls (e.g., threatened penalties from his wife, his job, and the courts) for him to maintain sobriety. AA helped to provide him with a supportive, nonthreatening peer group.

The patient later threatened to sign out of the hospital against medical advice. Because he was not clearly a danger to himself or others, the therapist was forced to allow him to leave. However, the family was informed of the patient's decision, and it was emphasized both to the patient and to the family that they could return for further treatment in the future.

PROGNOSTIC FACTORS

Outcome studies for the treatment of alcoholism differ in their criteria for success. Some use a unitary model (looking at abstinence alone), whereas others employ a multidimensional approach (looking at a number of areas of function [Babor et al. 1988]). Some of the factors that appear to influence prognosis include the presence of additional psychiatric illness, severity of antisocial tendencies (Rounsaville et al. 1987), socioeconomic stability, intelligence, positive family history for alcoholism, and psychological-mindedness. McLellan and colleagues (1983) demonstrated that alcoholic patients do best if the level of treatment provided matches their level of psychiatric difficulty. Those with moderate severity of psychiatric problems do better with inpatient treatment and with psychiatrically trained therapists; those with low psychiatric severity do well as outpatients and with counselors (McLellan 1986).

Another factor that affects outcome is the wide variability in therapeutic approach. As the research knowledge in the area increases, the complexity of the factors involved in the illness becomes more apparent.

As with psychotherapy in general, much research remains to be done in the area of alcoholism treatment. At this time, the psychotherapist needs to use a commonsense, practical approach based on knowledge of the disease and the particular patient's constellation of problems.

CONCLUSION

In summary, the individual psychotherapy of the alcoholic patient treated on the general psychiatric unit requires a focused yet comprehensive approach. The psychotherapist has to thoroughly assess the patient and then decide how to interweave the psychodynamic issues with the concrete tasks of recovery. In addition, a variety of treatment modalities need to be integrated into the patient's treatment, and the psychotherapist must take the role of coordinator of the treatment team. Although further systematic study is needed, many alcoholic patients appear to benefit from a targeted, compassionate psychotherapeutic relationship.

REFERENCES

American Psychiatric Association: Diagnostic and Statistical Manual of Mental Disorders, 3rd Edition, Revised. Washington, DC, American Psychiatric Association, 1987

Babor TF, Dolinsky Z, Rounsaville B, et al: Unitary versus multidimensional models of alcoholism treatment outcome: an empirical study. J Stud Alcohol 49:167–177, 1988

Bebbington PE: Efficacy of Alcoholics Anonymous: the elusiveness of hard data. Br J Psychiatry 128:572–580, 1976

Beck AT, Freeman A, et al: Cognitive Therapy of Personality Disorders. New York, Guilford, 1990

Ewing JA: Detecting alcoholism: the CAGE questionnaire. JAMA 252:1905–1907, 1984

Frances RJ: Update on alcohol and drug disorder treatment. J Clin Psychiatry 49 (suppl 9):13–17, 1988

Frances RJ, Allen MH: The interaction of substance-use disorders with non-psychotic psychiatric disorders, in Psychiatry, Vol 1. Edited by Michels R. New York, Basic Books, 1986, pp 1–13

Frances RJ, Borg LB: Treatment of anxiety in patients with alcoholism. J Clin Psychiatry (in press)

Frances RJ, Franklin JE: Concise Guide to Treatment of Alcoholism and Addictions. Washington, DC, American Psychiatric Press, 1989

Frances RJ, Khantzian EJ, Tamerin JS: Psychodynamic psychotherapy, in Treatment of Psychiatric Disorders, Vol 2. Edited by Galanter M, Karasu TB. Washington, DC, American Psychiatric Press, 1989, pp 1103–1111

Galanter M, Castaneda R, Franco H: Group therapy and self-help groups, in Clinical Textbook of Addictive Disorders. Edited by Frances RJ, Miller SI. New York, Guilford, 1991, pp 431–451

Heath AW, Stanton MD: Family therapy, in Clinical Textbook of Addictive Disorders. Edited by Frances RJ, Miller SI. New York, Guilford, 1991, pp 406–430

Helzer JE, Pryzbeck FR: The co-occurrence of alcoholism with other psychiatric disorders in the general population and its impact on treatment. J Stud Alcohol 49:219–224, 1988

Hesselbrock MN, Meyer RE, Keener JJ: Psychopathology in hospitalized alcoholics. Arch Gen Psychiatry 42:1050–1055, 1985

Hirsch SM, von Rosenberg R, Phelan C, et al: Effectiveness of assertiveness training with alcoholics. J Stud Alcohol 39:89–97, 1978

Intagliata JC: Increasing the interpersonal problem-solving skills of an alcoholic population. J Consult Clin Psychol 46:489–498, 1978

Kaufman E: A contemporary approach to the family treatment of substance abuse disorders. Am J Drug Alcohol Abuse 12:199–211, 1986

Kernberg OJ: Object Relations Theory and Clinical Psychoanalysis. New York, Jason Aronson, 1976

Khantzian EJ, Halliday KS, McAuliffe WE: Addiction and the Vulnerable Self. New York, Guilford, 1990

Leibenluft E, Goldberg RL: Guidelines for short-term inpatient psychotherapy. Hosp Community Psychiatry 38:38–43, 1987

Malan DH: The Frontier of Brief Psychotherapy. New York, Plenum, 1978

Malan DH: Toward the Validation of Dynamic Psychotherapy. New York, Plenum, 1980

Mann J: Time-Limited Psychotherapy. Cambridge, MA, Harvard University Press, 1973

Marlatt GA, Gordon JR (eds): Relapse Prevention. New York, Guilford, 1985

McCarrick AK, Rosenstein MJ, Milazzo-Sayre LJ, et al: National trends in use of psychotherapy in psychiatric inpatient settings. Hosp Community Psychiatry 39:835–841, 1988

McLellan AT: "Psychiatric severity" as a predictor of outcome from substance abuse treatments, in Psychopathology and Addictive Disorders. Edited by Meyer RE. New York, Guilford, 1986, pp 97–139

McLellan AT, Woody GE, Luborsky L, et al: Increased effectiveness of substance abuse treatment. J Nerv Ment Dis 171:597–605, 1983

Miller SI, Frances RJ, Holmes DJ: Alcoholism and psychotropic medication, in Handbook of Alcoholism Treatment Approaches. Edited by Hester RK, Miller WK. New York, Pergamon, 1989, pp 231–241

Musto DF: Evolution of American attitudes toward substance abuse. Ann N Y Acad Sci 562:3–7, 1989

Regier DA, Farmer ME, Rae DS, et al: Comorbidity of mental disorders with alcohol and other drug abuse: results from the Epidemiologic Catchment Area (ECA) study. JAMA 264:2511–2518, 1990

Rounsaville BJ, Dolinsky ZS, Babor TF, et al: Psychopathology as a predictor of treatment outcome in alcoholics. Arch Gen Psychiatry 44:505–513, 1987

Selzer ML: The Michigan Alcoholism Screening Test: the quest for a new diagnostic instrument. Am J Psychiatry 127:1653–1658, 1971

Sifneos PE: Short-Term Psychotherapy and Emotional Crisis. Cambridge, MA, Harvard University Press, 1972

Sifneos PE: Short-Term Psychotherapy: Evaluation and Technique. New York, Plenum, 1979

Vanicelli M: Group psychotherapy with alcoholics. J Stud Alcohol 43:17–57, 1982

Woody GE, McLellan AT, Luborsky L, et al: Severity of psychiatric symptoms as a predictor of benefits from psychotherapy. Am J Psychiatry 141:1172–1177, 1984

Patients With Eating Disorders

Bruce S. Rothschild, M.D.

INTRODUCTION

A variety of economic and social factors have contributed to an ever-shortening mean length of stay for psychiatric admissions. This belt-tightening has been felt across all psychiatric diagnoses, but it produces unique problems for specialty populations.

Eating disorders, primarily anorexia nervosa and bulimia nervosa, have become increasingly prevalent in our society. They bring with them problems of morbidity and mortality that require special attention. Anorexia nervosa is defined primarily by abnormally low body weight, most often accompanied by loss of menses. The characteristic psychopathological features are "fear of fatness" and a distorted body image. This disorder primarily affects postadolescent girls and young women. Its prevalence in this age range is 0.5%–1%. Bulimia nervosa is defined primarily by the *act* of frequent binge eating. A binge is defined as a large amount of food eaten privately in a discrete amount of time in an uncontrolled manner. A binge episode is most often accompanied by attempts to rid the body of unwanted calories through vomiting, laxative abuse, diuretics, or exercise. As in anorexia, there is a similar overconcern with body weight, shape,

---

Because the vast majority of patients with eating disorders are female, the female pronoun will be used in this chapter.

and calories. Prevalence rates in samples of college-age subjects have ranged from 3.8% to 13%.

When these symptom complexes are found together, the low body weight and the resulting biological consequences take diagnostic precedence over the binge-purge activity. Thus, a 5-foot, 2-inch 70-pound girl who does not eat during the day but has a binge followed by self-induced purging in the evening is diagnosed as having anorexia nervosa with bulimic features.

INDICATIONS FOR HOSPITALIZATION

The economic forces that have driven down the length of stay of psychiatric admissions have also made it more difficult to get patients admitted in the first place. Increased utilization review mechanisms have narrowed the gates through which patients can pass into psychiatric admission. It is not uncommon for a clinician to have to justify his or her reason for admission to a reviewer to get an admission authorized. Therefore, the clinician should be well versed in common indications for psychiatric admission for patients with eating disorders.

The most common reason a patient with anorexia nervosa needs to be admitted is that her weight has dropped below a critical weight range. The term "critical" here can have two meanings: first, the patient's weight may be medically critical if the patient is so emaciated she is at profound risk of imminent morbidity or mortality. Second, therapist and patient may have agreed to a critical weight range in therapy. In this case, a contract stipulates that the therapist is willing to continue to treat the patient as long as she keeps her weight above a certain number of pounds. This prudent outpatient policy helps protect the therapist against potential liability, and it serves to give the patient a clear, concrete message. If the patient subsequently is unable to keep her weight above this number, she also is clearly indicating that she is out of control and needs more intensive intervention or hospitalization.

Judy M., a 22-year-old college graduate with a 6-year history of anorexia nervosa, was self-referred for outpatient treatment. Her height was 5 feet 4 inches, and her weight was 101 pounds. Ms. M. would restrict her eating during the day and then eat excessive amounts of cereal in the evening. She was amenorrheic and visibly emaciated. Lab tests showed a mild elevation of her serum transaminases and a mild leukopenia.

Ms. M. entered treatment stating that she "wanted" to gain weight and sat attentively as her outpatient treatment plan was discussed. However, within the first few weeks of therapy, she increased rather than decreased her amount of exercise to 3 hours a day. She gave up her "cereal dinners" as recommended but did not replace them with other foods of equal caloric quantity. Her weight dropped to 97 pounds. Repeat lab tests showed worsening transaminases, mild hypoglycemia, and mild anemia.

A treatment agreement was made that Ms. M. would turn her weight loss around or she would need to go into the hospital. The following week her weight dropped to 95 pounds, and she was hospitalized.

Although all cases need to be individually assessed, Table 9–1 covers some general rules for indications for hospital admission.

An anorexic patient who is also engaging in purging behavior (e.g., vomiting, or using laxatives or diuretics) is at high risk for developing hypokalemic alkalosis or other metabolic abnormalities (Mitchell et al. 1983). Given the anorexic patient's poor nutritional status, she has limited reserves to weather these metabolic insults. The same metabolic consequences also apply to a bulimic patient who is vomiting and abusing laxatives and diuretics daily. Thus, clinicians should check lab results regularly.

The main criterion for admitting bulimic patients is that their bulimia is out of control. By definition, of course, bulimic behaviors *are* out of control. But once a patient has lost control to the extent of bingeing and purging 10 times a day, it is very unlikely that she will be able to turn it around outside of a structured inpatient setting.

Table 9–1.   General indications for hospitalization for patients with eating disorders

Weight loss > 20% ideal body weight	Excessive exercise in relation to general body state
Potassium < 3.0 mmol/L	
Binge-purge episodes > 5–10 times daily	Suicidality

Excessive exercise can also occasionally be a reason to seek admission. At our unit, we admitted a normal-weight male bulimic patient who was exercising so many hours daily that he developed foot ulcers and blisters and had recurrent abrasions on his lower back from doing more than 200 sit-ups at a time. The excessiveness of the exercising must be gauged in relation to the patient's general health status. For a severely starved anorexic person, climbing stairs for 5 minutes can be excessive.

Suicidality is the other main indication for admission of patients with eating disorders, although it more frequently accompanies the presentation of bulimic patients, probably as a result of their greater frequency of borderline features. Anorexic patients are also at risk. The mortality of eating disorder patients (approximately 1%) is accounted for by excessive starvation, metabolic complications, and suicide.

GOALS OF HOSPITALIZATION

Having determined that indications for admission are present, what are the goals that can reasonably be expected to be accomplished through hospitalization? Ideally, goals should be relatively concrete, practical, and attainable. The ability of the long-term admission to invoke changes in personality structure is uncertain at best and clearly not a practical goal of short-term hospitalization.

A determining factor of admission goals is the point at which hospitalization occurs in the course of the eating disorder. Goals for a patient with a long history of chronic anorexia nervosa and multiple past hospitalizations will be different from those for a young bulimic patient who is entering her first inpatient stay. In the former case, the exclusive goal may be that the patient return to the prearranged outpatient goal weight range. In the latter case, hopes will be brighter for a better prognosis, and goals may include complete cessation of bulimic behaviors. Potential goals of short-term admission for patients with eating disorders are perhaps best viewed as occurring hierarchically (Figure 9–1). The most basic goal is medical stabilization. Weight restoration and the normalization of eating behaviors are intrinsically bound to medical stabilization and are goals in and of themselves. A starved anorexic patient may be able to restore 10 pounds of weight over a 3- to 4-week admission. Normalizing the eating patterns of an out-of-control bulimic patient can satisfactorily result in abnormal lab results being corrected over the course of a short-term admission.

Moving up the "goal pyramid," the patient can be expected to learn more about eating disorders and nutrition through psychoeducation. Tied in with this behavior change and psychoeducation is the hope that the patient will be able to change entrenched patterns of thought concerning food and weight.

The intensity of the short-term hospitalization may help the patient *begin* to discover some of the issues driving her eating disorder. If there are negative psychosocial factors contributing to her disorder, the patient may, for example, be able to begin to implement life changes by finding a new job or ending a destructive relationship.

GENERAL MANAGEMENT

Before I address psychotherapeutic concerns, it is important to discuss some general management issues in the short-term hospitalization of eating disorder patients. Shorter lengths of stay and more stringent admission criteria have resulted in a physically as well as psychologically sicker population of patients. Medical stabilization thus takes precedence over other concerns early in the admission.

Most of the medical abnormalities (and even some of the psychologi-

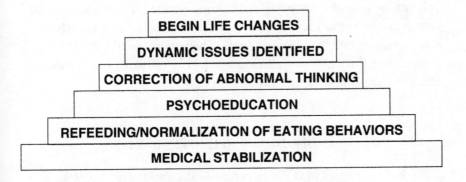

Figure 9–1. Hierarchical goal pyramid of eating disorder admissions.

cal ones) can be corrected with refeeding. It is sensible to begin starved anorexic patients on a 1,400-calorie diet and bulimic patients on an 1,800-calorie diet, although these should be adjusted to the patient's weight and medical condition. The refeeding of anorexic patients can then proceed at a more rapid pace. Calories can be increased by 300–500 calories every one-half to full week or so, resulting in an approximate weight gain of 3 pounds per week. Patients can be weighed two or three times weekly, preferably in the morning before breakfast, in nightclothes. During this period of refeeding, the patient should not be allowed to see her weight. Food is being prescribed for her just as medication would be, because she has shown that she cannot control her food intake in a medically healthy way.

The bulimic patient, or the anorexic patient with bulimic features, presents special challenges. Patients who purge should be on some type of observation status after meals. At a minimum, this could involve having the patient spend 1 hour in the dayroom after finishing her meal. Gradually, the patient may be able to assume more control herself and seek support from staff when necessary to avoid bingeing, exercising, and so on.

Building on this last concept, the hospitalization should be structured with a behavioral focus for the eating disorder patient. The patient's ability to achieve less restrictive nursing status, or more privileges, should be tied into pertinent behavioral goals. For instance, steady weight gain and the need for less redirection by the nurse observing meals would be used to advance the anorexic patient's status. Eating at a normal pace, complying with postmeal observations, and observing other unit protocols can be goals for lessening restrictions on the bulimic patients. Discharge is a powerful motivator for most hospitalized patients with eating disorders, especially anorexic patients. The patient should feel that she is progressing through her individualized hospital program toward discharge as her symptoms improve.

INDIVIDUAL PSYCHOTHERAPY

Now that I have outlined the structure of the short-term hospitalization for the eating disorder patient, I shall turn the focus of this discussion to the psychotherapy that is interwoven into this general fabric. Andersen

(1989) described a hierarchical approach to psychotherapy that progresses from supportive to cognitive, to insight-oriented, and then to existential. As the patient becomes physically and psychologically healthier, she is better able to tolerate different forms of psychotherapies. For the short-term psychotherapy of eating disorder inpatients, it is likely that only the first two approaches will be viable. If appropriate, a more insight-oriented and existential approach can take place over an extended period of time on an outpatient basis.

Early in the course of the hospital admission, patients are usually at their sickest. A starved anorexic patient is struggling with the refeeding process. The physiological sequelae of starvation result in a cold, thin, energy-depleted woman who has a poor ability to concentrate. A bulimic patient has been forced to give up her main coping patterns within the structure of the hospital; she is also struggling with having to eat three regular meals daily. Patients at this point are typically not ready to benefit from hour-long psychotherapy sessions. This is where the element of support is perhaps most necessary. Psychotherapy can best be received in more frequent doses of shorter duration. For the first few days or first week after admission, it is best that the clinician see the patient for 10–15 minutes on a daily basis. The primary focus should be on remaining supportive to the patient, hearing her complaints and difficulties, and giving reassurance that her symptoms will become easier to tolerate as treatment ensues.

Once the patient has become more acclimated to the behaviorally based milieu, has gained some strength and health, and is on her way in the refeeding process, psychotherapy can occur for longer periods of time. Seeing the patient after the first week for two or three 30- to 45-minute sessions weekly is typical.

Psychotherapy can now move from a primarily supportive emphasis to a more cognitive approach. Garner and Bemis (1985) have written an excellent chapter on cognitive therapy for anorexia nervosa, and much of what follows is taken from that source. Regardless of the etiological underpinnings in any patient's eating disorder, cognitive therapy is helpful in attacking the faulty thinking processes that help maintain the illness. In eating disorder patients, the primary abnormal belief is: "I must be thin." The patient brings to the treatment setting a number of errors of thinking that need to be addressed and modified.

Dichotomous reasoning is perhaps the quintessential distorted pattern of thinking in eating disorder patients. Otherwise known as black-or-white thinking, these patients are entrenched in rigid, absolute, and extreme thinking patterns. Dichotomous thinking is first evident in how they approach food. To anorexic patients, food is either good or bad, safe or unsafe. Eating one bite of a "forbidden" food is equivalent to losing control. Changes in weight are also seen through a black-or-white filter. The gain of even one-half pound cannot be easily distinguished from a gain of 50 pounds. All upward changes in weight, no matter how great or small, are considered to be bad or dangerous, whereas all weight loss is cheerfully accepted.

Dichotomous reasoning extends beyond the boundaries of food and weight and affects the patient's perceptions of herself and others. Family members may be perceived as all-harsh, all-angry, all-successful, all-failing. If a sibling is perceived as all-successful, the patient may latch onto thinness as an achievement. Conversely, a bulimic woman who sees herself as a total failure may use the "bad girl" identity of the bulimic patient to fulfill this prophecy. A patient who perceives her father as all-harsh may be reluctant to express unhappiness or anger to him. Of course, these patterns can also be seen in the patient's reactions to staff in the therapeutic milieu.

The perfectionism seen in anorexic patients can be understood as an outgrowth of black-or-white thinking. In scholastic or sports endeavors, striving for As or the perfect gymnastic routine can lead to a rigid life devoid of much joy or freedom.

Perfectionism can also affect the therapeutic process adversely. For the bulimic patient, having one slip such as a binge-purge episode can represent utter failure and hopelessness. These negative cognitions easily pave the way for repeated episodes, or for a nihilistic attitude.

Other cognitive distortions are commonly found in eating disorder patients. For example, emotional reasoning is the tendency to let emotions outweigh other evidence, such as responses from others and intellectual reasoning. "I feel fat [ugly, inadequate, etc.]" becomes synonymous with "I am fat," and other nonfeeling input remains insignificant.

Patients with eating disorders frequently use arbitrary inference, where comments or even glances by others may be misconstrued. For example, a friend tells an anorexic patient that she looks good. The patient infers the following: "I look good" means "I have gained some weight." "I've gained some weight" means "I'm getting fat." Then, "If I'm getting fat, I better skip my next couple of meals."

In selective abstraction, patients focus on details taken out of context. A woman perceives her shoulders as being broad, and so she sees herself as being big-boned or fat. It is difficult to control her negative body image, which is independent of her weight.

The process of therapeutic change begins with the patient monitoring her thinking and learning to recognize these cognitive distortions (Beck 1976). The patient is encouraged to articulate to her therapist the faulty beliefs that have been driving her emotional state and behaviors: "If I am thin, I will be happy;" "I have to binge once I have gone off my diet." Other cognitive interventions can then be employed to modify these faulty beliefs. For example, in decentering the patient evaluates a particular belief from the vantage point of other people's perspectives to assess its validity more objectively. Eating disorder patients are all too self-centered in their restricted and heightened concerns about themselves, to the point of shutting out the rest of the world (e.g., "If I gain 2 pounds, everyone will notice and make comments"). The patient can be asked if she notices others when they have gained 2 pounds.

Decatastrophizing is another technique. One could examine the validity of how life would change if the patient gained 2 pounds or took the risk of asking another person to go out and see a movie. The therapist can also help in challenging the "shoulds" (e.g., "I should avoid all fats;" "I should be the perfect daughter"). These expectations are bound to lead to feelings of failure and loss of self-worth. Reattribution techniques encourage the patient to distance herself from her faulty self-perceptions. This technique enables the patient to say, "I know I have anorexia nervosa, and so I can't be a good judge of my body size. I will have to trust my therapist on this one and stay within my goal weight range."

Complementing these cognitive strategies, there are a number of simple behavioral interventions that can be started in the inpatient setting. To combat faulty beliefs, patients can be encouraged to set up miniexperiments to provide empirical evidence to themselves. For example, an anorexic patient can be encouraged to eat a dessert three nights out of a given week and see what effect this addition to her diet has on her weight.

Distraction is a technique that is particularly useful to the bulimic patient. She should be taught to recognize her binge pattern, from the feelings that precede it to the actual bingeing and purging. Having a clearer appreciation of such an episode, she can practice strategies of distraction. She works on recognizing the binge feelings early enough in the cycle to intervene and then disrupts the pattern with a repertoire of alternative behaviors, such as taking a walk or talking to a friend.

For both anorexic and bulimic patients, the exercise of structuring time can be very important. This also serves as a distracting technique. In addition, it helps these patients devise a structure and a meaning that can help them combat the emptiness that many eating disorder patients feel. Weekend days in hospital can be especially useful in this regard.

Little mention has been made of insight-oriented dynamic psycho-therapy in this discussion. Through the goal pyramid of Figure 9–1, it can been seen as unlikely that major new insights will be achieved via inter-pretation and other psychodynamic interventions during short-term hos-pitalization. The short-term therapy models that I have been discussing are the most practical and indeed the most testable in empirical studies addressing the psychotherapy of these patients. Controlled studies have focused mainly on therapies whose approach can be specifically described in detail, such as through a treatment manual. For instance, comparative design studies have found cognitive-behavioral, behavioral, and interper-sonal therapy to be essentially equally effective (Fairburn 1988). However, in clinical practice, the boundaries between different forms of individual psychotherapy are not as firmly drawn as the theoretical and empirical literature would suggest. It is important for the clinician to have some familiarity with psychodynamic psychotherapy and to be able to recog-nize psychodynamic themes as they affect treatment.

Cathy L., a 30-year-old bulimic woman, came from a family in which most of the members had a major psychiatric disorder. She was, on the surface, overly compliant with treatment recommendations. However, Ms. L. continued to binge when unobserved and sheepishly reported these episodes to staff with a sly grin. In the context of her psy-choeducational and cognitive-behavioral treatment, she became aware that being sick was the way to get attention in her family and that giving up this behavior might result in the loss of care and attention from her parents. Ms. L.'s recognition of this dynamic enabled her to participate in cognitive-behavioral therapy more sincerely and to stop bingeing.

GROUP THERAPY

As hospital lengths of stay decrease and admissions and discharges increase, the psychiatrist faces additional administrative paperwork and less time for psychotherapy. Group therapy has been growing in popularity in response to these time and financial pressures and brings with it its own set of strengths and weaknesses.

Patients on a specialty eating disorders unit participate in groups with other patients with eating disorders. In these disorders of motivated behaviors, homogeneous groups may have therapeutic advantages. First, the patient feels that she is firmly understood by other group members who have shared similar difficulties. This helps reduce the patient's sense of shame or feelings of being uniquely alone with her "weird" behaviors. It also serves to lessen any adversarial component that may exist in the therapy. In addition to providing group support, other patients with eating disorders know when a group member is not being honest or is avoiding examining difficult issues.

To give an idea of the type of groups that are used in treating eating disorder patients, Table 9–2 is a list of the groups offered at the Eating Disorder Day Hospital at The Institute of Living. They are categorized

Table 9–2.   Typical groups in an eating disorders program

Psychologist	Registered Dietitian
Women's Group	Nutrition Group
Sexuality Group	Menu planning
Psychoeducation Group	Cooking Group
Social Worker	**Dance Therapist**
Family Issues Group	Body Image Group
Work issues	Exercise Group
"Play" therapy	Movement Group
Registered Nurse	Assertiveness training
Weight Group	Leisure and time management
Snack outing	Relaxation

according to the staff member who runs them, although for some groups, this is arbitrary. Some of these groups may overlap with those used on a general psychiatric unit and would obviously be appropriate for eating disorder patients in that setting. Others could perhaps be incorporated by interested staff members, particularly if eating disorder admissions were becoming more common on a particular unit.

Even when a homogeneous group is not available, group therapy on the general unit can be helpful. Again, the element of support is a key therapeutic factor. It is often difficult for other inpatients with affective disorders or schizophrenia to understand why the eating disorder patient is having problems with food and eating. The therapist must help the eating disorder patient feel understood and accepted by other group members. A caring psychoeducational approach is helpful here. Ultimately, the eating disorder patient's ability to bring her symptoms and feelings out in the open will help detoxify them.

FAMILY THERAPY

Much has been written on the role of family pathology in eating disorders, particularly anorexia nervosa. Most notable in this regard are the writings of Minuchin and colleagues (1978). Minuchin observed the following traits in the families of anorexic patients:

1. *Enmeshment.* There are poor boundary divisions between family members, so that the mother is typically overinvolved in the anorexic daughter's life;
2. *Overprotectiveness.* The anorexic patient is not allowed to venture out far enough to gain independence or real autonomy;
3. *Rigidity.* Families have a limited repertoire of abilities to relate, and a stereotypical approach to handling conflict;
4. *Lack of conflict resolution.* Problems are not truly worked out but rather "glossed over." According to this perspective, the sick child's symptoms take the focus off unresolved marital conflicts.

Russell and colleagues (1987) randomized discharged patients to either outpatient family therapy or individual supportive therapy. Anorexic patients with early onset (younger than age 19) and short duration of illness (less than 3 years) did better with family therapy than individual therapy. Therefore, the adolescent anorexic patient may be significantly influenced by family factors and respond best to family intervention. If the patient is still in her teenage years, it is crucial that family therapy at least be a part of (and often the major focus of) short-term hospital treatment. For the older and more chronic anorexic patient, the therapeutic effort may be to separate the patient from an overly dependent relationship with her family. For such a patient or for a bulimic patient, a more individual approach is probably warranted. The clinician should evaluate the importance of family dynamics on a case-by-case basis and intervene accordingly.

The initial meeting with the family provides an opportunity to make an assessment of the family situation. Individual family members, especially parents, need to be evaluated in terms of the role they might play in maintaining the patient's disorder. The family may see the patient as a "poor victim" and resist asking her to take more responsibility for her behavior. They may deny the problem (e.g., by saying "Everyone is trying to lose weight these days" or "Kick her out if she can't follow the rules"). Some parents are overly concerned and put their own lives on hold "until our daughter gets better."

All of the stereotypical postures mentioned here make sense in the anorexic family and can be seen as either contributing causes of, or different responses to, the primary problem. The clinician should avoid placing blame on any individual family member or members. Family patterns, like the disorder itself, are often deeply entrenched by the time the patient requires inpatient treatment, and goals should be limited. One strives for creating fluidity and a variety of responses where there was rigidity. One possible therapeutic strategy is to have parents attempt to swap roles. For example, an overly involved mother can *contribute* to making up some ground rules regarding the patient's behavior, perhaps during a weekend pass, and then be told not to get involved in the implementation of these. The more distant father can then be chosen to play the role of "enforcer" of the rules that the mother has had a more primary part in creating. This type of quick intervention, particularly as it continues into outpatient treatment, is often a helpful catalyst in demonstrating that the parents work together ineffectually. Follow-up visits can work on the concrete tasks of helping family members grow into new family roles and solidifying the marital dyad.

Knowing that there are no easy answers and that the struggle within the family sometimes continues for years, it is helpful to be able to refer family members to a support group. Groups that are specifically run for family members of eating disorder patients are becoming increasingly popular and at times are held down the hall when groups for the patients themselves meet. In addition, the excellent book by Siegel and colleagues (1989) for family members struggling with a relative who has an eating disorder can be routinely recommended to families.

MEDICATIONS

Medications can play an important role in the treatment of eating disorders. Studies have documented the efficacy of tricyclic antidepressants (Hughes et al. 1985), monoamine oxidase (MAO) inhibitors (Walsh et al. 1988), and fluoxetine (Freeman et al. 1988) in treating bulimia. Antidepressant agents appear to decrease the frequency of binge-purge cycles, even in patients without a concurrent major depressive episode. If a patient has failed a psychotherapy trial, the addition of an antidepressant can be clinically helpful in its psychopharmacological properties as well as providing new hope to the patient. Many hospitalized bulimic patients will fit this pattern, so it is likely that many will be started on a medication during the hospitalization. At times, explaining the different side effect profiles of two or three medications and letting the patient contribute to the decision of which agent would be best to start with gives her a feeling of control and respect.

THE SPECIALIZED EATING DISORDER UNIT

It is often easier and more effective to treat these patients on a unit that specializes in eating disorders. Beyond the varying abilities of the primary clinicians, the most critical difference between specialized and general units is the staff. The treatment of eating disorder patients often goes more smoothly when conducted by a team of individuals who have experience with and an interest in treating this population. On a general unit, time that could be spent in psychotherapy often has to be spent putting out fires (e.g., "The patient isn't eating again") or teaching various multidisciplinary team members how to approach the patient.

However, managed care may not always allow for such an admission, even if a facility is available. Eating disorder services are considered long-term treatment (often a minimum of 1 to 2 months), and third-party payors may not be willing to use them. It may also make sense to avoid admitting to a specialty service if the eating disorder (often bulimia) is not the primary diagnosis, but rather a symptom of a borderline patient.

The eating disorder patient on a general unit may feel out of place, misunderstood, and not taken seriously. These feelings further contribute to an already existing sense of hopelessness, self-denigration, and anger, and can cause the patient to close up in a therapeutic situation. A primary task of the therapist on the general unit is to search for these responses, empathize with them, and then create the milieu of support and understanding necessary for the patient to trust and disclose.

COMORBIDITY

Eating disorders tend to "travel" with other Axis I and Axis II diagnoses, and it is especially important to ask specifically about certain symptoms (e.g., in the mental status examination). Once the diagnosis of comorbid disorders is made, a rational treatment plan, including psychotherapeutic focus, can be devised.

Major Depression

The most common comorbid diagnosis in patients with eating disorders, especially bulimia, is major depression. Piran and colleagues (1985) found a lifetime prevalence of major depression in 36% of bulimic patients. The diagnosis of depression in this patient population is challenging at times. The anorexic patient who is starved and the bulimic patient who is vomiting several times a day can experience low mood, low energy, and sleep difficulties as physiological consequences of altered metabolism. These symptoms typically resolve with medical stabilization. Esteem is often chronically poor in patients with eating disorders. Often patients carry a "rule out" diagnosis of major depression for several weeks until their physiology has begun to normalize.

Even in the absence of a formal diagnosis, however, the signs and symptoms can and should be addressed in psychotherapy from early in the admission, for they are very real to the patient. As part of a psychoeducational approach, the patient can be told that depressive symptoms are often a result of the starved state and may resolve as the patient becomes physically healthier. An ongoing effort must be made to assess the progress of these symptoms. Psychotherapeutically, this contributes to the patient's sense of being cared for by the therapist.

It is often helpful to broaden the cognitive therapy focus in these patients so that they become more aware of their negative self-image, self-blaming tendencies, and negative interpretation of events.

Substance Abuse

The comorbidity of substance abuse with eating disorders, especially bulimia nervosa, is becoming more and more prevalent. In one study, Marcus and colleagues (1988) found 50% of the female patients being treated on a substance abuse unit to have a diagnosable eating disorder. Patients are admitted to the hospital with multiple impulses out of control, so it may be difficult to identify the primary diagnosis. Given short lengths of stay, it is important to begin to aggressively treat each problem as soon as possible. If a substance abuse problem is identified, a consultation by a chemical dependency specialist is helpful. Hospitals often run special groups for people with alcohol and drug abuse problems, and patients can attend these during their inpatient stay. It is the role of the primary clinician to integrate these treatments into the patient's individual psychotherapy so that she does not experience her different problems as being fragmented. Active contact with these other therapists will enable one to interweave common themes into the therapy.

Patients with both eating disorders and substance abuse problems often have the concern that "If you take away all my crutches, I will crumble." This does not seem to be borne out. Patients who are motivated to get well quickly recognize that they feel better in a sober and nutritionally healthy state. They are then able to focus on their underlying feelings, and the stage is set for a relatively quick discharge and follow-up outpatient psychotherapy.

Obsessive-Compulsive Disorder

Whereas chemical dependency seems to occur with greater frequency in bulimic patients, we are increasingly aware of the comorbidity of obsessive-compulsive disorder (OCD) with anorexia nervosa. Kasvikis and colleagues (1986) found adult women with OCD to have an increased incidence of prior anorexia (15%). In general, anorexic patients tend to display traits of perfectionism, rigidity, and compulsivity. However, true OCD also occurs in this patient population, and clinicians must ask the right questions to elicit the diagnosis. The occurrence of food and eating rituals is part of the anorexic disorder and in isolation should not be used to make an OCD diagnosis. However, patients who wash their hands or bodies excessively, check the stove, lights, and doors excessively, or have nonfood-related obsessive thoughts may have OCD.

Because the patient is removed from many of the environmental stimuli of home, OCD symptoms often spontaneously improve in the hospital and may not need acute intervention. In these cases, the patient should be referred for appropriate follow-up therapy as an outpatient. Patients who remain symptomatic in the hospital require support and understanding from the staff, as well as a modified behavioral plan of exposure and response prevention.

Axis II Disorders

Some would argue that eating disorders do not exist in isolation outside of personality disorders. The stereotypical anorexic patient follows the pattern of the Cluster C-type personality disorders in DSM-III-R (American Psychiatric Association 1987). Anorexic patients tend to be perfectionistic, compulsive, rigid, resistant to change, passive and ultimately passive-aggressive. They appear on the surface to be perfectly compliant and are often overachievers. Underneath, of course, there exists untapped anger, frustration, and sadness.

A psychoeducational approach is a useful first step to take in a short-term therapy. The patient can see that her compulsive and perfectionistic traits have both positive and negative ramifications; the same drive and stick-to-itiveness that resulted in her being an A student are now contributing to her rigid, relentless pursuit of thinness. It is often helpful to use a touch of humor when focusing on trait patterns. Although the therapist might not be able to do much to change these generally stable characteristics, recognizing them and developing the ability to "lighten up" when the patient is feeling caught in old patterns is a worthwhile goal.

Group therapy can be a useful adjunct for the personality disorder component of patients with such dual diagnoses. Themes of passivity, shyness, avoidance, and dependency can be quickly recognized in the group setting. Other patients, particularly those who are more outspoken, can be helpful in identifying these traits and perhaps offering useful suggestions.

Lastly, the anorexic patient's overcontrol around food can be seen as a reflection of her feeling very much out of control in other aspects of her life. Therefore, it may be necessary for the clinician to take over temporary control of the patient's nutritional needs; but it is equally important to help the patient take on more control over other aspects of her life. In the setting of short-term hospitalization, this could take the form of sharing the decision-making process regarding nonfood-related issues with the patient (e.g., through passes or visits). Overtly giving the patient permission to say "No" to the requests of other patients or of family members can help break the rigid pattern of superficial overcompliance. Another helpful milieu intervention is to have the patient accept a position of leadership in patient government and to work actively with her to combat the perfectionistic expectations she will develop for herself in that role.

The stereotypical bulimic patient fits the pattern of Cluster B-type personality disorders. There is a large, albeit controversial overlap between bulimia nervosa and borderline personality disorder. Each disorder can exist in isolation of the other; each can contain only traits of the other; or the two can coexist as comorbid conditions. Bulimic patients often have poor impulse control across a variety of behaviors, including sexual promiscuity. They may be histrionic, needy, and overly sensitive to perceived rejection. They may participate in antisocial activities, such as stealing (food and other items), drug abuse, and job abandonment. Occasionally there may be a history of self-mutilating behavior and suicide attempts.

One risks the Pandora's Box scenario with these patients, who tend to have tumultuous backgrounds, largely unmet narcissistic needs, and histrionic presentations. Therefore, in the short-term setting, it is more helpful to adopt a "sealing over" approach. Recognizing and empathizing with the fact that the patient has undergone many injustices in her life is crucial. However, the clinician can stress to the patient that it is impossible to resolve these lifelong, complex issues in the setting of short-term hospitalization. Given the time limitations, there is more to be gained from focusing on real-life issues.

A reality therapy approach described by Glasser (1965) can be useful. Responsibility is focused back on the patient for situations in which she repeatedly finds herself, such as being badly treated or rejected. One can extend the behavioral approach of the patient beyond the eating disorder treatment. Strict limits with clear-cut repercussions that are proactively elucidated are useful. The treatment team's ability to positively reinforce healthy changes and behaviors in the patient is equally important.

CONCLUSION

It is easy for the therapist treating patients with eating disorders to become frustrated and discouraged. The limitations built into short-term hospitalization can compound these feelings of therapeutic pessimism.

Having a preliminary familiarity with these disorders and their treatment is the first step in helping effect change in the patient. It is important to set realistic goals in the short-term setting. This will ensure an element of success at the outcome of treatment, which can provide a sense of accomplishment to both patient and therapist. The patient can then use this achievement to enhance her motivation and confidence in pursuing further growth on an outpatient basis.

REFERENCES

American Psychiatric Association: Diagnostic and Statistical Manual of Mental Disorders, 3rd Edition, Revised. Washington, DC, American Psychiatric Association, 1987

Andersen AE: Prescribing psychotherapy: lesson 17. Directions in Psychiatry 9:3–7, 1989

Beck AT: Cognitive Therapy and the Emotional Disorders. New York, International Universities Press, 1976

Fairburn CG: The current status of the psychological treatments for bulimia nervosa. J Psychosom Res 32:635–645, 1988

Freeman CP, Morris JE, Cheshire KE, et al: A double-blind controlled trial of fluoxetine versus placebo for bulimia nervosa. Paper presented at the Third International Conference on Eating Disorders, New York, April 1988

Garner DM, Bemis KM: Cognitive therapy for anorexia nervosa, in Handbook of Psychotherapy for Anorexia Nervosa and Bulimia. Edited by Garner DM, Garfinkel PE. New York, Guilford, 1985, pp 107–146

Glasser W: Reality Therapy: A New Approach to Psychiatry. New York, Harper, 1965

Hughes PL, Wells LA, Cunningham CJ, et al: Treating bulimia with desipramine: a double blind study. Arch Gen Psychiatry 43:182–186, 1985

Kasvikis JG, Tsakiris F, Marks IM, et al: Women with obsessive-compulsive disorder frequently report a past history of anorexia nervosa. International Journal of Eating Disorders 5:1069–1075, 1986

Marcus R, Halmi K, Gallagher T: Eating disorders in substance abusers. Paper presented at the annual meeting of the American Psychiatric Association, Montreal, Canada, 1988

Minuchin S, Rosman BL, Baker L: Psychosomatic Families: Anorexia Nervosa in Context. Cambridge, MA, Harvard University Press, 1978

Mitchell JE, Pyle RL, Eckert ED, et al: Electrolyte and other physiological abnormalities in patients with bulimia. Psychol Med 13:273–278, 1983

Piran N, Kennedy S, Garfinkel PE, et al: Affective disturbance in eating disorders. J Nerv Ment Dis 173:395–400, 1985

Russell GF, Szmukler GI, Dare C, et al: An evaluation of family therapy in anorexia nervosa and bulimia nervosa. Arch Gen Psychiatry 44:1047–1056, 1987

Siegel M, Brisman J, Weinshel M: Surviving an Eating Disorder: New Perspectives and Strategies for Family and Friends. New York, Harper & Row, 1989

Walsh BT, Gladys M, Roose SP, et al: Phenelzine vs placebo in 50 patients with bulimia. Arch Gen Psychiatry 45:471–475, 1988

CHAPTER 10

Treating Concurrent Medical and Psychiatric Illness

Stephen A. Green, M.D.

The inextricable link between mind and body is a reality of medical practice. Despite long-standing belief in the Cartesian philosophy that separated mental activities from physiologic events, there is now an acceptance of the influence of emotions on the onset and course of illness (Engel 1977, 1980; Reiser 1975). This, of course, has implications for diagnosis and treatment (Engel 1980), including the recognition that one's psychological response to physical illness may facilitate or hinder coping (Green 1985). Broader acceptance of the biopsychosocial medical model has also sensitized the medical profession to the widespread concurrence of medical and psychiatric illness (Hall et al. 1978, 1980; Knight and Folstein 1977; Maguire and Granville-Grossman 1968; Moffic and Paykel 1975; Robbins and Regier 1991; Rodin and Voshart 1986; Strain 1982; Strain et al. 1981; Von Korff et al. 1987).

Recognition of this indisputable comorbidity has prompted a group of contemporary clinicians to work toward the reaffirmation of psychiatry's medical underpinnings. This has resulted in a progressive reuniting of the divergent "psychotherapeutic" and "biologic" spheres within the field, as well as a more direct involvement of psychiatrists with the families, physicians, and primary care staff of medical patients. This so-called remedicalization of psychiatry has spawned the new field of medical psychiatry, a most effective model for attending to concurrent medical and mental disorders, particularly on the inpatient unit.

Medical Psychiatry

As presented by Stoudemire and Fogel (1988), medical psychiatry defines the role of the psychiatrist as "a medical specialist who assumes primary clinical responsibility for the diagnosis and treatment of psychiatric disorders in the medically ill" (p. 208). The authors discuss the medical psychiatrist's specific skills, attitudes, activities, and knowledge base, including:

1. Responsibility for ongoing psychiatric care of patients, as opposed to serving as a consultant to other medical specialists;
2. Assumption of ongoing medical care of patients, which requires regular performance of physical and neurologic examinations, an ability to interpret basic and specialized laboratory tests, knowledge of the applications of basic neurodiagnostic tests to neuropsychiatric conditions, and an appreciation of the many psychiatric manifestations of medical illness;
3. The ability and experience to appreciate diagnostic and therapeutic implications of the frequent overlap between psychiatric and neurologic diseases;
4. A comprehensive knowledge of psychopharmacology (which requires understanding the psychiatric side effects of medical drugs, the interaction between psychotropic agents and the many drugs used to treat common medical diseases, and an ability to use psychopharmacologic agents in seriously medically ill patients) and the expertise to appropriately utilize electroconvulsive therapy (ECT); and
5. A comprehensive knowledge of therapeutic modalities used to treat maladaptive illness behaviors and to foster coping skills, such as brief psychodynamic psychotherapy and behavior therapy techniques.

In addition to redefining the role of practitioners, the evolving field of medical psychiatry has also prompted administrative and organizational changes in the psychiatric inpatient setting. The most obvious demonstration of this change has been the development of the med/psych unit.

Between one and two dozen such units currently exist in major American teaching hospitals; early prototypes included those at Mount Sinai Hospital (Goodman 1985) and at Brown University (Fogel et al. 1985). The latter was established, in part, to provide for the treatment of problem cases followed by the department's consultation-liaison service.

Medical psychiatry is also practiced de facto by many private practitioners who have their primary clinical base in general hospitals and/or by those who identify themselves as consultation-liaison psychiatrists (Stoudemire and Fogel 1988). This fact is evident in the definitive changes in the orientation of the general psychiatric unit, which has progressively moved toward the more traditional medical model of diagnosis and treatment (Asch 1987) and now admits patients previously referred to specialized med/psych units. Patients with significant medical issues—delirium, behaviorally complicated dementia, psychiatric complications of neurologic disease (e.g., parkinsonism, head trauma, cardiovascular accident), eating disorders with significant medical complications, chronic pain, paroxysmal behavioral disorders, somatoform disorders, and physical illness combined with complex family or psychosocial problems that interfere with the patient's ability to cooperate with necessary treatment—are no longer classified into the three categories proposed by Fogel and Stoudemire (1986) as solely appropriate for a med/psych unit. Such patients are now treated on a general inpatient unit. This has necessitated that psychiatrists become adept at treating the common and often severe medical illnesses that frequently affect their patients. This parallels the role of the skilled surgeon who simultaneously manages surgical and medical issues.

Samuel K., a 35-year-old attorney, was brought to the psychiatric emergency room by the police after attacking his longtime lover with a hammer. Mr. K. had demonstrated increasingly bizarre and confused behavior in recent months, which prompted his precipitous resignation from a prestigious firm after several reprimands for uncharacteristically shoddy performance. He also developed a concern that friends and family members "no longer held my interests dear," and he became increasingly withdrawn and isolated from his widespread social network. Though Mr. K. had never previously exhibited violent behavior, he had the reputation of being "an ugly drunk" during a long siege with alcohol abuse. This behavior ceased when he joined Alcoholics Anonymous (AA) and stopped drinking in his late 20s.

At admission, Mr. K. was openly suspicious of all patients and ward personnel and exhibited marked cognitive deficits, including diffuse memory impairment and disorientation to time. He had a vague memory of the events surrounding his admission, but he did not understand why his lover wore a cast on his fractured hand, nor did he believe that he was responsible for the injury. Mr. K. reported increasingly intrusive suicidal thoughts, including a plan to tranquilize himself and then jump to his death from a tall building, but said he did not understand why "my outlook is so morbid." Physical examination revealed a frail, debilitated appearance (which he attributed to a history of intermittent diarrhea over several months) and oral thrush. Past history revealed the presence of major depressive illness in three of Mr. K.'s close relatives, and his earlier bout with alcoholism. Laboratory testing revealed—for the first time, according to his lover—that Mr. K. was HIV positive.

The comprehensive evaluation and treatment of Mr. K.'s biopsychosocial problems is a complicated if not daunting task, yet his is an increasingly common type of case seen on psychiatry wards of general hospitals. Myriad questions immediately emerge in planning his overall care. What is his primary problem? Is his HIV status the predominant (and possibly exclusive) cause of his behavior? Is he experiencing sequelae of previous alcohol abuse? What will be the lasting effects of his recent decline on family and social relationships and on his professional life? Will his physical status interfere with the somatic treatment of his psychiatric symptoms? What are the legal implications of this decompensation? Will Mr. K. comply with treatment, or does he want to die?

In fact, none of these questions can be answered without constant attention to the interplay between Mr. K.'s medical and psychological issues, which is so intricate that his care demands simultaneous attention to his physical and mental health. It is first necessary to determine Mr. K.'s multiaxial DSM-III-R diagnoses (American Psychiatric Association 1987) on Axes I through V and use that assessment as the basis of a broad-based treatment plan, but this is only a necessary first step. Optimal treatment requires a biopsychosocial approach based on the principles of medical psychiatry, which involves appropriate modifications to the therapeutic milieu and its treatment programs.

THE THERAPEUTIC MILIEU

Treatment Philosophy

Though a physician was usually "the ultimate arbiter of treatment" in the traditional therapeutic milieu (Asch 1987, p. 161), this was an ineffective model for dealing with medically ill patients. Consultants from other medical specialties typically ordered diagnostic procedures and therapeutic regimens after little if any consultation with the psychiatric treatment staff, often creating a situation that undermined patients' psychiatric care. Splitting, and subsequent intrastaff struggles, could arise over issues such as the use of prn analgesics, a patient's absence from ward activities because of diagnostic testing or restricted physical activity (e.g., bed rest), and disagreement over whether the etiology of an individual's complaints (e.g., pain) was "psychological" or "organic." A patient might also act out psychological conflicts via noncompliance with a prescribed medical regimen. The resulting physical deterioration fueled the struggle between the ward staff and consulting specialists, further detracting from the patient's psychiatric and medical treatment. Patients who developed severe medical illnesses were generally transferred to medical wards until they stabilized. This prevented effective psychiatric treatment and sometimes aggravated patients' psychopathology.

> Lorraine L., a 21-year-old student, presented to the Emergency Room because of repeated fainting episodes which she attributed to "emotional fatigue." She voluntarily accepted admission to the psychiatric unit after relating a history of periodically "being too nervous to eat" when stressed by difficulties in her recent marriage. Ms. L.'s initial response to treatment was positive; however, as couples meetings with her husband became increasingly intense, her physical status declined. It was eventually discovered that Ms. L. had been hiding food in her room and periodically purging the meals she had consumed.
>
> Because of a cardiac arrhythmia presumably secondary to hypokalemia, Ms. L. was eventually transferred to the medical service, where she quickly responded to treatment. When she returned to the psychiatric unit, she became increasingly resistant to exploring conflicts and again began restricting her diet. This effectively shifted the focus of care exclusively to her physical condition by necessitating her transfer to the

medical service on four separate occasions. Ms. L. ultimately refused psychiatric treatment and left the hospital against medical advice.

Effectively treating the medically ill patient can only occur when the unit's treatment philosophy employs *a multidisciplinary approach that consistently addresses psychiatric and medical issues.* This focus permits the integration of a variety of professional disciplines in a collaborative fashion, enabling them to provide comprehensive care for patients' physical and emotional needs. Lacking that cooperation, medical responsibility for patients becomes fragmented and ultimately detracts from psychiatric care.

In Ms. L.'s case, optimal treatment would require the use of psychotherapy as well as behavioral and medical interventions. All treatment would be administered by the same staff, with the periodic assistance of medical consultants. Ms. L.'s hypothetical treatment plan would include:

1. A balance of supportive and insight-oriented psychotherapy;
2. A behavioral treatment plan, with designated rewards (e.g., privileges, passes) based on graduated weight gain;
3. Medical attention (e.g., assessing her fluid and electrolyte balance; cardiac monitoring) as needed;
4. Regular consultation with experts from other medical specialties; and
5. A series of couples meetings.

Comprehensive treatment of this type requires input, information sharing, strategy planning, and implementation by all components of the staff—physicians, nurses, social workers, and ancillary workers, such as occupational and recreational therapists, dietitians, and rehabilitation personnel.

An inpatient unit committed to this medically oriented multidisciplinary treatment approach has specific requirements that differentiate it from the general psychiatric ward. The staff must be adequately trained in medical issues so they may feel comfortable and competent regarding the overall management of patients. This requires familiarity with the diagnosis and treatment of common medical conditions, and the clinical sense to recognize when help from an expert consultant is needed. In this environment, a patient's *psychiatric and medical* status must be assessed daily on ward rounds. In addition, this multidisciplinary approach can only occur within a setting that permits adequate medical monitoring.

This approach requires an open, collegial relationship with medical and surgical services within the hospital, primarily for consultation, but also for the extreme instance when transfer is required (e.g., fulminant infection in an immunosuppressed patient, or pronounced cardiac instability). It also requires access to diagnostic procedures frequently employed when treating patients with complex medical issues, including sophisticated imaging techniques (e.g., computed tomography [CT] scan, magnetic resonance imaging [MRI]), and the ability to monitor serum levels of psychiatric and nonpsychiatric medications (Stoudemire and Fogel 1988). There are also certain physical necessities for a unit that applies a multidisciplinary philosophy to the treatment of patients with concurrent medical illness. In addition to modern, well-supplied examination rooms, the ward (or a designated number of beds) must be equipped with bedside oxygen, intravenous setups, respiratory therapy equipment, and (in some instances) a cardiac monitor.

Administrative Organization

The shift toward treating patients with concurrent medical illness has highlighted the importance of the general hospital psychiatric unit's administrative organization. This first requires two things: the administrative leadership of a medical director who is ultimately responsible for all psychiatric and medical care on the inpatient unit, whether he or she is the physician of record for all patients or oversees the care rendered by other attending physicians; and multidisciplinary treatment teams specifically geared to the practice of medical psychiatry.

The medical director has diverse functions concerning medical needs idiosyncratic to patients admitted to the mental health unit, including

1. Assessing possible causes of an individual's behavior (e.g., impulsive, disorganized), which include long-standing psychiatric disorders (e.g., bipolar illness) and/or organic conditions (e.g., HIV encephalopathy);
2. Determining the ward's physical and personnel capabilities, as they apply to each patient's medical issues; and
3. Coordinating a comprehensive biopsychosocial assessment, via dis-

cussion with the patient's medical doctors, psychotherapists, and members of the inpatient nursing staff, to review diagnostic strategies and particular treatment needs (e.g., scheduling hemodialysis).

Betty E., a 27-year-old nurse with a history of juvenile diabetes, was admitted to the psychiatric service following a serious suicide attempt with an insulin overdose. In addition to her long-standing bout with major affective illness, she was notorious for noncompliance with her medical regimen, which necessitated numerous medical admissions to bring her dangerously high blood sugars under control. In addition, Ms. E. had twice attempted suicide while hospitalized by slashing her wrists. The unit director reviewed Ms. E.'s clinical needs with the head nurse, who arranged for extra staffing, a free seclusion room, and active involvement by the hospital's dietary service. The medical director discussed these arrangements with the patient's internist, who coordinated her transfer from the medical ward where she had been under constant one-to-one observation since admission.

A second role of the medical director is to coordinate an individual's overall treatment, which involves judgments concerning administration of the multidisciplinary approach. Different therapeutic interventions, both medical and psychologic, are required during different periods of a patient's hospitalization. It is ultimately the responsibility of the medical director to determine the focus of treatment during the patient's hospital course.

Keith M. was a 55-year-old male admitted to the hospital because of acute mental status changes that included disorientation, memory deficits, and the delusion that he had been followed to Washington, DC, by "federal agents" after his reentry into the country through the Miami airport. Mr. M. had a long history of alcohol abuse, complicated by head trauma from two motor vehicle accidents and numerous falls. However, he had never previously exhibited paranoid ideation. The initial phase of his treatment consisted of a diagnostic workup, a thorough medical and neurologic evaluation that included blood and radiologic studies, and medical management for possible withdrawal symptoms.

The primary responsibilities of the nursing staff involved supportive care, orienting Mr. M. to his surroundings, and assisting him in his activities of daily living, while continually monitoring his medical condition. Mr. M.'s workup determined that his symptoms were due solely to the acute and chronic effects of alcohol. He progressively recompensated, at which time the focus of treatment shifted to confronting the patient about his alcohol abuse, involving him in regular AA meetings in the hospital, and requiring his family to attend a series of meetings with the social worker.

Three weeks after admission, Mr. M. was transferred to an inpatient alcohol rehabilitation facility. The medical director determined how and when to implement these different phases of Mr. M.'s treatment, by involving colleagues from other medical specialties in the patient's care, and coordinating this treatment with the work of ward personnel from all professional disciplines.

In addition, the medical director has a central role in facilitating a comprehensive educational program on the inpatient unit, as well as throughout the hospital. This is particularly important in the treatment of psychiatric patients with concurrent medical illness, as this is an area frequently neglected by training and continuing education programs. In addition to providing daily instruction concerning these issues on ward rounds and in multidisciplinary team meetings, the medical director helps plan a broad-based didactic program that addresses clinical situations frequently encountered by mental health personnel (e.g., psychiatric manifestations of endocrinologic disorders, etiology of dementia, drug interactions between psychotropics and common medications), procedures for common medical emergencies (e.g., seizure disorder, blood sugar abnormalities, cardiac arrhythmias), and idiosyncratic patient care issues, as illustrated by the following case.

Brian W., a 19-year-old college sophomore, was transferred to the mental health unit from the Oncology Service when he became precipitously suspicious, then menacing toward caretakers he had known for a period of months. He had been receiving a second course of chemotherapy for an osteosarcoma that had earlier necessitated the amputation of his leg, when he became acutely psychotic and threatening. After transfer to the Psychiatry Service, Mr. W. was medicated with neuroleptics and immediately placed in an opened seclusion room, where he remained for a period of time uncharacteristically long for a patient on the unit.

Following discussions with the nursing coordinator, the medical

director concluded that staff members were reluctant to involve themselves actively with Mr. W., an avoidance not felt to be caused by
countertransference issues of dealing with a dying patient or one who
was potentially violent. It was ultimately discovered that staff members
were concerned that they would be unable to monitor safely the medical
impact of Mr. W.'s chemotherapy regimen, as they were uneducated
about its side effects. There was, for example, a shared fantasy among
many ward personnel that his antimetabolites were responsible for his
paranoia. When the medical director recognized the root of the therapeutic impasse, he arranged for an oncologist to conduct an inservice
program on the fundamentals of chemotherapy. This cognitive training,
effected via an educational program, greatly reduced the staff's collec-
tive resistance toward Mr. W. They began to respond to his psychotic
behavior as they would with other patients, promoting his rapid clinical
improvement.

Finally, in addition to the medical director's usual administrative
duties, he or she has specific responsibilities related to patients with
concurrent psychiatric and medical illness. For example, these individuals
often have unusual needs concerning length of stay and utilization review
criteria (Fogel and Stoudemire 1986), requiring the medical director to
coordinate decision making with members of other clinical departments
and the hospital's administrative hierarchy, and to actively discuss these
issues with third-party payors.

Medical psychiatry cannot be successfully implemented without a
multidisciplinary team structure that regularly facilitates active, ongoing
interaction among professional disciplines on the inpatient unit. This
treatment philosophy provides the flexibility required for comprehensive
assessment and treatment of all patients; however, as I have indicated, it is
essential when working with patients who have concurrent medical illness, as they routinely require rapid modifications to their therapeutic
regimen, and careful aftercare planning through a network of medical and
mental health resources that work in conjunction with the inpatient unit.

Andrea F., a 72-year-old woman with long-standing arteriosclerotic
disease, was admitted to the Psychiatry Service because of severe depression. She had insidiously developed increasing neurovegetative symptoms during the previous 6 months, which had initially been attributed

to progressive debilitation from her heart disease. However, Mrs. F.'s husband arranged for a psychiatric evaluation because she began having "crying spells like she did during the change of life," when she had been treated as an outpatient with unknown medications for a major depression.

At the time of her current admission Mrs. F. appeared emaciated and sickly, exhibited severe psychomotor retardation, and was practically mute. Clinical evaluation and laboratory testing suggested malnutrition secondary to anorexia, and the initial treatment focused on monitored feeding and hydration. The medical and nursing staffs worked closely together to achieve this end, with consultation from the hospital's dietary department. Mrs. F.'s cardiovascular status was simultaneously assessed by her internist. Blood testing suggested that she had not been taking her prescribed digoxin; an electrocardiogram, echocardiogram, electroencephalogram, and CT scan of her head did not indicate acute pathology. Her cardiovascular status was judged to be stable, despite a heart rhythm of "atrial flutter/fibrillation," and mild cerebral atrophy presumably secondary to arteriosclerotic changes consistent with the two myocardial infarctions she had had earlier. Mrs. F.'s overall medical status was guarded.

Despite close attention by the nursing staff, Mrs. F. remained extremely withdrawn, initiating no spontaneous activity (including eating) without direct and active prompting. The multidisciplinary team felt discouraged, fearful of "losing the patient" without more aggressive treatment. The nursing staff increased the acuity of her care, essentially providing one-to-one interaction throughout her waking hours. Despite the staff feeding Mrs. F., she continued to lose weight and remained dehydrated. At the urging of the nursing staff, her meals were supplemented by carefully monitored intravenous feedings, which stabilized her fluid and electrolyte balance but not her inanition.

Further discussion among the nursing and medical staff members of the multidisciplinary team produced a consensus for intensified treatment of Mrs. F. Options for somatic interventions were presented to the medical director, who agreed that the time required to reach a therapeutic blood level with antidepressant medications argued against their use. After consultation with her cardiologist, the medical director decided to treat Mrs. F. with a psychostimulant (methylphenidate). The patient had a positive response to the medication, with diminished psychomotor withdrawal, slightly improved independent functioning, and (most importantly) considerably improved nutritional status.

At this point in Mrs. F.'s care, the treatment team was able to shift from a medical to a more psychotherapeutic stance. Mrs. F. was asked to attend ward activities, in an attempt to provide structure and support and to build the alliance that would permit talking therapy. Unfortunately, she had little positive response to any of these interventions, and in fact began to regress. This prompted discussion of additional somatic interventions, which resulted in the recommendation to use ECT. Mrs. F.'s treatment again shifted back to a more medical approach, focused on the workup for ECT, as well as a coordinated discussion with her internist and cardiologist concerning possible contraindications to this course. The decision was made to proceed with ECT, which caused progressive affective improvement over a 2-week period. Mrs. F. became mildly confused, again requiring increased efforts from the nursing staff to provide assistance with activities of daily living and additional structure during this period of disorientation.

As Mrs. F.'s disorganization remitted, she was again reintegrated into the various activities of the therapeutic milieu. Her adaptation was much improved from the previous attempt, though she still resisted talking openly about her recent decline. It was therefore decided to involve her in more concrete treatment programs, particularly occupational therapy, as she enjoyed the relationship with personnel in that group. In the context of working on individual and group projects, Mrs. F. became progressively more revealing about some psychosocial stressors that had contributed to her decompensation. Her comfort in discussing these matters increased, and she was successfully encouraged to explore them in individual therapy with her psychiatrist and with various members of her multidisciplinary team. A measure of her ability and willingness to do so was her eventual active participation in group psychotherapy. As she continued to improve, the focus of treatment shifted to discharge planning. Members of the Social Service Department became more involved with Mrs. F. and her husband, both to provide guidance and appropriate reassurance to the couple concerning the transition to home and to help arrange for Mrs. F.'s psychiatric aftercare.

Mrs. F. made excellent progress during her 6-week hospitalization. The multidisciplinary team's ability to effectively share and continually reassess essential clinical data created a therapeutic environment that permitted rapid, pragmatic therapeutic responses to the changing clinical status of her psychiatric and medical needs—which were essentially interdependent.

PSYCHOTHERAPY

General Principles

Fundamental changes in the therapeutic milieu, along with the movement toward briefer hospitalizations, has limited the practice of long-term, insight-oriented inpatient psychotherapy and placed greater reliance on a panoply of treatments (e.g., group psychotherapy, family therapy, and psychoeducation programs). This increased flexibility facilitates planning of a comprehensive psychotherapeutic regimen that simultaneously focuses on the patient's major psychopathology, as well as any abnormal emotional response that may have been precipitated by a concurrent physical illness.

> Theodore C., a 53-year-old salesman with non-insulin-dependent adult-onset diabetes, was admitted to the Psychiatry Service because of mild confusion and progressive neurovegetative symptoms that had interfered with his ability to work. As a college student, Mr. C. had been successfully treated for a dysthymic disorder with individual and group psychotherapy. He never required antidepressant medication, which was significant given the prevalence of alcohol abuse and major affective illness among his paternal relatives. At age 46, Mr. C. had a mild, uncomplicated heart attack that responded well to treatment. However, he began to experience transient cerebral ischemic attacks 4 years later, and his current depression began soon after the last of these episodes. After an extensive medical and psychological evaluation, Mr. C. was diagnosed as follows:

> Axis I: (1) r/o Organic mood disorder
>   (3) r/o Major depression
> Axis II: (1) Obsessional and passive-dependent traits
> Axis III: (1) Diabetes mellitus
>   (2) s/p Myocardial infarction
>   (3) Transient cerebral ischemia

Like many psychiatric patients with concurrent physical illness, Mr. C.'s clinical issues are complex. Determining the type and role of psychotherapy in a treatment approach that integrates psychological and medical interventions requires evaluation of three broad areas. First, it is necessary to assess the psychodynamic and psychogenetic issues contributing to a patient's clinical decompensation. For example, in Mr. C.'s case, it is important to determine whether the recent stressor of declining health reactivated the unconscious conflicts that contributed to the dysthymic episode of his youth. If so, psychotherapy would be more exploratory, focusing on a central conflict (e.g., dependency concerns related to his compromised physical functioning, reflecting similar issues precipitated by the move away to college). On the other hand, if Mr. C.'s diagnostic workup suggested a major depressive episode similar to those of other family members, pharmacotherapy would be indicated in combination with the psychotherapeutic work.

Second, the patient's personality structure must be carefully evaluated when planning a psychotherapeutic regimen, as it has considerable implications concerning whether the approach should be anxiety suppressing or anxiety provoking. Axis II traits also affect a person's ability to psychologically cope with physical illness (Bibring 1965; Kahana and Bibring 1964), a common focus of treatment with medically ill patients.

Finally, there must be a careful assessment of the patient's illness dynamics, the idiosyncratic meaning an individual assigns to a particular illness during a particular phase of the life cycle (Green 1985). This entails a biopsychosocial evaluation of the patient, with a comprehensive assessment of his or her physical pathology and an analysis of how it affects and is affected by psychosocial issues.

For example, in addition to Mr. C.'s concern about his current physical well-being, his response to repeated transient ischemic attacks (TIAs) included disturbing ruminations about his future life. His repeated statements about his mortality were unusual, given his age and the fact that his medical illness was not immediately life-threatening. He also expressed concern that he would be unable to provide for his family and that he would be deprived of the opportunity to watch his children grow to maturity. Each of these issues was addressed in his overall psychotherapeutic treatment.

Mr. C.'s workup determined that his mental status changes had a mixed etiology. Neurologic assessment, including brain imaging and neuropsychological testing, indicated mild, bilateral cerebral ischemia in the frontal cortices, most probably secondary to small vessel changes consistent with diabetes mellitus. Psychiatric assessment, based on clinical evaluation and psychological testing, suggested a major depression characterized by neurovegetative symptoms and some degree of pseudodementia. His biologic depression was aggravated by a depressive response (Green 1985) to the progression of his diabetes. Mr. C.'s multiple diagnoses—organic mood disorder and major depression—required a multifaceted treatment approach that stressed varied interventions during different phases of his hospitalization.

Mr. C. was prescribed nortriptyline, chosen because of its relatively low anticholinergic effects. His initially low dose, designed to minimize any potential for aggravating his organic deficits, was gradually increased until his neurovegetative symptoms, particularly social withdrawal, remitted. As his therapeutic alliance with individual staff members increased, Mr. C. became more interactive, particularly in group psychotherapy and occupational therapy.

When Mr. C. had returned to his premorbid state, the staff initiated an insight-oriented approach to his psychotherapy, focusing on several areas. The first was his long-standing dependency issues, including a review of his depressive episode earlier in life, and exploration of ongoing difficulties in Mr. C.'s relationship with his father. This work primarily occurred on an individual basis with his psychiatrist and other mental health personnel on his treatment team. Second, there was considerable discussion of the patient's concern about the effects of his chronic medical illness. Mr. C. began to grieve his loss of health, by assessing his current physical limitations, then addressing his "worst fears"(i.e., that he would first become impotent and then eventually "a senile fool").

Initial discussion with his therapist was expanded to couples work, which allowed Mr. C., for the first time, to share these feelings with his wife. In addition to the mutual support provided by these meetings, they also provided a forum to plan concretely for (potential) future issues (e.g., financial concerns, the prospect of severe debility due to multiple strokes, and the possibility of his sudden death). The social worker began meeting regularly with Mrs. C. to provide her additional support. Coincident with this intensive psychotherapeutic experience was careful and constant monitoring of Mr. C.'s medical condition, which was reassuring to the C.s as they became increasingly cognizant of the relationship between his physical and emotional condition. Shortly before discharge, Mr. and Mrs. C. began attending an education group conducted by the Endocrinology Service that presented an overview of the impact and effects of diabetes mellitus, distributed and discussed literature about the illness, and kept the couple apprised of support resources in the community.

Mr. C.'s case is an excellent illustration of how the interplay between psychiatric and medical disorders affects an individual's psychotherapeutic treatment. Aspects of Mr. C.'s psychosexual development, his probable biologic predisposition to depression, and his emotional reaction to a chronic illness all contributed to a distinctive clinical presentation that warranted a similarly distinctive psychotherapeutic regimen. The case highlights some common psychotherapy issues that arise in patients with concurrent medical and psychiatric illness, such as conflicts over dependency and feelings of anger and/or guilt toward caretakers (Stoudemire and Fogel 1986), the need to grieve over loss of one's health (Green 1985), and the relationship of dependency to the sick role (Parsons 1951). In addition to addressing one's major psychiatric disorder, working through these various issues often becomes a central psychotherapeutic goal when treating patients with concurrent medical illness.

Pathologic Illness Responses

Certain individuals develop diagnosable psychiatric disorders solely because of their inability to effectively grieve the losses incurred by ill health. For many reasons, they are unable to recognize, feel, or come to terms with some or all of the emotions precipitated by medical illness. They may completely deny their feelings or, more commonly, may experience one emotion to the relative exclusion of all others. In effect, these patients get stuck in a particular stage of the grief process, become consciously or unconsciously preoccupied with the feelings characteristic of that phase, and consequently do not attain an emotional resolution regarding their loss of health. Rather, they develop an abnormal psychological reaction to illness, usually characterized by excessive denial, anger, anxiety, depression, or dependency (Green 1985).

Randolph A., a 40-year-old widower, was a midlevel manager diligently working his way up the corporate ladder while supporting three young

children. In addition to family responsibilities and professional obliga-
tions, Mr. A. devoted considerable time to a flourishing relationship
with a 32-year-old co-worker whom he hoped to marry. His past history
was significant for the unexpected death of his mother, from a cerebro-
vascular accident, when he was 13 years old.

Mr. A.'s life changed dramatically when he had a mild heart attack
while driving to work. After surviving the immediate threat of death, his
initial anxiety was progressively supplanted by a growing sense of helplessness. The death of his mother at an early age sensitized Mr. A. to loss,
and specifically affected his psychological development by enhancing
dependent yearnings. Moreover, because she died of a cardiovascular
illness, he more closely associated his heart disease with his mother's
sudden demise. He also identified with his children's concerns, as he,
too, had experienced the anxiety that comes from recognizing that one's
future depends on the welfare of a single parent.

Mr. A. became angry and anxious when he considered the impact of
his illness on his career and on the developing relationship with his
girlfriend. All these factors contributed to a heightened affective response to his physical impairment, which interfered with his ability to
resolve the intense feelings precipitated by his heart attack. As a result,
Mr. A. became increasingly anxious and dependent on others.

Because of an inability to effectively grieve his loss of health, Mr. A.
experienced a continuing emotional distress that negatively affected his
physical well-being. His excessive helplessness resulted in treatment noncompliance that, in conjunction with his heightened anxiety, caused an
intermittent cardiac arrhythmia. Worry about "my declining health" further impeded his return to routine functioning, as he became progressively negativistic and passive. This type of abnormal psychological
response to physical illness signals the need for medical psychotherapy, a
specialized form of psychotherapeutic intervention that primarily addresses the patient's emotional life as it relates to his or her physical
welfare. Medical psychotherapy is based on "the communicated understanding between physician and patient concerning the biologic, psychologic, and social aspects" of the individual's illness (Goldberg and Green
1985, p. 174).

Medical psychotherapy is utilized for crisis situations (e.g., acute
onset of illness) or chronic conditions (e.g., persisting illness) and can

take a supportive or introspective approach. Just as illness dynamics determine whether a patient has a healthy emotional adaptation to illness as opposed to pathologic denial or crippling anxiety, these dynamics also dictate the psychotherapeutic treatment of the abnormal illness response that occurs. Medical psychotherapy designed to facilitate grief work is indicated in patients with a demonstrated ability to work through the powerful emotions accompanying loss of health. On the other hand, this insight-oriented approach may be contraindicated in patients who are obviously overwhelmed by their current affective state. The latter group benefits from measures that support adaptive ego functioning, such as supplying an obsessional patient with extensive information about his or her day-to-day condition. The expert knowledge of clinicians concerning the substantive and temporal course of grief work is counterproductive if it prompts them to doggedly confront the defensive structure and maladaptive behaviors of psychologically immature individuals. Attempts to pressure patients through the various stages of grief is more likely to foster a clinical regression—often seen, for example, in individuals with traditional psychosomatic ailments (Sifneos 1973) and psychophysiologic disorders (Sifneos 1972–1973).

There are also clinical situations where patients' emotional distress is so extreme that psychotherapeutic interventions alone fail to ameliorate their level of dysfunction. When individuals experience severe affective turmoil or exhibit a pathologic denial that inhibits the emotional and/or intellectual appreciation of an illness, then pharmacotherapy is indicated. Psychoactive medications may then be employed as the primary treatment modality (e.g., prescribing major tranquilizers for delirium or a postoperative psychosis) or adjunctive to psychotherapy (e.g., utilizing minor tranquilizers to control the anticipatory anxiety exacerbating an individual's angina).

When treating medical and surgical patients unable to contend with the emotions precipitated by illness, the clinician's most important decision concerns a clear delineation of therapeutic goals. The physician must choose between commending and encouraging the patient's usual style of emotional functioning, or pursuing a more analytic path. The former approach, which attempts to foster an atmosphere of support and reassurance that can then be exploited to enhance the clinician's positive influence, may or may not include the use of psychoactive medications. The latter course, which helps the patient work through the conflictual feelings precipitated by his or her illness, is based on the principles of brief psychodynamic psychotherapy as described by Davanloo (1980), Malan (1976), and Sifneos (1972).

The decision as to whether a patient with an abnormal illness response requires introspective (i.e., anxiety-provoking) investigation of his emotions, or is more in need of reassurance and support (i.e., anxiety-suppressing) treatment, is founded on the systematic evaluation of objective clinical findings. The most fundamental of these is an accurate DSM-III-R multiaxial psychiatric diagnosis, particularly as it applies to major mental illness. For example, medically ill patients with major depression require initial supportive interventions (usually somatic treatments) to alleviate their symptoms (Cohen-Cole and Stoudemire 1987; Rifkin et al. 1985). When patients do not exhibit evidence of significant Axis I pathology, the most useful criteria for determining the type of medical psychotherapy required are their level of ego functioning (Vaillant 1977) and the maturity of object relationships. Other important parameters parallel the more rigid selection criteria for brief psychotherapy proposed by Sifneos (1972).

Medical psychotherapy is not confined to individual treatment but can occur in the context of family therapy, couples work, or group psychotherapy, each of which may be anxiety suppressing or anxiety provoking. Couples work is indicated when a patient's abnormal illness response causes increasing distance in the relationship, possibly threatening its viability. The treatment helps to improve communication between spouses, either by discussing generalized problems (e.g., a mutual withdrawal caused by smouldering resentments) or specific issues (e.g., decreased sexual intimacy due to the transient impotence caused by a husband's diabetes). Couples work provides support during the crisis of illness, allows for mutual exploration of the resulting (often unstated) emotions, and can serve an important educational role concerning specific medical issues.

Group therapies can be useful in helping patients work through fundamental psychological issues. Insight-oriented work has traditionally been used in the treatment of classic psychosomatic illnesses (Stein 1971) and has been effective in helping patients adjust to terminal illness (Spiegel 1979; Spiegel et al. 1989; Yalom and Greaves 1977). Groups are also effective as a supportive form of medical psychotherapy. Information sharing helps diminish feelings of alienation and isolation by bolstering patients' interpersonal contact and providing psychological support (Bilodeau and Hackett 1971). Groups also foster a generalized acceptance of emotional expression (Adsett and Bruhn 1968; Stein 1971) and may be particularly useful in helping patients facilitate or reestablish social skills that have been compromised by depression secondary to their medical illness. This often occurs in the context of discussing common medical experiences (e.g., amputation, myocardial infarction, or the impact of a mastectomy or colostomy [Slaby and Glicksman 1985]).

Though anxiety-suppressing and anxiety-provoking therapies are both founded on psychodynamic principles, each has distinctive behavioral and cognitive attributes that can be used to considerable advantage with patients with combined psychiatric and medical illness. Supportive treatment, in particular, often occurs within a clinical framework quite removed from psychodynamic therapy. Useful behavioral interventions include relaxation protocols and desensitization (e.g., to treat excessive anxiety) or positive and negative reinforcement (e.g., to deal with excessive regression). Cognitive therapy is useful for many depressed patients who have low self-esteem associated with illness (Beck 1969; Lewinsohn 1974). Moos and Schaefer (1984) describes a specific cognitive approach, based on crisis theory, for treating patients unable to cope with the impact of physical illness. He outlines two sets of treatment goals for these individuals—illness-related tasks (e.g., dealing with pain and incapacitation, and dealing with the hospital environment) and general tasks (e.g., preserving a reasonable emotional balance, and sustaining relationships with family and friends). The treatment includes fundamental interventions of supportive therapy (e.g., education, reassurance, and abreaction) effected via cognitive, problem-solving techniques.

REFERENCES

Adsett C, Bruhn J: Short-term group psychotherapy for myocardial infarction patients and their wives. Can Med Assoc J 99:577–581, 1968

American Psychiatric Association: Diagnostic and Statistical Manual of Mental Disorders, 3rd Edition, Revised. Washington, DC, American Psychiatric Association, 1987

Asch S: The psychiatric inpatient unit: 1947 to 1986. Psychiatr Clin North Am 10(2):155–164, 1987

Beck A: Depression: Clinical, Experimental and Theoretical Aspects. New York, Harper & Row, 1969

Bibring G: Psychiatry in medical practice in the general hospital. N Engl J Med 254:336–372, 1965

Bilodeau C, Hackett T: Issues raised in a group setting by patients recovering from myocardial infarction. Am J Psychiatry 128:73–78, 1971

Cohen-Cole S, Stoudemire A: Major depression and physical illness. Psychiatr Clin North Am 10(1):1–17, 1987

Davanloo H (ed): Short Term Dynamic Psychotherapy. New York, Jason Aronson, 1980

Engel G: The need for a new medical model: a challenge for biomedicine. Science 196:129–136, 1977

Engel G: The clinical application of the biopsychosocial model. Am J Psychiatry 137:535–544, 1980

Fogel B, Stoudemire A: Organization and development of combined medical-psychiatric units, part 2. Psychosomatics 27(6):417–420, 1986

Fogel B, Stoudemire A, Houpt J: Contrasting models for conjoint medical and psychiatric inpatient treatment: psych/med vs. med/psych. Am J Psychiatry 142:1085–1089, 1985

Goldberg R, Green S: Medical psychotherapy. Am Fam Physician 31(1):173–178, 1985

Goodman B: Combined psychiatric-medical inpatient units: the Mount Sinai Model. Psychosomatics 26(3):179–189, 1985

Green S: Mind and Body: The Psychology of Physical Illness. Washington, DC, American Psychiatric Press, 1985

Hall R, Popkin M, DeVaul R, et al: Physical illness presenting as psychiatric disease. Arch Gen Psychiatry 35:1315–1320, 1978

Hall R, Gardner E, Stickney S, et al: Physical illness manifesting as psychiatric disease: analysis of a state hospital inpatient population. Arch Gen Psychiatry 37:989–995, 1980

Kahana R, Bibring G: Personality types in medical management, in Psychiatry and Medical Practice in a General Hospital. Edited by Zinberg N. New York, International Universities Press, 1964, pp 108–123

Knight E, Folstein M: Unsuspected emotional and cognitive disturbance in medical inpatients. Ann Intern Med 87:723–724, 1977

Lewinsohn P: A behavioral approach to depression, in The Psychology of Depression. Edited by Friedman R, Katz M. Washington, DC, Winston-Wiley, 1974

Maguire G, Granville-Grossman K: Physical illness in psychiatric patients. Br J Psychiatry 114:1365–1369, 1968

Malan D: The Frontier of Brief Psychiatry. New York, Plenum, 1976

Moffic H, Paykel E: Depression in medical inpatients. Br J Psychiatry 126:346–353, 1975

Moos R, Schaefer J: The crisis of physical illness: an overview and conceptual approach, in Coping with Physical Illness, 2: New Perspectives. Edited by Moos R. New York, Plenum, 1984, pp 3–25

Parsons T: The Social System. Glencoe, IL, Free Press, 1951

Reiser M: Changing theoretical concepts in psychosomatic medicine, in American Handbook of Psychiatry, Vol 4. Edited by Reiser M. New York, Basic Books, 1975, pp 477–500

Rifkin A, Reardon G, Siris S, et al: Trimipramine in physical illness with depression. J Clin Psychiatry 46:4–8, 1985

Robbins L, Regier D (eds): Psychiatric Disorders in America: The Epidemiologic Catchment Area Study. New York, Free Press, 1991

Rodin G, Voshart K: Depression in the medically ill: overview. Am J Psychiatry 143:696–705, 1986

Sifneos P: Short-Term Psychotherapy and Emotional Crisis. Cambridge, MA, Harvard University Press, 1972

Sifneos P: Is dynamic psychotherapy contraindicated for a large number of patients with psychosomatic diseases? Psychother Psychosom 21:133–136, 1972–1973

Sifneos P: The prevalence of "alexithymic" characteristics in psychosomatic patients. Psychother Psychosom 22:255–262, 1973

Slaby A, Glicksman A: Adapting to Life-Threatening Illness. New York, Praeger, 1985

Spiegel D: Psychological support for women with metastatic carcinoma. Psychosomatics 20:780–787, 1979

Spiegel D, Bloom J, Kraemer H, et al: Effect of psychosocial treatment on survival of patients with metastatic breast cancer. Lancet 2:888–891, 1989

Stein A: Group therapy with psychosomatically ill patients, in Comprehensive Group Psychotherapy. Edited by Kaplan H, Sadock B. Baltimore, MD, Williams & Wilkins, 1971

Stoudemire A, Fogel B: Organization and development of combined medical-psychiatric units: part I. Psychosomatics 27(5):341–345, 1986

Stoudemire A, Fogel B: The emergence of medical psychiatry: a provocative viewpoint. Psychosomatics 29(2):207–213, 1988

Strain J: Needs for psychiatry in the general hospital. Hosp Community Psychiatry 33:996–1002, 1982

Strain J, Leibowitz M, Klein D: Anxiety and panic attacks in the medically ill. Psychiatr Clin North Am 4:333–350, 1981

Vaillant G: Adaptation to Life. Boston, MA, Little, Brown, 1977

Von Korff M, Shapiro S, Burke J, et al: Anxiety and depression in a primary care clinic. Arch Gen Psychiatry 44:152–156, 1987

Yalom I, Greaves C: Group therapy with the terminally ill. Am J Psychiatry 134:396–400, 1977

CHAPTER 11

Adolescent Inpatient Psychotherapy

Marcia Slomowitz, M.D.

In recent years, several trends have led to the expansion of acute inpatient services for children and adolescents. Data on the limits of long-term residential treatment for severely disturbed children decreased clinicians' enthusiasm for long-term care (Lewis et al. 1980). Insurance companies provided benefits for inpatient treatment, in the belief that these costs could be controlled by limiting the length of stay (Geraty 1989). The acute inpatient unit began to be seen as one site of treatment along a continuum of treatment modalities with specific goals and treatment capacities.

In 1980, 81,532 children under age 18 were admitted to psychiatric beds. Of this number, 67% were ages 15 to 17, 28% ages 10 to 14, and 5% under age 10. Thus, the vast majority of hospitalized children were adolescents. Twenty percent were hospitalized in state or county hospitals and 21% in private psychiatric hospitals. The number of episodes of hospitalization for children 18 and under increased in 1985 to 109,941. The major growth was in the number of admissions to general hospitals without psychiatric units (Kiesler and Simpkins 1991). In 1980, the length of stay for the majority of these patients (87%) was 90 days or less (Milazzo-Sayre 1986). Commercial insurance was the primary source of payment for 50%–75% of adolescent patients admitted to private facilities between 1970 and 1980, with Medicaid and Medicare becoming increasing sources of payment in general hospitals and county hospitals (Thompson et al. 1986).

Over the past 20 years, there has been a shift in the diagnosis and symptoms of the children admitted, with an increase in patients with depression and violent behavior. Between 1970 and 1980, the diagnosis of affective disorders in 10- to 18-year-olds increased in non-Federal general hospitals, state and county hospitals, and private psychiatric hospitals. In reviewing trends in violence among psychiatrically hospitalized adolescents ages 12 to 17 from 1969 to 1979, one-half of the boys exhibited extremely violent behavior in both years, whereas the proportion of girls with violent behavior increased significantly from 12% to 48% (Inamdar et al. 1986).

Equally important changes are seen in the families of the children hospitalized. In 1975, 70% of the parents of school-age children in one institution were intact two-parent families; by 1985, this number fell to 30%. Increased numbers of foster parents were noted, as were nontraditional family constellations with homosexual or bisexual parents (Jemerin and Philips 1988).

In the 1950s and 1960s, the predominant model for adolescent treatment was long-term treatment predicated on a psychoanalytic model. Because the treatment goals were to effect substantial changes in the patient's character structure, the average length of stay was from 2 to 4 years. The hospital served as a secondary conflict-free home in which the child could develop more normally. Diverse groups of adolescents were treated in these settings, including those with severe personality disorders and major mental illnesses such as schizophrenia.

More recently, because of shortening of important stays, models for short-term treatment have been developed. Instead of lengthy reconstructive work, attention is focused on an in-depth assessment of the child and the family, then linking them with outpatient services to provide continuity of care. Tasks of treatment include stabilizing the tumultuous events surrounding the crisis, assessing the developmental strengths and weaknesses of the adolescent and parents, and beginning the inpatient treatment program and developing aftercare plans (Parmelee 1986). The latter might include individual or group therapy, family therapy, and education. The hospital thus responds to the crisis situations of adolescents and families and provides the groundwork for further care. The outpatient site becomes the place where reconstructive work can be done (Goodrich 1987).

THE DEVELOPMENTAL NEEDS OF ADOLESCENTS

Fundamental to understanding the role of inpatient treatment (and of psychotherapy as part of the treatment) is an appreciation of the developmental issues of adolescence.

The developmental phase of adolescence encompasses growth and maturation physically, cognitively, and socially. The physical changes—and the responses to them—are the most dramatic. The intensification of sexual urges, coupled with growth, lead to possibilities of adult sexual gratification not heretofore available to the child. Developing sexuality fills the child with pride at his or her new capacities (Galatzer-Levy 1991).

Cognitive changes bring about a sense of history about the child's place in the world (i.e., that he or she has both a past and a future; Galatzer-Levy and Cohler 1990). The child thinks of him- or herself as an emerging adult, in the process of becoming (Galatzer-Levy 1991).

The worldview of an adolescent is substantially different from that of grade school-age youngsters. Younger children follow rules to gain adult approval. Adolescents use their own principles, which may come into conflict with community or parental rules. As they develop intellectually, they use more sophisticated defensive styles.

Socially, adolescents begin to move away from the protection of the family to the world outside, seeking out friendships. The egocentricity of childhood evolves into a reciprocity of relationships. Such relationships compensate for the loss of the family and provide a means to become part of a larger group. Ideally, adolescents begin to develop loyalty, intimacy, and a sense of mutuality in their relationships. This implies a capacity for dealing with others in a cooperative, nonmanipulative, and respectful fashion. The development of empathy marks another milestone.

Failure to advance along expected developmental tracks can lead to crises precipitating hospitalization. The adolescent phase of life brings with it predictable tasks to be accomplished. Social and academic expectations may exceed the capacity of some adolescents to cope. If earlier childhood years were problematic, those difficulties will be added on to the new demands. Families that had been at ease with the younger child may respond differently to their more sexual youngster.

In psychotherapy, the task of the clinician is to understand the meaning of the individual's and family's behavior in the context of their developmental timetable. The psychiatric treatment of adolescents takes into account the developmental levels of an individual, understanding how far along patient and family may be in any particular sequence.

INDICATIONS FOR HOSPITALIZATION

The Joint Commission on Accreditation of Hospitals (1974), the American Medical Association (1972), the American Psychiatric Association (1976), and the American Academy of Child and Adolescent Psychiatry (1989) have defined admission criteria for children and adolescents in psychiatric settings. The following are guidelines summarized from their criteria:

1. The adolescent's behavior or threatened behavior indicates that his or her life or that of someone else is in danger and that the family or other support system cannot provide safety. This may include episodes of drug use or psychosis in which the adolescent's high level of unpredictability creates the potential for life-threatening behavior.
2. The adolescent must have a psychiatric disorder, and the psychiatric disorder must be of such severity as to cause impairment of daily functioning in two important areas of the adolescent's life (i.e., school performance, social interactions, or family relationships).
3. The adolescent has had a prolonged period of disturbing and disruptive behavior for which outpatient treatment was either unsuccessful or refused. Examples of such behavior include physical or intense verbal arguments with family and friends, truancy, school failure, drug and alcohol abuse, running away, promiscuity, and increasingly withdrawn behavior.
4. The adolescent may have been in outpatient treatment for a protracted period of time, and the treatment has stalemated. The clinician may suggest to the adolescent and family that hospitalization can help break through the therapeutic impasse.
5. The court may mandate hospital treatment (Parmelee 1986).

Additionally, beyond the symptomatic behavior of the adolescent, the proposed inpatient treatment must be relevant to the problems diagnosed and adjudged likely to benefit the patient. Other available but less restrictive treatment resources must be considered inappropriate to the patient's needs or have been attempted and proven unsuccessful (American Academy of Child and Adolescent Psychiatry 1989).

There is controversy as to whether adolescents should be treated on general psychiatric units or on specialized adolescent units. Adult inpatients are seen as either harmful influences and poor role models (Easson 1969) or as adult figures that recreate a sense of community or family (Bond and Auger 1982). Most of the clinical reports describe adolescent-adult wards (Beskind 1962; Elliott et al. 1980; Fineberg et al. 1980). The majority of the reports were written when lengths of stay were much longer than they are today.

One outcome study compared adolescents hospitalized on mixed adult-adolescent wards with no specific services to adolescents on mixed ward with special services, and then to adolescents hospitalized on specialized adolescent units. The presence of special services was associated with better outcome whether the patients were on all-adolescent or mixed wards. Data were gathered from clinical sites, and patients were not assigned or matched in any way.

Consistent with these findings, a policy statement from the American Academy of Child and Adolescent Psychiatry (1989) states:

> Unless there are compelling clinical reasons to the contrary, or serious limitations in availability, children and adolescents younger than 16 years of age should be admitted only to programs that are designed for children and adolescents and physically distinct from programs for adult psychiatric patients. Adolescents 16 and older may be admitted to adult units for valid clinical reasons, but should be treated in a program specifically designed for hospitalized adolescent psychiatric patients. (pp. 1–4)

Thus adolescents are hospitalized for containment and provision of intensive, comprehensive treatment. Within this context, the psychotherapies employed serve to arrest and forestall further developmental deviation. Ultimately, the hope is that adolescents will renew their capacity to grow and develop and to learn how to approach and change difficult situations (Galatzer-Levy 1991).

PSYCHOTHERAPY CONSIDERATIONS

Many adolescents begin their hospital stay with mistrust and skepticism. They complain that parents forced them into the hospital against their will. Frequently, this stance represents bravado overlying an awareness of failure and a feeling of helplessness. To overcome this resistance, the clinician must engage the adolescent around issues of concern to the inpatient. Agreement on goals of the hospitalization and for individual psychotherapy is important in the development of the alliance. Articulating these goals provides a sense of meaning and order to the psychotherapy while enhancing the adolescent's sense of competence and mastery (Parmelee 1986). For this reason, it is also important to negotiate the rules of psychotherapy, including frequency, duration, and compliance with sessions. The following clinical vignette illustrates the issues.

> Sherri J. was a 16-year-old admitted after an overdose of aspirin. She adamantly stated that she was fine and needed no help. The psychiatrist learned she had been rejected by her boyfriend and felt abandoned by her parents because of their apparent lack of concern about this event.
>
> Sherri and the psychiatrist began their work together with an agreement that the overdose was a response to her disappointments and that this was a matter to be taken seriously. They developed a plan in which Sherri and the psychiatrist would talk about what triggered the overdose and how to prevent another one. Sherri also wanted her family to understand her feelings about their behavior, so family psychotherapy sessions were initiated.

Adolescents are concerned about independence, but they are still dependent on their families for a variety of needs. It is therefore predictable that they will test their psychiatrists to see if they are really interested in them and their problems, or if the therapists are the agents of their parents. They will look for evidence that therapists wish to censor or judge them, much as others in their life may do. They will be rightfully wary of being traumatized again by adults, and they therefore may be reluctant to be forthcoming in psychotherapy.

Therapists can facilitate the development of a relationship with the youngster through active participation. At times, therapists may alternately act as sounding boards for future plans, address specific vocational or educational issues, give direct advice, and provide information on sex (Jaffe 1991). They can wonder out loud how they might feel if they were in the patient's position. They can also acknowledge issues common to adolescents as they grow up.

An objective of the psychotherapy in short-term inpatient care is to help adolescents tolerate emotional stresses and develop stronger and more effective defenses against anxiety. Unconscious conflicts need not be explicitly interpreted. The focus is on the here-and-now conflicts in real life, helping patients to reach effective solutions and master difficult situations. Adolescents are offered a chance of a new kind of relationship, rather than the distorted and anxiety-ridden ones they may have with their parents. As with other inpatient populations discussed in this book, psychotherapy is more clearly thought of as reeducative and supportive, rather than as uncovering or exploratory (Hersov and Bentovim 1985).

Psychotherapy emphasizes self-development and competent function, not conflict resolution (Jaffe 1991). The following clinical example highlights this issue.

> Carol S. was a 15-year-old hospitalized because of recurrent depression and anxiety that persisted after 6 months of outpatient treatment. Her symptoms were of sufficient severity to lead to her refusing to go to school and withdrawing from her peers. The psychiatrist and outpatient therapist understood the symptoms in terms of apprehension about her attractiveness, her dating, and her burgeoning sexual interest. Carol and her psychiatrist developed a plan in which she would try to understand her experiences with other patients on the unit in order to feel less overwhelmed by interpersonal issues and to enhance her competence in interactions with her peers.

Some of these adolescents can express affect only through physical behavior, aggressively and impulsively. Psychotherapy helps them learn to identify their feelings and communicate them verbally (Marohn 1991).

> Joe T. was a 17-year-old admitted to the hospital because of recurrent anger, depression, and threats of violence at home. He was failing the 10th grade. As a child, he was subjected to physical abuse by his drunken father. In the hospital, Joe frequently had his feelings hurt and retaliated

with angry threats toward staff and other patients. Individual and group psychotherapy interventions repeatedly focused on Joe's behavior and his feelings, helping him to identify the feelings that occurred before he became angry. He was asked to imagine how others felt when he yelled at them and was given suggestions in what he might say instead of threatening others.

Three types of verbal interventions have been described based on the level of self-organization. (Although these interventions are not designed specifically for adolescents, they are useful ways to think about the kinds of psychotherapeutic interventions available.)

1. Pacification, the provision of a soothing and consistent environment, is useful when an adolescent lacks the capacity for self-reflection.
2. Unification requires that the therapist present him- or herself as a real, responsive person who is able to help the patient reestablish stability when self-cohesion is disrupted.
3. Optimal frustration is used when self-cohesion is stable, but a patient needs help functioning realistically, without self-sustaining illusions.

Adolescents may shift between needing these three types of interventions, and the therapist must maintain empathic contact by understanding and intervening accordingly (Gedo and Goldberg 1973; Jaffe 1991). The next vignette illustrates the use of these interventions.

Leo B. was a 15-year-old hospitalized for depression. He also had a learning disorder and problems with academic performance. The psychiatrist listened to Leo's plans to develop competence in school, admiring his ability to struggle nightly with his learning problems. Leo began to tolerate his dysphoric feelings about school while developing coping strategies to improve his academic skills. However, after several days in the hospital, he was taunted by a patient and withdrew, refusing to go to school. The psychiatrist correctly suspected that Leo's burgeoning but fragile self-esteem was damaged by the taunting.

Therefore, the therapist shifted her stance and reminded Leo that even though his feelings were hurt, he was capable and could continue with his plans. This intervention allowed Leo to regain his self-esteem and continue thinking about his coping strategies.

Successful treatment also requires that therapists develop and sustain good working alliances with parents. Although adolescents may complain bitterly about their parents, they are also loyal. Most parents are concerned about their child's welfare. Therapists cannot assume that parents understand either their adolescents' psychology or the therapeutic process. They must start from the beginning, assuming that parents do not know, and make clear exactly what will happen and why.

Acknowledging that one's child is in serious psychological difficulties is painful and frightening. Parents will be concerned about why the problem occurred, what they have done, and what the future holds for them and their child. Additionally, parents often feel both angry at their youngster and relieved that the hospitalization will provide them with some respite.

The therapist must maintain alliances with both the adolescent and his or her parents (Galatzer-Levy 1991). As with individual therapy, the terms of family therapy must be negotiated. Parents and child must agree on the need for family therapy. The goals and content of the therapy, and the frequency and duration of sessions, must be negotiated (Parmelee 1986). In particular, failure to agree on treatment goals of hospitalization can lead to interrupted treatment (Galatzer-Levy 1991).

Steve E. was a 13-year-old hospitalized for severe depression. His parents were divorced. He lived with his mother and saw his father twice a month. Steve's parents still fought over their son's care, leaving Steve to feel hopeless and helpless.

Steve and the psychiatrist agreed to meet to discuss the boy's feelings about his parents' divorce. The psychiatrist recommended meeting with Steve's parents to address caretaking issues. However, at the meeting, the parents stated that they wanted Steve to be "cured," and they refused to address other issues. Each parent blamed the other for Steve's problems. Subsequently, Steve's mother withdrew him from the hospital.

IMPLEMENTATION OF A PSYCHOTHERAPY PROGRAM

The components of a program for hospitalized adolescents include a therapeutic milieu, psychotherapies, and psychopharmacology.

Therapeutic Milieu

The milieu acts as a matrix to hold together the entire treatment program. It is a structured environment that provides a variety of human relationships and opportunities for new learning. Its aims are many: to meet adolescents' needs for respect, appreciation, approval and praise; to reduce anxiety, guilt, and conflict; and to strengthen competence and facilitate development of new coping strategies (Berlin et al. 1984).

The milieu is the same as with adults, but the structure may be different. Most adolescent programs are highly structured; for instance, patients attend school for two significant parts of the day. There are unit rules on behavior and explicit consequences for violating the rules. Some treatment programs utilize a token economy or a point system, either for all patients or for selected ones.

School is a major component of an adolescent treatment program. Many patients are academically behind by several grades. The school staff and structure must contain and decrease the adolescents' symptomatic behavior during class time so they can learn. Within this environment, adolescents can achieve and enhance their sense of competence. The school program should emphasize acquiring skills, enhancing confidence, and improving social behavior. The teacher may become a key person in the therapeutic program, as many adolescents model themselves after this individual (Goodrich 1987; Hersov and Bentovim 1985).

> Lisa F. was a 14-year-old hospitalized for depression and recurrent suicidal thinking. Because of attentional and learning difficulties, she was only in the sixth grade. Lisa, anticipating continued academic failure, initially refused to go to school. The teacher approached her and together they negotiated a school plan she could accomplish. Lisa attended the school program and developed a close relationship with the teacher. With encouragement by the teacher, she began to speak up in class. She gained confidence from this, becoming more outgoing on the patient unit and in her individual psychotherapy sessions.

Psychotherapies

Individual, family, and group psychotherapies are all components of the overall treatment plan. In this section, I illustrate how each psychotherapeutic modality can be used to treat common presenting problems of hospitalized adolescents.

Often adolescents present with severe depression and suicidal feelings accompanied by low self-esteem and self-worth. The following is an example of the use of individual psychotherapy for this constellation of symptoms.

Alice N. was a 16-year-old living with her mother. Her father had died 2 years before of cancer. Alice had become progressively more isolated and withdrawn since her father's death, and this worsened when her older brother went off to college. In the hospital, Alice began to talk about her grief about her father's death and her mother's unavailability. Because her brother was the only person she could talk to, she had felt bereft, hopeless, and angry since his departure.

Alice's therapy consists of daily sessions to help gain control of her suicidal feelings and to begin to believe that psychotherapy could be useful to her. By the time of her discharge, she was still depressed but more optimistic about working out her problems.

Family psychotherapy can address the family system's functioning and the effect on the family of an individual's illness. The next example illustrates the use of family psychotherapy for a psychotic adolescent.

Tonya V. was a 16-year-old living with her parents. She was hospitalized because of unusual behavior involving elaborate rituals to "ward off the devil." She had homicidal feelings about a schoolmate and stated, "The voices want me to kill her." A preliminary diagnosis of schizophrenia was made.

As Tonya's behavior changed only gradually over the course of a year, her parents were stunned and saddened by the knowledge of the diagnosis. Family sessions dealt with the impact of a psychotic child on the entire family, including accommodations the parents and siblings might need to make. Tonya's parents were educated about the course of the illness and their daughter's need for medication.

Group psychotherapy offers particular advantages to hospitalized adolescents. Frequently, they experience isolation, loneliness, and anger; they have poor social skills, sexual concerns, and conflicts about authority and parents; and they are concerned about intimacy and dependency. All of these issues can be addressed in psychotherapy groups. These groups can also capitalize on the importance of the peer group for adolescents.

In psychotherapy groups, adolescents can learn about maladaptive behavioral and interpersonal patterns. The group can offer observations on here-and-now behavior, and the patients can learn how their behavior prevents them from developing optimal interpersonal relationships. Also, the group can enhance adolescents' ability to relate to one another during the hospitalization and thus provides instruction on posthospital social behavior.

Additionally, groups provide an antidote to social isolation and loneliness. Patients see that others have similar problems with family, friends, school, or the legal system. The experience of sharing personal events and feeling understood can lead to enhanced self-esteem and improved social skills. Adolescents can thus develop skills in empathic understanding of human beings, an important ingredient of satisfying social relationships.

> Paul C. was a 14-year-old mandated to the hospital because of recurrent running away, truancy, stealing, and substance abuse. His parents were divorced, and he had lived in multiple foster homes. He was angry and severely depressed.
>
> While in the hospital, Paul continued to state that he had no problems and that he was doing his time until released. He was unengaged in treatment. Another teenager in one of the psychotherapy groups began to talk about what it was like for him to be shuffled from foster home to foster home. They then discussed their drinking and how out of control it had become. Paul subsequently became involved in the treatment program and began to turn his life in another direction.

Psychopharmacology

The role of psychotropic medication in treating adolescents has changed substantially. Controversy surrounding the contemporaneous use of medication with psychotherapy appears to be subsiding (Sholevar 1989).

The clinician should initiate medication only after discussing with both the adolescent and his or her family how a particular medication will affect specific target symptoms. These discussions should take place in both family and individual settings. The target symptoms need to be described in terms the adolescent can understand, and the advantages of the medication in treating them should be clearly explained. Adolescents are likely to deny they have a medical problem or a need for medication. Therefore, the more clearly the patient sees his or her symptoms as problematic, and the more he or she appreciates that medication offers relief, the more likely the patient is to comply.

The potential side effects of medications must be clearly acknowledged and outlined. Adolescents are integrating a new body image. The possibility of side effects may make them feel out of control and frighten them away from the medication.

As part of the psychotherapy, the adolescent and his or her parents should be educated about the nature of the specific disorder to be treated. For example, an adolescent with attention-deficit hyperactivity disorder should have the biologic basis of the disorder explained. The family and the adolescent may have misconceptions about the etiology of the illness (e.g., that it is "badness," "oppositionalness," or "craziness"), and these beliefs should be explored. Much of the work may revolve around unraveling the complex relationships between distractibility, low self-esteem, dysphoria, and interpersonal problems that are an outcome of attention-deficit hyperactivity disorder, for example (Hendren 1991).

Medication can provide an excellent battleground for struggles within the family. Such conflicts most likely mimic other such problems at home and offer an opportunity for beginning a discussion between adolescent and parents on issues of autonomy and independence. Clarification of the meaning of the medication to the adolescent and his or her family will prove useful.

Clearly, there is increased use of psychotropic medication on inpatient units. This increase reflects a growth in the knowledge and practice of pediatric psychopharmacology. But it also reflects the need for more rapidly effective methods of modifying disordered behavior as staff members attempt to manage a more acutely disturbed patient in a shorter period of time. As the number of highly disruptive and agitated adolescent patients increases, pressure mounts from inpatient staff to begin or increase medication to contain the behavior. Under these circumstances, it is easy to see how controlling the adolescents can take priority over helping them to gain their own self-control (Jemerin and Philips 1988).

Sam S. was a 13-year-old referred for hospitalization because of behavioral problems. At the time of his hospitalization, he appeared oppositional and mildly depressed while denying any significant problems. In the classroom, Sam had difficulty attending to tasks and intruded into the work of others. In individual psychotherapy, he was easily distractible. In addition to individual, family, and group psychotherapies, Sam was begun on stimulant medication. Conner's rating scales (1973) were completed twice a week by Sam's mother, teacher, and primary mental health worker.

Once stimulants were initiated, Sam's psychotherapist noted that he was less distractible and could talk about emotionally arousing topics for longer periods of time. His mother found him to be less oppositional, both in family therapy and on weekend passes at home. Sam became less intrusive on the unit and made friends. His teacher developed a school program including individual time with her, and this program was shared with the teacher at his school in the community. Sam's aftercare plans included outpatient individual and family therapy, in addition to continuation of his medication (Hendren 1991).

CONCLUSION

The psychotherapy of adolescents on short-term inpatient units offers the opportunity to quickly identify and stabilize the problems of youngsters in crisis. Using a developmental framework, the therapist's task is to help the individual regain competence and set the stage for further psychotherapeutic work to follow. A complete psychotherapy program for hospitalized adolescents will contain a variety of treatment modalities, including individual, family, and group psychotherapies, in addition to milieu therapy and an educational program.

REFERENCES

American Academy of Child and Adolescent Psychiatry: Policy Statement on the Inpatient Hospital Treatment of Children and Adolescents. Baltimore, MD, American Academy of Child and Adolescent Psychiatry, June 1989

American Medical Association: Peer Review Manuals, I and II. Chicago, IL, American Medical Association, 1972

American Psychiatric Association: Manual of Psychiatric Peer Review. Washington, DC, American Psychiatric Association, 1976

Berlin IN, Critchley DL, Rossman PG: Current concepts in milieu treatment of seriously disturbed children and adolescents. Psychotherapy 21(1):118–131, 1984

Beskind H: Psychiatric inpatient treatment of adolescents: a review of clinical experience. Compr Psychiatry 3(6):354–369, 1962

Bond TC, Auger N: Benefits of the generic milieu in adolescent hospital treatment. Adolesc Psychiatry 10:360–372, 1982

Conners CK: Rating scales for use in drug studies with children. Psychopharmacol Bull (spec ed) 1973, pp 24–34

Easson WM: The Severely Disturbed Adolescent: Inpatient Residential and Hospital Treatment. New York, International Universities Press, 1969

Elliott K, Stein BA, McKeough M: Adolescents in a general hospital psychiatric unit. Can J Psychiatry 25:545–552, 1980

Fineberg BL, Sowards SK, Kettlewell PW: Adolescent inpatient treatment: a literature review. Adolescence 15(60):913–925, 1980

Galatzer-Levy R: Considerations in the psychotherapy of adolescents, in Adolescent Psychotherapy. Edited by Slomowitz M. Washington, DC, American Psychiatric Press, 1991, pp 83–100

Galatzer-Levy R, Cohler B: The Essential Other. New York, Basic Books, 1990

Gedo J, Goldberg A: Models of the Mind. Chicago, IL, University of Chicago Press, 1973

Geraty R: Administrative issues in inpatient child and adolescent psychiatry. J Am Acad Child Adolesc Psychiatry 28(1):21–25, 1989

Goodrich W: Long-term psychoanalytic hospital treatment of adolescents. Psychiatr Clin North Am 10(2):273–287, 1987

Hendren RL: Psychotherapy of adolescents with attention-deficit disorder, in Adolescent Psychiatry. Edited by Slomowitz M. Washington, DC, American Psychiatric Press, 1991, pp 123–142

Hersov L, Bentovim A: In-patient and day hospital units, in Child and Adolescent Psychiatry: Modern Approaches, 2nd Edition. Edited by Rutter M, Hersov L. Oxford, England, Blackwell Scientific, 1985, pp 766–779

Inamdar SC, Darrell E, Brown A, et al: Trends in violence among psychiatrically hospitalized adolescents: 1969 and 1979 compared. Journal of the American Academy of Child Psychiatry 25(5):704–707, 1986

Jaffe CM: Psychology psychoanalytic approaches to adolescent development, in Adolescent Psychiatry. Edited by Slomowitz M. Washington, DC, American Psychiatric Press, 1991, pp 13–40

Jemerin JM, Philips I: Changes in inpatient child psychiatry: consequences and recommendations. J Am Acad Child Adolesc Psychiatry 27(4):397–403, 1988

Joint Commission on Accreditation of Hospitals: Accreditation Manual for Psychiatric Facilities Serving Children and Adolescents. Chicago, IL, Joint Commission on Accreditation of Hospitals, 1974

Kiesler CA, Simpkins C: Changes in psychiatric inpatient treatment of children and youth in general hospitals: 1980–1985. Hosp Community Psychiatry 42:601–604, 1991

Lewis M, Lewis DO, Shanok SS, et al: The undoing of residential treatment: a follow-up study of 51 adolescents. Journal of the American Academy of Child Psychiatry 19:160–171, 1980

Marohn RC: Psychotherapy of adolescents with behavioral disorders, in Adolescent Psychotherapy. Edited by Slomowitz M. Washington, DC, American Psychiatric Press, 1991, pp 143–161

Milazzo-Sayre LJ: Use of inpatient psychiatric services by children and youth under age 18: United States, 1980 (Mental Health Statistical Note No 175, Publ No ADM-886-1451). Rockville, MD, U.S. Department of Health and Human Services, April 1986

Parmelee DX: The adolescent and the young adult, in Inpatient Psychiatry: Diagnosis and Treatment, 2nd Edition. Edited by Sederer LI. Baltimore, MD, Williams & Wilkins, 1986, pp 280–295

Sholevar P: Psychodynamic child and adolescent psychiatry: an introduction. J Am Acad Child Adolesc Psychiatry 28(5):655–656, 1989

Thompson JW, Rosenstein MD, Milazzo-Sayre LJ, et al: Psychiatric services to adolescents: 1970–1980. Hosp Community Psychiatry 37(6):584–590, 1986

Geriatric Patients

David Bienenfeld, M.D.

INTRODUCTION

Through the 1980s, significant attention was devoted to the psychiatric needs and capacities of the aging population. Nonetheless, psychotherapy with older people has remained underutilized. Many psychiatrists, having received little training in the theory and technique of geriatric psychotherapy, spend little time practicing it. Limited Medicare reimbursement for psychotherapy, sensory impairments, physical ailments, and complicated social structures all serve to discourage the psychiatrist from delivering psychotherapeutic services to aging patients. Countertransference issues including fear of one's own mortality and unresolved parental conflicts may constitute further impediments (Wheeler and Bienenfeld 1990). All of these factors are magnified in the inpatient setting, where rapid treatment is a major goal and the therapist may fear that psychotherapy with a depressed 70-year-old could extend the patient's length of stay unacceptably.

Nonetheless, there is empirical evidence of the efficacy of psychotherapy in the treatment of geriatric patients (Gallagher and Thompson 1983; Lazarus et al. 1987; Yesavage and Karasu 1982). The capacity of psychotherapy to solidify the gains of pharmacotherapy and milieu therapy, and to extend recovery and prevent relapse, applies equally at all ages. In this chapter, I outline a conceptual framework for defining the clinical problems of geriatric inpatients and a model for assessment and treatment planning. I then describe techniques of individual therapy, family therapy, and group therapy with hospitalized elderly patients.

THE DEVELOPMENTAL PERSPECTIVE

Attempts to generalize about the psychology of old people frequently fail in the face of the psychological diversity elders exhibit. Older individuals differ more from one another than the "average" 80-year-old differs from the "average" 30-year-old (Bienenfeld 1990b). The psychotherapeutic enterprise is, in general, a process of constructing a coherent story of the patient's current state. Regardless of age, the story is most coherent, and thereby most therapeutically powerful, when it is longitudinal in perspective. With the aging patient, the task of weaving the historical tapestry is more complicated but no less important.

Frameworks that examine the nature of psychological development in adult life first came to prominence in the 1950s with the influential publications of Erik Erikson (1959), who described eight life crises from birth to senescence: basic trust versus basic mistrust, autonomy versus shame and doubt, initiative versus guilt, industry versus inferiority, identity versus identity diffusion, intimacy versus isolation, generativity versus self-absorption, and integrity versus despair. Although other theorists have proposed alternative formulations to Erikson's attractive but simple schema (Bowlby 1988; Vaillant 1977), successful clinicians are generally guided by the principle that early life dispositions are influenced by the environment at all ages, and that the manifestations of personality and pathology in old age are the product of lifelong development and contemporary stressors (McCrae and Costa 1984).

Formulated most generically, individuals are born with certain temperamental traits. Early upbringing influences the manifestations of these traits and shapes whether they become sources of strength or distress. Relationships with individuals and social structures through childhood, adolescence, and adulthood help determine one's vulnerability to stressors (Bowlby 1988).

The stressors attendant to aging in modern society are abundant. Friends become disabled; some die. Children grow up and move away. Retirement from formal employment is almost universal. The body often ails or fails. The clinician must be aware, however, that these stressors do not dictate psychopathology. Retirement is a death knell for some, a new beginning for others. Widowhood may bring despair or relief. Effective psychotherapy with an elderly patient mandates not only an identification of the stressors, but a productive curiosity about what developmental threads in the patient's history have made the stressors pathogenic.

Similarly, only some fraction of those who become symptomatic in the wake of these losses and threats will require hospitalization. Hospitalization may be necessitated by the severity of the emotional response, as is the case with the forced retiree who becomes suicidally depressed. Physical incapacity may be not only the cause of the emotional distress, but also the factor requiring inpatient treatment when, for example, crippling arthritis induces intense anxiety about bodily deterioration and also prevents the patient from attending outpatient therapy. The integrity of the support network also determines whether a stressor results in hospitalization. For example, a married man may be able to endure the depression following the death of a close friend, whereas a widower may require admission to the hospital (Tourigny-Rivard 1991).

Evaluation of the Elderly Patient

It is a basic principle in all of geriatric medicine that evaluation is at least as important as diagnosis. For the older individual who cannot climb a flight of stairs, it is certainly important to know if the cause is congestive heart failure, osteoarthritis, or a hip fracture. The treatment for each of the etiologic conditions is generally well defined. However, an assessment of the patient's situation is more important than diagnosis for setting therapeutic goals, determining prognosis, and implementing a comprehensive plan. Does the patient's home have bathrooms only on the second story? Are family members available to provide postdischarge assistance? What is the patient's nutritional status? What are his or her financial resources? What is his or her cognitive status?

The answers to these questions have little or no bearing on the dosage of digoxin or the placement of the hip prosthesis. However, they may influence the choice of treatment strategy. The patient who has considerable social and instrumental support (i.e., transportation, home care, etc.) may receive a complicated medication regimen. The elder who lives alone may appropriately be treated with a simpler regimen that may be less effective or have more side effects. The answers have every bearing on the quality of life that can be expected as a result of the hospital treatment.

They may determine whether this patient is more likely to return home or be transferred to a long-term care setting.

The centrality of assessment in the evaluation of the geriatric patient is even more pronounced in the case of psychiatric disorders. Goal setting must precede the selection and implementation of specific hospital therapies, and assessment is the groundwork on which the goals are set (Finkel and Andrle 1990). If, for example, the patient has sufficient financial resources and mobility to engage in continuing outpatient psychotherapy, it may be advisable to aim to uncover psychodynamic issues that could not be completely resolved prior to discharge. For a patient with a similar degree of suffering who cannot return for intensive follow-up therapy, a more appropriate goal would entail symptom resolution without addressing his or her underlying psychological vulnerability.

The following example of a format for comprehensive assessment of the hospitalized geropsychiatric patient makes the process efficient and comprehensible for physician, patient, and caregivers (Goldstein 1990):

1. Elicit the patient's understanding of the chief complaint and the clinical features of the current problem. Identify whether it was the patient's choice to come for treatment or somebody else's.
2. Review the patient's relevant physical, laboratory, and radiologic findings. Decide if further medical evaluation should precede psychiatric intervention. Remain aware of medical conditions and treatments that can influence the outcome of the psychiatric therapies.
3. Assess the patient's functional capacities. Physical activities of daily living include ambulation, bathing, and elimination. Instrumental activities of daily living include using the phone, choosing appropriate clothing, and cooking. Note impairments that compromise function, including incontinence, sensory deficits, and cardiopulmonary disease.
4. Investigate the patient's living environment and situation. Relevant dimensions include not only housing, but also the nature and reliability of the patient's support system, educational and socioeconomic background, and financial resources.
5. Review the patient's strengths and adaptive capacities. The elicitation of a developmental history allows staff to review adaptation to past life crises and to understand the values and priorities to which the patient adheres. By eliciting a narrative of how the patient coped with a

divorce, a major illness, or the death of a friend, the therapist obtains data that are likely to be valuable in helping the patient find the internal resources to adapt to the stressor precipitating the current problem.

6. Repeat the assessment of the presenting problem, functional capacities, perceived deficits, and recognized strengths with the patient's family or other caregivers. Observation of the interaction of patient and caregivers provides data for which there are no substitutes.

This review allows therapist and patient to arrive at a formulation of the presenting problem, in preparation for planning the psychotherapy. The specific content of the formulation will be shaped by the therapist's theoretical model. Because the emotional and behavioral problems of elderly patients are so intricately connected with the biological substrate and the social environment, the formulation usually needs to be broader in scope than what is customary for younger patients; an individually centered psychological formulation with passing reference to somatic and social factors is insufficient for defining the problems of most elders in the psychiatric hospital unit.

With the results of the assessment framed in a comprehensive formulation of the presenting problem, therapist and patient can set appropriate goals for the inpatient treatment generally and for the psychotherapy specifically. In the hospital setting, symptom reduction or relief is the primary goal. Depending on the patient's strengths, resources, and situation, this relief may come through mastery of a stressor or through acceptance of its inevitability—through confrontation with a threat or through avoiding it in the first place. Goals should not be limited to the patient as an individual, however. Because older hospitalized patients generally depend on a social matrix for recovery and survival, the physician must also be mindful of setting and working toward social and family goals (Finkel and Andrle 1990; Finkel et al. 1982). The therapist can use the hospital setting to effect a reduction in family tension or collusion. Social goals, such as environmental manipulations, may not belong in the realm of psychotherapy proper, but the clinician's role in implementing these goals becomes a relevant factor in the psychotherapy. This is true, for example, when the psychiatrist is instrumental in arranging a nursing home placement while at the same time helping the patient who is angry about the physical disability that necessitated the placement in the first place.

The assessment and goals then determine the choice of therapeutic modality. For the patient with intact cognition and a substantial range of adaptive defenses, for whom goals include a return to home, insight-oriented psychotherapy might be a logical choice. If the major problem is family disruption deriving from maladaptive communication about the meaning of the presenting symptoms, family therapy is indicated. When insight is limited and adaptation to disability is the goal, supportive psychotherapy is appropriate. For the patient with some resistance to self-observation for whom an increase in the productivity of interpersonal communication is a desired goal, group psychotherapy may be the primary modality. Table 12–1 summarizes a framework for planning psychotherapeutic interventions in the hospital.

Table 12–1. Planning scheme for inpatient psychotherapies

Modality	Nature of problem	Insight and motivation	Therapeutic goals
Focal psychotherapy	Adjustment to discrete stressor (e.g., death of spouse)	High	Resolution of focal conflict
Supportive psychotherapy	Generally chronic and severe psychiatric disability, acutely exacerbated (e.g., acute medical illness in patient with chronic dysthymia)	Low	Reduction in maladaptive responses; resolution of disabling symptoms
Family therapy	Family disruption causing, or caused by, psychiatric illness in identified patient (e.g., return home of divorced daughter)	Moderate	Restoration or establishment of family as effective support for patient
Group psychotherapy	Maladaptive interpersonal behavior or communication (e.g., alienation of environmental caregivers)	Moderate	Reinforcement of adaptive interpersonal skills

Source. Adapted from Wheeler and Bienenfeld 1990.

TECHNICAL ASPECTS

Features of Geriatric Psychotherapy

Elicitation of History

Although the general principles of obtaining a chief complaint and present history are independent of the patient's age, the elicitation of the history from an elderly patient often requires some expansion of the technical repertoire. Some of the reasons are obvious: The older patient may speak more slowly or have sensory impairment that affects the pace of the diagnostic conversation. The susceptibility of older depressed individuals to cognitive interference ("pseudodementia") can confront the therapist with factual deficits that must be filled from external sources, usually family.

More subtle, but also more insidious, is the problem of engaging the patient in a psychologically centered conversation. The geriatric patient of the 1990s was raised during the Great Depression and pre-World War II era, when words such as "depression" and "anxiety" were not part of everyday conversation and popular culture was only minimally influenced by psychological notions. Additionally, the image of psychiatric treatment, in the minds of this cohort, consists of the state hospitals of the 1940s and 1950s, contributing to a justifiable fear of a clinical conversation with a psychiatrist.

Here, the physician must take the initiative—reading the observable affect, making empathically educated guesses, and reflecting to the patient in a way that guides the conversation to the internal state. Everyday words, such as "nervous" and "worried," are safer openers than jargon such as "depressed" or "anxious." Commonly, the patient may respond to the opening inquiry by relating the external facts of his or her arrival at the hospital. The therapist can then encourage a more introspective focus with a response such as, "It sounds as if that scared you," or "You sound frustrated."

A similar manifestation of this cohort effect is the tendency of many of today's older people to speak in "organ language." The geriatric patient who says, "I have a lump in my throat" may mean the statement more literally than a younger person. The therapist is then obliged to translate,

"Does that mean you feel as if you could cry?" By bridging the linguistic and perceptual gap across the cohorts, the therapist not only encourages the patient's curiosity about his or her feelings and thoughts, but also demonstrates that the therapy is a setting where emotions are tolerated and understood.

Integration of Somatic Therapies With Psychotherapy

Empirically, the vast majority of psychiatrically hospitalized elderly patients will be receiving psychotropic medications. Some thought in each case to the relative roles of the psychotherapy and pharmacotherapy in the treatment strategy serves a clarifying role for both patient and therapist. Because the first task of crisis intervention is relief of immediate distress, medication can serve an invaluable function by relieving the pressure of overwhelming anxiety, exhausting insomnia, or psychotic thinking (Kahana 1987). This relief not only allows the patient to "settle into" the psychotherapeutic process, but it also promotes the image of the physician as a caring person who comprehends and believes the patient's sense of distress.

It is rare for the aging psychiatric patient not to be receiving several medications for somatic conditions at the time of admission. The patient's experience with these agents contributes to his or her expectations of the medications the psychiatrist will prescribe. Resentment at taking antihypertensives that "do nothing but make me go to the bathroom" is likely to reduce the patient's tolerance for medications that take weeks to work and have significant side effects. Experience with analgesics that work quickly and predictably may result in unrealistic expectations of more subtly acting psychotropics.

Older patients, even more than younger ones, may lump together all "nerve pills" as sedatives that can remove psychological distress. The physician is obligated to explain to the patient the purpose for and realistic expectations of the medication, and the same is true for the psychotherapy. It can be helpful for the patient to hear a formulation such as this:

> This antidepressant will probably help with the problems of sleep, appetite, and energy we've talked about. In time, it should also help with those terrible blue feelings that feel like they just fall on you from outside. But it's not going to help with the things that make you unhappy, like your

feeling so useless since you retired or the tension that's been between you and your daughter for years. The medicine can help with the depression, while we use the psychotherapy to address your unhappiness.

In subsequent conversations, the patient may need to work through his or her own solution of the mind-body dilemma, a lifelong task that assumes particular importance with increasing age. The definition of major depression as a "chemical imbalance," for example, is a useful simplification that can reduce self-blame and facilitate recovery. It may also focus the patient's curiosity about biological determinants of his or her feelings about the possibility of emotional integrity in the face of physical deterioration.

Reminiscence

The pressure of impending mortality is one of several factors contributing to an almost ubiquitous feature of the presentation of many older individuals—reminiscence. Far from being a pathological feature of late-life narcissism, reminiscence is a manifestation of the process of life review that is a necessary tool for the resolution of the crisis of integrity versus despair (Butler 1963). In the hectic pace of the inpatient unit, stories of the "good old days" may understandably be viewed as resistances to the therapeutic task at hand, but they are in fact a response to the developmental challenge.

Reminiscence constructs an autobiography. Whether objectively accurate or factually distorted, it serves the function of putting the past in order, so that the patient's present circumstance may be placed into historical perspective (Bienenfeld 1990b). An attitude on the part of the physician and the staff that allows for reminiscence, without fostering confusion of past and present, conveys to the patient a sense of appreciation for his or her historical continuity, diminishing some of the threat posed by the pace of change that the psychiatric hospital unit encourages.

Psychotherapeutic Modalities

Focal Psychodynamic Psychotherapy

As discussed in previous chapters, focal psychodynamic psychotherapy is an insight-oriented modality, which aims at resolution or decreased intensity of contemporary manifestations of core conflicts or deficits. Techniques of confrontation and clarification focus the patient's attention on the historical continuity of the present problem and allow him or her to analyze the effectiveness of defensive strategies (Wheeler and Bienenfeld 1990). At first blush, the therapist may be discouraged by the prospect of addressing a focal problem from within the context of decades of entrenched patterns of defense. Paradoxically, however, focal psychotherapy with elderly patients affords unique leverage. These same decades of experience provide therapist and patient with a broad range of coping mechanisms brought to bear in different situations. The therapist can highlight these for the patient and engage him or her in the exercise of recalling them as potential solutions to the current problem.

> Dorothy A. was a 63-year-old woman admitted after an overdose on sleeping pills. She denied any suicidal intent, claiming that she was "just trying to get some rest." The therapist inquired about her need for rest, and Mrs. A. responded with a description of the stressors in her life. Her husband was alcoholic; though never abusive, he generally ignored her. Her son had been born with a serious cleft palate and was borderline mentally retarded. Mrs. A. perceived him as seriously disabled. Her husband saw the son as lazy and constantly berated him for his irresponsibility and inability to keep a job. Mrs. A. and her husband frequently argued about their son. One of these arguments preceded the overdose, and it was from this tension that she wanted "a rest." She agreed at this point that part of her had wanted to die, but that she also felt obligated to stay alive to protect her son.
>
> Mrs. A. then freely associated to how much she missed her older sister, who had died several years earlier. Their father had been alcoholic, occasionally abusive, but usually absent. Their mother had died when Mrs. A. was 12. She described her mother in uniformly positive terms. After her mother's death, Mrs. A. was raised by her sister, whom she quite clearly and consciously idealized. In adulthood, they saw each other almost daily. Mrs. A. would recite her troubles to her sister, who would sometimes offer advice or concrete help but mostly just listened.
>
> The therapist focused with Mrs. A. on her emotional state when she and her husband argued about their son. She was able to articulate a sense of powerlessness and loneliness. Mrs. A. agreed that her sister had been able, by her mere presence, to alleviate such feelings after their

mother's death and through their contacts in their adult lives. After her sister's death, Mrs. A. became more protective of her son; she concurred with the therapist's formulation that she identified with her son's disabilities, to the point of exaggerating them. Additionally, protecting her son provided her with a sense of self-worth (albeit a fragile, ambivalent one). Having brought this overidentification to awareness, Mrs. A. was able to consider options that would foster her son's autonomy without threatening her own sense of psychological integrity.

In family meetings, Mrs. A. was able to adopt a more realistic stance with her son. She also began to attend Al-Anon meetings before discharge, and she made a friend who she said "kind of reminds me of my sister."

In this therapy, the core issues of self-deficit were tacitly acknowledged by the physician in his formulation of the current problem but were not overtly addressed. Attention was directed instead at how the patient felt she was falling apart without the selfobject cohesiveness her sister had afforded. The motivations behind her maladaptive efforts at coping were clarified, and more productive options were entertained and attempted.

Supportive Psychotherapy

When the capacity or motivation for insight is limited or when the ego functions are tenuous, supportive therapy is more useful than insight-oriented modalities. In supportive psychotherapy, as described elsewhere in this book, the most adaptive of the patient's available defenses and coping strategies are identified and reinforced. In the words of Bellak and Small (1978), the therapist aims for "understanding nearly everything and doing only the little that makes a difference" (p. 192).

Whereas focal psychotherapy aims at mobilizing repressed or neglected defenses in the service of coping with contemporary challenges, supportive psychotherapy is indicated when the patient relates a history of a more limited range of coping capacities. Typically, it is applicable in the case of the aging patient who has coped for many years in similar fashion and who now faces any of the losses that are common in late life.

Simon B., who was 74 at the time of his hospital admission, had been a successful executive who never tolerated anything less than perfection from his employees. He had sold his business at a substantial profit at age 68 but had never truly enjoyed his retirement. Complications of his diabetes accumulated, and his wife died 2 years prior to his admission. Because of his prickly personality, neither of Mr. B.'s sons would take him in when he became physically unable to live alone, and in-home nursing was a short-lived experiment as he fired one nurse after another for "incompetence." Six months prior to admission, he was admitted to one of the most exclusive long-term care facilities in the area, though one where on-site psychiatric consultation was not available. There, Mr. B.'s pattern of antagonism with caregivers continued to the point where psychiatric hospitalization was requested by his primary physician and the Director of Nursing at the nursing home.

On initial evaluation, Mr. B. freely expressed his disdain for the notion of psychiatric hospitalization. He immediately demonstrated with the hospital staff the behavior that had resulted in his referral. He insisted on having his meals served in his room; he complained of the inadequacy of the beds, the mediocrity of the food, and the incompetence of the housekeepers. He rang his call bell several times an hour and berated the psychiatrist for the "paltry" half-hour daily visits that did nothing to alleviate his ill-defined suffering.

At first, the therapist attempted to engage Mr. B. in a focal psychotherapy, focusing on the loss of control forced by his illness and his widowhood. Mr. B. would have none of this "voodoo." The psychiatrist recognized in his own frustration a projection of his patient's feelings and made the decision to use this dynamic cluster to therapeutic advantage. "Mr. B.," he began, "you're accustomed to doing business, and doing it well. Up to now, you've generally held most of the cards. Now, the business is getting yourself taken care of, but you've got fewer cards to play. Let's see what kind of profit you can cut from the capital at hand."

Identifying the hospital staff as the agents of the medical authority that Mr. B. respected, the psychiatrist worked with him on operationalizing his wishes and identifying those that could be met in the environment. Physician visits were scheduled and maintained at exactly 30 minutes. Nursing staff came to his room the first 5 minutes of every hour and at no other times. Adequate medications for sleep and pain were provided; most prn medications were converted to scheduled ones. Mr. B.'s self-defeating outrage was contained to an ego-syntonic bluster that was tolerable to staff of the acute hospital and the nursing home. Their staff was invited to come in for predischarge planning to learn the care plan and its philosophy.

Family Therapy

Stereotypes of elders, particularly older psychiatric patients, as existing in isolation from their families are quite inconsistent with demonstrable reality. Of all men over age 65, at least 75% are married and living with their wives. The same is true of 30% of older women. Three-quarters of Americans over 65 have at least one living child (Storandt 1983). These families are not just statistical entities; family members provide 80%–90% of personal care, medically related services, and instrumental assistance such as transportation, shopping, and home maintenance for aged relatives. Twice as many elders live with their families as live in institutions (Brody 1986). It is often through the intervention of family members that older patients are brought to clinical attention. Because families are such a crucial element of the social environment, the effective hospital treatment of geriatric patients mandates competence in family therapy.

The model described by Herr and Weakland (1979) applies family systems theory to the management of the problems of older adults and their families. It includes definition of the problem, establishment of goals, and planning of interventions.

On initial contact with the family, the therapist allows each member to feel entitled to discuss the problem and share in its resolution. Definition of the problem is a crucial step. Systems theory views the identified patient as the weak link in a stressed chain. In the evaluation session, each member is allowed to present his or her own formulation of the nature of the presenting problem. Although this step is part of any family therapy, it assumes particular features in the case of the elderly identified patient. Because the children and their respective spouses no longer live with the identified patient and often have independent contact with him or her, they have often drawn independent (and often incompatible) conclusions about the nature of the problem. Care must be taken to avoid indications of siding with one person or faction against others. The therapist listens for common threads in the often divergent stories and presents a single formulation that is acceptable to all members. He or she must generally stress the shared nature of the burden.

Just as the conduct of individual psychotherapy pays heed to the patient's coping with prior life crises, family therapy with the elderly patient demands attention to the family's history of coping and adaptation. The therapist should elicit some of the family's history (noting how family members have related to each other in the past), what the unspoken expectations are, and what implicit rules of communication apply.

> Elmore C., who had smoking-induced chronic lung disease, had been hospitalized with pneumonia 1 year prior to admission, when his wife died suddenly of a stroke. Over the succeeding year, Mr. C. complained about the lack of attention and caring from his children and seemed to deteriorate physically. He was admitted to the hospital after cutting his wrists superficially, "to end the suffering." In the family evaluation session, Mr. C.'s son characterized his father as "manipulating" the family with his suicide gesture. Mr. C.'s daughter and son-in-law voiced their bitterness that his pulmonary illness was self-induced and deserved no pity. Mr. C. himself said that this was just the sort of disrespect he had to put up with.
>
> Inquiring about the family's coping with the death of Mrs. C., the therapist discovered that Mr. C. had not attended the funeral and that no real conversation about Mrs. C.'s death had ever taken place among all involved parties ("We just don't talk about stuff like that"). The therapist pointed out that the current squabbling may have been their way of talking about it, but it wasn't leading anywhere. All members of the C. family quickly and eagerly began to talk about their respective experiences of grief.

Problems must then be specified as precisely as possible. For example, "my children don't respect me" is not a problem that can be addressed effectively. To reformulate the worry as "My children don't call or visit as often as I'd like" makes the applicable goals self-evident.

Goals should then match the identified problems and be as realistic and as small in scope as possible. The guiding question posed to each family member should be, "What is the smallest change that would give you a sense of progress toward resolution of this problem?" The patient may acknowledge that hearing from at least one of the children daily would help him or her feel less isolated. The division of problems and goals into such small units allows the family members to experience some success and relief even in the time-limited setting of hospital therapy.

The planning and implementation of interventions begins with a review of solutions the family has already attempted. Most people, after all, come to need hospitalization only after exhausting most other attempted solutions. Particularly with elders and their adult children, it is the intended solutions themselves that precipitate the emotional decompensations resulting in hospitalization. The adult child may perceive the parent as failing and endangered and force a "solution" of bringing the parent into his or her own home. Chaos is the understandable result, as the reluctant parent is thrown into close quarters with an adult daughter and son-in-law and adolescent grandchildren.

The interventions appropriate to hospital family therapy are generally behavioral in nature, though there is some room for modifications in attitude, expectations, and communication. Unlike outpatient family therapy, the inpatient setting does not usually allow the family to implement the solutions between sessions, return, and then review results and modify further. Because the therapist is usually limited to two or three sessions, he or she must formulate interventions that will be implemented after discharge. Ideally, the therapist will be the one to meet with the family after discharge to continue the therapy; if not, he or she must ensure adequate follow-up and communicate fully with the outpatient family therapist.

Termination of the inpatient family therapy should therefore include review of how progress toward the established goals will be monitored within the family as well as professionally. The therapist will continue to remind the family that they have considerable power in alleviating the problems that brought the older patient to the hospital.

Family Therapy for Relatives of Patients With Dementia

Behavior resulting from dementing illnesses is a frequent precipitant for hospitalization of aged individuals. It is almost always family members who bring their cognitively impaired relative to clinical attention, and it is axiomatic that clinicians provide these relatives with education and with assistance in finding placement and instrumental services. Less obvious, however, is the need for family intervention at a psychotherapeutic level. Although depression and other psychiatric symptoms are common among relatives and others who are caregivers, they occur in proportion to the subjectively perceived burden posed by the demented patient, not the objectively measured level of instrumental need (George and Gwyther 1986).

In addition to evaluating the problem-solving capacity of the family, the therapist is well advised to inquire about the family's perception of the illness and the relative it afflicts. Because affective burden drains energy from the implementation of solutions, addressing emotional issues augments the efficacy of problem-solving interventions (Schmidt et al. 1988). Commonly, old issues of resentment over parental inattention or rivalry among siblings, dormant for decades, will emerge as a parent becomes forgetful and confused, making demands on the adult children. The experience of caring for a familiar body as the identity of the person inside fades with each passing month is so strange that family members need to have the opportunity to share it with each other, in a psychotherapeutic context.

Group Psychotherapy

There are some particular advantages that group psychotherapy offers in the treatment of elderly patients. The threat of social isolation is an ingredient of the presentation of many elders. Group therapy offers not only a chance for contact with others but also a forum to shed maladaptive social skills and adopt more effective ones. Resistance to accepting observations from younger therapists is common; group therapy offers peer feedback, which is often more readily accepted. One vehicle of social interaction is the exchange of information. Older patients are often better sources of information for each other than the therapist can be, advising each other about bus schedules and bargain outlets. In the process of helping each other, group members can achieve a sense of self-esteem that helps to repair the worthlessness that is a frequent component of many late-life psychiatric disorders.

Although many believe that groups composed of older patients alone offer many advantages over age-integrated groups, this choice is rarely available in the hospital setting. If there is no separate geriatric psychiatry unit, there are not likely to be enough older patients on a general adult unit to comprise a workable group. Given the practical necessity of such integration, the therapist must keep in mind that cohorts of different ages subscribe to different rules of social behavior and communication. Colloquial expressions exchanged freely among those in their 20s and 30s may need to be translated for those in their 60s and 70s. It is a delicate technical line for the therapist to tread while watching for signs that the older members are "tuning out" because the conversation is too fast, without seeming condescending as he or she attempts to draw them back into the process. A useful maneuver is for the therapist to summarize the group issue and ask the older members for reflections on how they dealt with such problems in the course of their own maturation.

Given these obstacles, there are advantages to exploit from having patients of different ages in the same psychotherapy group. Groups foster considerable regression and mobilize active expressions of transference almost regardless of setting and composition. When an older patient and a younger one engage in a dyadic reenactment of their respective parental and filial relationships, the therapist can exploit the opportunity to show each the potency of the perceptual template that transference forges, and to encourage perceptions that obviate repetitive maladaptive responses. The reminiscence that is a ubiquitous feature of geriatric psychotherapy can be used to particular advantage. The older patient can learn to frame reminiscences in a way that engages rather than bores others, thereby obtaining gratification and mirroring. At the same time, younger patients can get a glimpse of the longitudinal nature of psychological growth, bringing a different perspective to their own psychotherapeutic work in the hospital and beyond (Butler 1975).

The therapist who attempts to "work through" individual losses of older group patients may find him- or herself trapped by the multitude of losses that color late life. More productive is an approach that acknowledges existential vulnerability to loss and focuses on attitudes and behaviors that facilitate coping with the inevitable (Bienenfeld 1988, 1990a).

Principles of behavioral and cognitive therapies may be productively applied in group settings (Liberman 1970). Role-playing scenarios are used to reenact situations resembling those precipitating the admission, typically interactions with family members. As the scenario is played out, the patient identifies the moment when behavior and communication become irresistibly influenced by anxiety. Group members help identify the expectations and perceptions that produce the anxiety and assist the patient in arriving at more effective coping mechanisms (Foster and Foster 1989).

Thomas E. was a 35-year-old man who had been divorced twice and had great difficulty holding jobs. Lois F. was a 64-year-old woman whose depressive symptoms were linked to her disappointment with the turmoil in her children's lives. As Mr. E. was describing in group a disagreement with his boss that resulted in his most recent job termination, the therapist asked Mrs. F. to role-play Mr. E.'s employer. The group members, with minimal guidance from the therapist, were able to identify Mr. E.'s parental transference to his supervisor and Mrs. F.'s provocation of him by subtle attempts to induce guilt.

Summary

Regardless of setting, therapy with the aging patient makes the most sense when the current problem is viewed from a developmental perspective. Temperamental predispositions are carried by the patient through countless situations and relationships, each of which exerts some modifying influence. The therapist attempts to define the circumstances precipitating the hospitalization from within this longitudinal framework.

The assessment of the geriatric patient entails much more than diagnosis and psychodynamic formulation. Social supports, financial resources, physical environment, and a host of other influences are as important as internal psychic resources in strategizing a patient's therapeutic goals.

Individual psychotherapy with aging patients in the hospital is not only possible, but immensely useful. Focal psychotherapy and supportive psychotherapy are guided by the same principles as they are in younger patients, although the themes at issue vary with age, and technical adjustments facilitate their effectiveness. Family and group therapy can be conducted with the depth of "true" psychotherapy, and elderly patients benefit from them in a way that complements the progress made in individual psychotherapy.

Above all, the harried inpatient psychiatrist does well to avoid the trap of therapeutic nihilism with the aged patient. Constraints of time and reimbursement are undeniable; but equally undeniable is the observation that psychotherapy in the hospital makes all other progress deeper and more enduring.

REFERENCES

Bellak L, Small L: Emergency Psychotherapy and Brief Psychotherapy. New York, Grune & Stratton, 1978

Bienenfeld D: Group psychotherapy with the elderly in the state hospital, in Group Psychotherapies for the Elderly. Edited by MacLennan BW, Saul S, Weiner MB. New York, International Universities Press, 1988, pp 177–187

Bienenfeld D: Other psychotherapies, in Verwoerdt's Clinical Geropsychiatry, 3rd Edition. Edited by Bienenfeld D. Baltimore, MD, Williams & Wilkins, 1990a, pp 223–233

Bienenfeld D: Psychology of aging, in Verwoerdt's Clinical Geropsychiatry, 3rd Edition. Edited by Bienenfeld D. Baltimore, MD, Williams & Wilkins, 1990b, pp 26–44

Bowlby J: Developmental psychiatry comes of age. Am J Psychiatry 145:1–10, 1988

Brody EM: The role of families in nursing homes: implications for research and public policy, in Mental Illness in Nursing Homes: Agenda for Research. Edited by Harper MS, Lebowitz BD. Washington, DC, U.S. Department of Health and Human Services, 1986, pp 159–180

Butler RN: The life review: interpretation of reminiscence in the aged. Psychiatry 26:65–76, 1963

Butler RN: Psychiatry and the elderly: an overview. Am J Psychiatry 132:893–900, 1975

Erikson EH: Identity and the Life Cycle. New York, International Universities Press, 1959

Finkel SI, Andrle TE: Treatment planning, in Verwoerdt's Clinical Geropsychiatry, 3rd Edition. Edited by Bienenfeld D. Baltimore, MD, Williams & Wilkins, 1990, pp 197–203

Finkel SI, Stein E, Miller N, et al: Special perspectives on treatment planning for the elderly, in Treatment Planning in Psychiatry. Edited by Lewis JM, Usdin G. Washington, DC, American Psychiatric Association, 1982, pp 377–433

Foster RP, Foster JR: Group therapy with geriatric patients, in Group Psychodynamics: New Paradigms and New Perspectives. Edited by Halperin DA. Chicago, IL, Year Book Medical, 1989, pp 297–310

Gallagher DE, Thompson LW: Effectiveness of psychotherapy for both endogenous and non-endogenous depression in older adult outpatients. J Gerontol 38:707–712, 1983

George LK, Gwyther LP: Caregiver well-being: a multidimensional examination of family caregivers of demented adults. Gerontologist 26:253–259, 1986

Goldstein MZ: Evaluation of the elderly patient, in Verwoerdt's Clinical Geropsychiatry, 3rd Edition. Edited by Bienenfeld D. Baltimore, MD, Williams & Wilkins, 1990, pp 47–58

Herr JJ, Weakland JH: Counseling Elders and Their Families: Practical Techniques for Applied Gerontology. New York, Springer, 1979

Kahana RJ: Geriatric psychotherapy: beyond crisis management, in Treating the Elderly With Psychotherapy. Edited by Sadavoy J, Leszcz M. Madison, CT, International Universities Press, 1987, pp 233–264

Lazarus L, Groves L, Guttman D, et al: Brief psychotherapy with the elderly: a study of process and outcome, in Treating the Elderly With Psychotherapy. Edited by Sadavoy J, Leszcz M. Madison, CT, International Universities Press, 1987, pp 265–293

Liberman R: A behavioral approach to group dynamics, I: reinforcement and prompting of cohesiveness in group psychotherapy. Behavioral Therapy 1:141–175, 1970

McCrae RR, Costa PT: Emerging Lives, Enduring Dispositions. Boston, MA, Little, Brown, 1984

Schmidt GL, Bonjean MJ, Widem AC, et al: Brief psychotherapy for caregivers of demented relatives: comparison of two therapeutic strategies. Clinical Gerontologist 7:109–125, 1988

Storandt M: Family therapy, in Counselling and Therapy With Older Adults. Edited by Storandt M. Boston, MA, Little, Brown, 1983, pp 57–65

Tourigny-Rivard MF: Acute care inpatient treatment, in Comprehensive Review of Geriatric Psychiatry. Edited by Sadavoy J, Lazarus LW, Jarvik LF. Washington, DC, American Psychiatric Press, 1991, pp 583–602

Vaillant GE: Adaptation to Life. Boston, MA, Little, Brown, 1977

Wheeler BG, Bienenfeld D: Principles of individual psychotherapy, in Verwoerdt's Clinical Geropsychiatry, 3rd Edition. Edited by Bienenfeld D. Baltimore, MD, Williams & Wilkins, 1990, pp 204–222

Yesavage JA, Karasu TB: Psychotherapy with elderly patients. Am J Psychother 36:41–55, 1982

CHAPTER 13

Patients With Severe Personality Disorders

Andrew E. Skodol II, M.D.
John M. Oldham, M.D.

Patients with severe personality disorders frequently require hospitalization (Skodol et al. 1983). Inpatient treatment is often necessary for such a patient because of exacerbations in psychopathology and psychosocial crises that disturb and threaten the patient's social and therapeutic environments. These may in turn lead to life-threatening, self-destructive behavior. Economic exigencies of mental health care in the 1990s, as well as lack of convincing evidence of the superiority of long-term hospitalization (Rosenbluth and Silver 1992), indicate that short-term hospitalization will increasingly play a crucial role in the care of patients who have severe personality disorders.

Our purpose in this chapter is to provide guidelines for the short-term hospital care of these patients. Included in this discussion are indications and goals for hospitalization; suggestions for individual, group, family, and psychopharmacologic intervention; special considerations in inpatient treatment; and guidelines for discharge planning.

Hospitalized patients with severe personality disorders are often diagnosed as having multiple co-occurring personality disorders. Borderline personality disorder is most common; but patients may also meet criteria for paranoid, narcissistic, schizotypal, or antisocial personality disorders. Perhaps surprisingly, patients with one or more of these traditionally more severe personality disorders may exhibit features of histrionic, avoidant, dependent, obsessive-compulsive, or passive-aggressive personality disorders as well. In fact, in our experience, the severity of personality disturbance is often directly correlated with the number of DSM-III-R Axis II disorders (American Psychiatric Association 1987) that can be diagnosed.

Clinicians routinely do not diagnose more than one Axis II disorder in their patients. They usually focus on the one that they consider the most prominent, serious, or relevant to their treatment approach. It is unlikely that each Axis II diagnosis represents a distinct disorder in patients with severe personality disturbance. They are more likely to be manifestations of more fundamental, underlying psychopathological disturbances (e.g., in impulse control, mood regulation, or behavioral inhibition [Siever and Davis 1991]) that differ from each other on variables such as severity, stage of illness, aspect of functioning affected, or co-morbid Axis I disorder. Implications of the co-occurrence of particular combinations of Axis II disorders are discussed below in the subsection on Differential Diagnosis.

Kernberg's (1975, 1984) concept of borderline personality organization cuts across numerous DSM-III-R categories and would almost always apply to patients with personality disorders necessitating hospitalization. These patients have distorted concepts of self and others that lead to chaotic interpersonal relations, and they use primitive defenses such as splitting, projective identification, and acting out. In these patients, overall ego weakness contributes to intolerance of anxiety, poor control of impulses, and lack of capacity to be invested in issues other than those of immediate self-interest.

INDICATIONS FOR HOSPITALIZATION

The most common and significant indication for hospitalizing a patient with a severe personality disorder is high suicide risk. Hospitalization can also be indicated for other reasons, such as diagnostic purposes. Other reasons for hospitalization may be to treat superimposed Axis I disorders, to prevent other forms of self-damaging or other-menacing behaviors, to stabilize family or other social or occupational situations in times of crisis, to consult and assist in difficult or problematic ongoing outpatient treatment, or to establish outpatient treatment in previously untreated patients or patients who have prematurely interrupted their treatment.

Suicide Risk

Patients with severe personality disorders, particularly those with borderline personality disorder, are prone to impulsive suicide attempts. These are often in response to frustration, disappointment, loss, or fear of abandonment. Patients with borderline personality disorder frequently develop major depressive episodes, often in response to negative life events (Perry et al. 1992). The combination of an impulsive personality style and major depression can be lethal.

Patients with severe personality disorders often use suicidal threats, gestures, or attempts in an effort to manipulate or control important people in their lives—lovers, parents, therapists, and others. Such behavior may be part of a general wish to abdicate responsibility for themselves, regress, and be taken care of by others. In the case of bona fide suicidality, the patient should be admitted to the hospital for self-protection. Furthermore, hospitalization indicates that the therapist is concerned with the patient's welfare and can and will set limits on his or her behavior. Hospitalization can be involuntary, if necessary, as a demonstration that the therapist can tolerate the patient's anger. In the case of manipulative suicidal behavior, hospitalization is usually considered countertherapeutic, because it promotes regression and irresponsibility.

The task, then, is to distinguish real suicide risk from manipulative threat. Patients with impulsive personality traits and superimposed major depressive episodes should be considered at high risk. In less clear-cut cases, the indications for hospitalization vary according to the extent of the evaluator's prior experience with the patient and understanding of the patient. With a patient involved in an ongoing therapeutic relationship, knowledge of the patient's past behavior is influential. A patient who chronically uses the threat of suicide as an interpersonal device is likely to continue in this pattern, but not invariably so. A patient can often come to an agreement with the therapist that he or she will not act on self-destructive impulses and will let the therapist know if he or she is losing control. In any case in which the therapist has reason to doubt or distrust the patient's honesty, ability to maintain self-control (e.g., because of frequent drug or alcohol intoxication), investment in his or her own welfare, or relatedness to the therapist, hospitalization is the preferred choice. For patients with whom the therapist has had little contact, hospitalization should be used to *assess* suicide risk. Patients who survive a bona fide suicide attempt should be hospitalized for further evaluation.

> Mary R. called the psychiatrist who was covering for her doctor, who was on vacation. She related how much she missed her thrice-weekly sessions and admitted that she had been having thoughts of hurting herself. In fact, while on the phone Ms. R. was holding a razor blade she had bought that morning and touching the edge to the skin on her wrists, legs, and chest. The previous night, after several drinks at a neighborhood bar, she had walked across Central Park and along FDR Drive to the Triboro Bridge, before returning to her apartment at about dawn.
>
> The covering psychiatrist convinced Ms. R. to meet him at a nearby hospital emergency room. There, exhibiting little resistance, she agreed to be hospitalized.

When a therapist decides not to hospitalize a patient with a personality disorder who has made an unambiguous suicide threat or gesture, he or she should have a clear therapeutic rationale, which is then documented in the patient's chart. The therapist should also have an explicit understanding with the patient that there are limits to the threats or gestures that can be tolerated in the interests of the patient's overall treatment and that recurring threats or gestures will result in hospitalization.

> Joan D. described the previous night's encounter with her new boyfriend to her longtime therapist. Ms. D.'s boyfriend had apparently suggested that they have sex and had begun to touch and kiss her when she broke from his arms yelling "I can't, I just can't!" She ran into her bedroom, opened the window, and sat on the sill, saying "Don't come near me!" with panic in her eyes. After about 15 minutes of her boyfriend's coaxing and promising that he would make no more advances, Ms. D. relented and let herself be led by the hand back to the living room couch. The man stayed awake all night and insisted he accompany her the next morning to her therapy session.

The therapist did not hospitalize Ms. D. because he recognized her behavior as one of many ways in which she escaped the "threat" of intimacy, and because he knew that she commonly wished to regress and have others protect and take care of her. However, he also made it very clear to Ms. D. that if she seemed unable to control the impulse to place herself in dangerous circumstances, he would not hesitate to hospitalize her.

Differential Diagnosis

As we mentioned earlier, patients with severe personality disorders can present with a complicated psychopathological picture encompassing many DSM-III-R Axis I and Axis II categories (Skodol and Oldham 1991). Although the essential interrelationships between these descriptive syndromes is still poorly understood, clinical heterogeneity often has significant implications for treatment or prognosis.

Axis I disorders that may co-occur with severe personality disorders include organic mood disorder, intoxication and withdrawal (i.e., from alcohol or other substances), alcohol or other psychoactive substance abuse or dependence, major depression, bipolar disorder (I and II), dysthymia, cyclothymia, schizoaffective disorder, panic disorder, social phobia, obsessive-compulsive disorder, posttraumatic stress disorder, anorexia nervosa, bulimia, and various dissociative, somatoform, and impulse control disorders not otherwise specified (NOS). Some of these syndromes require specialized psychosocial or pharmacologic interventions, and combinations of Axis I and Axis II disorders may present special clinical challenges.

Barry W., a 35-year-old businessman, was admitted to the hospital following an overdose of sleeping pills, 1 month after he was indicted for involvement in a money-laundering scheme.

The history revealed that Mr. W. was the only child of parents who were described as self-centered, demanding, critical, rejecting, manipulative, controlling, and exploiting. He had had chronic low self-esteem and social isolation since childhood. After 2 years in college, he joined the family business and became a workaholic, never taking even a single vacation in 10 years.

Mr. W. described intense anxiety in most social situations because he feared humiliation. Throughout his adult life, he had periods of binge eating, alternating with periods of self-starvation, with resultant weight fluctuations between 300 and 160 pounds. On admission he complained of severely depressed mood accompanied by a host of vegetative signs. Regarding his illegal activities, which had profited him several hundred thousand dollars, he claimed to be "only trying to make a living."

A consultant administered a structured diagnostic interview, which revealed that Mr. W. had recurrent major depression, social phobia, bulimia nervosa, and avoidant, schizotypal, histrionic, narcissistic, and borderline personality disorders. A trial of a monoamine oxidase inhibitor (MAOI) and possible long-term hospitalization were recommended.

Accumulating data suggest that the course of treatment of Axis I psychopathology is often adversely affected by the presence of a concomitant Axis II disorder (Reich and Green 1991). Therefore, cases that fail to respond to the usual outpatient management or that follow an unusual clinical course may be candidates for hospitalization to clarify Axis II status.

In addition to comorbid Axis I and Axis II disorders, patients can also present with features of several Axis II disorders. Mixed personality disorders require special considerations in treatment as well. The borderline patient with paranoid personality psychopathology may be particularly prone to transference regression into brief psychosis; the narcissistic personality with antisocial elements may prove unable to communicate with sufficient honesty to participate in the treatment contract. The patient with schizotypal features may be too aloof to form a therapeutic alliance; the dependent patient may be resistant to sharing responsibility for the treatment; the passive-aggressive or self-defeating patient may have the need to defeat the therapist or undermine the success of the therapy. Again, untoward events in the course of treatment may necessitate hospitalization for differential diagnostic purposes.

Because the hospital milieu includes many people, it provides an opportunity to observe a patient's interpersonal relationships (or object relations) firsthand. Although short-term hospital units are not designed to bring out the patient's most extreme behavior, the inpatient setting nonetheless provides a wealth of data for diagnostic purposes.

Treatment of Episodes of Axis I Disorders

An acute episode of an Axis I disorder such as major depression, alcohol abuse, or bulimia often precipitates the hospitalization of a patient with a severe personality disorder. Symptomatic episodes often result from psychosocial crises, which themselves result from maladaptive interactions between the patient and his or her social support systems. Therefore, the symptomatic treatment of acute Axis I disorders is a legitimate goal of brief hospitalization. Common pharmacologic treatments and their limitations are discussed later in this chapter.

Self-Damaging or Other-Menacing Behavior

Patients with severe personality disorders often engage in behaviors, besides suicidal behaviors, which may cause very serious negative consequences to themselves or others. It is the therapist's obligation to intervene, with hospitalization if necessary, to prevent a patient from doing irreparable harm to him- or herself by engaging in excessive drug or alcohol use, impulsively quitting schools or jobs, bingeing and purging, starving, gambling or giving away a family's assets, having high-risk sexual liaisons, and so on. It is also necessary to intervene when a patient who lacks sufficient capacity for self-control threatens to harm other people. Because prediction of violence can be quite difficult, it is again better to err on the side of safety, whenever there is any doubt. Persons who have acted violently in the past are obviously at high risk for repeat acts.

Ray B. was a 28-year-old man who was evaluated by a prison psychiatrist shortly after his arrival at a large city's correctional facility. He had been arrested by a plainclothesman for taking part in a drug deal. Mr. B. felt that he had been an undeserving victim and vowed violent retribution to the police, prosecutors, and judges involved.

Mr. B. had a history of physical abuse as a child, lifelong social isolation, and prior arrests for robbery and assault. During one previous imprisonment, he had been transferred to a maximum security psychiatric ward following an assault on a guard. In speaking of his past history of violence and his current homicidal desires toward law enforcers in general, he exhibited no fear of consequences, guilt, or remorse. The psychiatrist transferred Mr. B. to the prison hospital for further evaluation.

Stabilization of Psychosocial Crises

Crises often complicate the lives of persons with severe personality psychopathology. These patients' maladaptive and inflexible interpersonal styles alienate significant others, friends, employers, and family members, with a resultant loss of interpersonal or economic support. Psychosocial crises frequently precipitate the development or exacerbation of additional psychopathology, which in turn causes further deterioration in the social network and eventually leads to hospitalization. In these instances, the goal of hospitalization is to stabilize the patient's social system. Hospitalization may enable a patient's family to regroup before withdrawing all support and abandoning a needy patient, or before needlessly and destructively enmeshing with the patient by taking over all responsibility. In this role, the hospital functions as a holding unit, enabling equilibrium to be reestablished between the patient and his or her social system.

James R. was a 29-year-old man who had lived at home until the past year and was in his second year of an MBA program. One night, his girlfriend announce that they should "see other people." Mr. R. reacted with shock and dismay, jumped into his car, and drove to his parents' home. There, in an agitated and tearful state, he told his mother what had happened.

Although his parents supported him financially, Mr. R. never felt satisfied with the attention he received from them. In the middle of his story, the phone rang. When his mother did not immediately end the call, Mr. R. flew into a rage. He pounded his fist on the kitchen table, then swept a setting of dinnerware to the floor. He then walked to the counter and picked up a large knife. His mother ran from the room and out of the house. Mr. R. became calmer and went outside. His mother insisted that he leave before she would come back into the house.

The next day, Mr. R.'s psychiatrist received a phone call from Mr. R.'s parents, who after discussing the previous night's incident threatened to cut off support for their son's therapy, apartment, and education. The incident, which had not been the first, appeared to be the last straw. The psychiatrist convinced the parents and Mr. R., who was now feeling suicidal, that a brief stay for Mr. R. in the hospital would be helpful. The parents agreed to postpone making any final decisions.

Crises in Psychotherapy

The outpatient treatment of demanding patients can be stressful for both the patient and the therapist. Patients may respond to the prospect of intimacy or responsibility with acting-out behavior or by psychotic transference regressions. Therapists may experience profound countertransference reactions of anger or despair. At times, psychotherapy crises develop, and the treatment requires the consultative assistance of the inpatient hospital unit. The hospital staff can evaluate the adequacy of the treatment, take over during a particularly stressful time, and assist patient and therapist in reestablishing the alliance and in reassessing goals and techniques. In some cases, a new treatment plan or a new therapist is needed.

Establishing Outpatient Treatment

Many patients with severe personality disorders may enter treatment for the first time via the inpatient service. Following an episode of depression or substance abuse, a psychosocial crisis, or a suicide attempt, the patient may confront the destructive consequences of his or her problematic personality for the first time. After a diagnostic assessment, institution of specialized treatment such as a substance abuse program or pharmacotherapy, and determination of a suitable psychotherapeutic modality, attempts can be made for the patient to begin outpatient treatment with a therapist who is a good "fit."

GOALS FOR HOSPITALIZATION

The goals for short-term hospitalization should be consistent with the indications. In contrast to long-term hospitalization, short-term inpatient treatment provides no opportunity for therapeutic regression or change in personality structure. Stabilization has been the term most often used to refer to the short-term hospital process.

Active suicidal or other self-damaging behavior or aggressive behavior toward others can be prevented and diagnostic questions clarified. Superimposed Axis I syndromes can be treated with medications, and specialized treatment programs initiated when indicated. Family interventions and interventions with others in the patient's social environment can be geared toward reestablishing a reasonable status quo with a minimum of catastrophic losses. Outpatient therapy can be begun or renewed with new insight, direction, and enthusiasm. The patient should be discharged as soon as possible after the goals of the hospitalization have been achieved. He or she should not be allowed to become excessively dependent on the hospital.

SUGGESTIONS FOR TREATMENT

The optimal treatment setting for the short-term hospitalization of patients with personality disorders is a highly structured unit, with clear goals and procedures. The unit should have well-defined limits for ensuring appropriate behavior. Staff should use treatment contracts to ensure compliance and to provide unambiguous consequences for dysfunctional behavior (Gunderson 1984). It is probably advantageous to limit the number of difficult, provocative, or challenging patients hospitalized on a given unit at one time.

Treatment should be multimodal and include individual, group, and family therapy, as well as psychopharmacology as indicated (Oldham and Russakoff 1987). As we have mentioned, referrals can be made to drug abuse counselors or Alcoholics (or Gamblers, Narcotics, Overeaters, etc.) Anonymous. (Specific chapters on the various forms of psychotherapy employed on the inpatient psychiatric unit are included elsewhere in this book.)

A member of the inpatient staff should assume primary responsibility for treatment of a hospitalized patient in ongoing outpatient therapy, when possible. This prevents the patient from using the hospital to obtain more from his or her outpatient therapist; provides for a fresh, objective look at the patient; and enables new pharmacologic intervention without concern for its effects on the ongoing therapeutic transference (or countertransference).

Individual Psychotherapy

Individual psychotherapy may be psychodynamic, interpersonal, behavioral, or cognitive. Psychodynamic therapy during a time-limited inpatient stay would be largely supportive and would focus on solving current problems, strengthening adaptive functioning, and avoiding regression. Attempts to act out, split staff, or be manipulative would be dealt with largely by confrontation and environmental approaches (i.e., constant observation or transfer out of the facility by contract agreement) rather than by interpretation (Waldinger and Gunderson 1984, 1987).

Because maladaptive interpersonal behaviors are a sine qua non of severe personality disturbance, Benjamin (in press) has outlined an interpersonal treatment approach based on her model of interpersonal behavior—the structural analysis of social behavior (SASB). The treatment emphasizes

1. Forming a working alliance;
2. Identifying patterns of interpersonal interaction and their origins for a patient;
3. Blocking maladaptive patterns;
4. Giving up underlying wishes and challenging fears; and
5. Learning new, more adaptive patterns.

Behavioral techniques are now being developed for certain severe personality disorders, including borderline personality disorder. Linehan (1987) employs dialectical behavior therapy (DBT) to treat borderline patients with suicidal behaviors. DBT uses traditional behavioral techniques such as exposure, skills training, contingency management, and cognitive modification to help patients manage suicidal and avoidance behaviors, regulate their emotions, and increase their frustration tolerance. Linehan has found the treatment to be acceptable to patients and to decrease the severity of parasuicidal behaviors and the length of inpatient hospitalization.

Cognitive therapy has also been adapted for the treatment of patients with personality disorders (Beck and Freeman 1990; Young 1987). For example, distorted beliefs that are common among borderline patients and may be addressed by cognitive therapy include 1) "the world is dangerous," 2) "I am powerless and vulnerable," and 3) "I am unacceptable." Taken together, these beliefs lead to vacillations between extreme dependency and inappropriate autonomy (Shea 1991). Another target of cognitive therapy is dichotomous thinking, referred to in psychodynamic terms as splitting. Other goals for patients with borderline personality disorder are to increase emotional stability and impulse control and to firm up a patient's sense of self or identity. A patient with antisocial personality disorder may be taught to more carefully consider the consequences of his or her actions. Because personality patterns are deeply ingrained, cognitive therapy of patients with severe personality disorders is likely to be a much longer process than for patients with anxiety or depressive disorders. However, if it is focused on a specific set of circumstances that precipitated a hospitalization, cognitive therapy may be very useful in resolving a particular crisis.

Group Therapy

Group therapy for patients with severe personality disorders has a long history, especially in hospital settings (Clarkin et al. 1991). Group therapy can be useful by diluting typically intense transference reactions, by providing the opportunity for identification with many persons, and by providing the patient with feedback about his or her behavior that is sometimes more acceptable than if it had emanated from an individual therapist. Peer pressure is useful in limit setting, and group support is helpful in times of severe depression. The group experience demands that the patient display appropriate social behavior and maintain appropriate degrees of involvement with others.

Family Therapy

Because of the growing appreciation of the psychopathology in families of patients with severe personality disorders, especially borderline personality disorder, there is a clear rationale for family intervention. Psychopathology in family members ranges from frank Axis I and II disorders to physical and sexual abuse, neglect, or overprotection of the patient.

Family intervention can be useful in helping a patient separate and individuate from an overinvolved family. Families can be taught to recognize patterns of interaction that may lead to suicide attempts or other acting-out behaviors. Families can be taught appropriate techniques of discipline and limit setting. Finally, intervention may be critical to stop ongoing physical or sexual abuse.

> Barbara S. was a 23-year-old unemployed woman who lived at home with her parents and was hospitalized for repeated episodes of cutting herself with a razor. She was extremely meek and childlike, spoke in a squeaky, whining voice, and seemed virtually always on the verge of tears.
>
> Family evaluation revealed very overprotective parents who did everything for Ms. S., including buying her clothes, doing her laundry, and making her bed. During the family session, her father sat next to her, holding her hand. At one point, he got up from his chair, got on his knees in front of her, and put his head in her lap. Family intervention consisting of limiting the father's visitation while Ms. S. was hospitalized and educating the parents about their overinvolvement. Arrangements for follow-up family therapy in conjunction with individual therapy were made prior to Ms. S.'s discharge.

Psychopharmacology

Advances in psychobiology and psychopharmacology have made medications a common adjunct and often an integral part of the treatment of severe personality disorders. The three principal targets of psychopharmacologic intervention are affective symptoms, psychotic symptoms, and impulsive aggressive behavior (Coccaro and Kavoussi 1991).

Affective symptoms.   Disturbances in mood can take many forms in persons with severe personality disorders. Some patients, such as those with borderline personality disorder, have generalized mood instability characterized by rapid shifts in and out of depressed or anxious states. Although emotional instability is not a diagnosable syndrome in and of itself, mood-stabilizing medications such as lithium and carbamazepine have been found to be useful for modulating rapidly shifting moods.

Severe personality disorders are commonly accompanied by diagnosable mood disorders, especially when affected patients are in need of hospital treatment. Patients with major depressive episodes require intervention with antidepressant drugs. Studies have shown that MAOIs are generally more effective in treating depressive episodes in borderline patients than are tricyclic antidepressants (TCAs), particularly when the depression is characterized by "atypical features," such as rejection sensitivity and reversed vegetative signs (Cowdry and Gardner 1988; Liebowitz and Klein 1981; Parsons et al. 1989). Recently, fluoxetine has been shown to be beneficial in reducing depressive symptoms (Cornelius et al. 1990).

Psychotic symptoms. Borderline personality disorder is often accompanied by transient, stress-related, "quasi-psychotic" cognitive-perceptual distortions (Zanarini et al. 1990), which may fall short of DSM-III-R definitions of psychosis. Low-dose treatment with neuroleptic medications such as thiothixene, haloperidol, or thioridazine has been demonstrated to be effective on a wide range of mild, "psychotic" symptoms, such as suspiciousness, ideas of reference, odd communication, and illusions (Goldberg et al. 1986; Soloff et al. 1989). Patients with Cluster A paranoid or schizotypal personality disorders would therefore also be candidates for neuroleptic treatment.

> Roberto P. was a 33-year-old man who was admitted to the hospital after he threatened to kill his boss. The boss had come to the defense of a co-worker, who Mr. P. thought was purposefully "baiting" him and otherwise going out of his way to give him a hard time.
>
> Mr. P. had a lifelong history of impulsivity. As a teenager, he had been in frequent fights and had abused drugs. As an adult he commonly walked away from jobs when he felt mistreated, and he had frequent extramarital affairs. He also described himself as a very moody person and claimed that it was during periods of depression that he became sensitive and easily provoked to anger.
>
> Following a negative neurological workup, Mr. P. was started on 2 mg of thiothixene tid. He felt calmer and became engaged in the treatment milieu. Later in the hospital course, he was also started on lithium carbonate, which seemed to dampen his mood swings. Mr. P. also continued in outpatient therapy, in which he tried to understand why he felt so sensitive and in which he learned to "think before reacting."

Impulsive aggressive symptoms. Lithium (Links et al. 1990; Sheard et al. 1976), carbamazepine (Cowdry and Gardner 1988), and fluoxetine

(Coccaro et al. 1990; Cornelius et al. 1990) have all been shown to reduce impulsive behaviors. Thus, these medications should be considered in the management of behavioral dyscontrol, including self-injurious behaviors (Markovitz et al. 1991).

Other symptoms and syndromes. Because patients with personality disorders may also present with other Axis I syndromes, psychopharmacology may play an even broader role. Patients with bulimia may require treatment with MAOIs; those with obsessive-compulsive disorder may warrant trials of fluoxetine or clomipramine; and those with panic disorder may need TCAs. On a cautious note, alprazolam has been found to increase behavioral dyscontrol in persons predisposed to loss of impulse control (Gardner and Cowdry 1985).

In Chapter 2, the integration of psychotherapy and psychopharmacologic treatment is discussed. In the short-term inpatient setting, as we have mentioned, treatment of persons with personality disorders is best assumed by an inpatient therapist not involved in the long-term outpatient care of the patient. In these instances, interference with intensive psychotherapy is usually minimal, because the psychotherapy itself is brief, targeted, and crisis-oriented. In instances when the treating psychiatrist also continues with primary responsibility for the patient during a brief hospital stay, the key to protecting a viable, exploratory psychotherapy is clear communication to the patient that medication is prescribed for a specific reason (symptom or syndrome). It is also necessary to let the patient know that continued psychological growth and personality change require his or her active effort and sense of responsibility.

SPECIAL CONSIDERATIONS

It is certainly not easy to treat patients with severe personality disorders on a short-term inpatient unit. These patients are among the most difficult and challenging inpatients, and it is often impossible to achieve the goals of hospitalization within strict time constraints.

Borderline psychopathology can make each step of the hospitalization process taxing. A sullen patient admitted involuntarily to the hospital from an emergency room after a failed suicide attempt is unlikely to provide a wealth of helpful information. Dramatic and emotional patients inhibit assessment, because they are difficult to focus or render the clinician unable to distinguish exaggeration from fact. All statements may be made in the extreme (i.e., the result of characteristic black-and-white, all-or-nothing thinking). Splitting may also lead to apparent contradictions.

Once on the ward, such patients can be very disruptive. They can provoke continuous anxiety among staff members with suicide threats and may pit staff members against one another in a characteristic good-bad split. They may entice other patients to use drugs, go AWOL from the hospital, or attempt suicide. These patients may monopolize staff time and energy to the detriment of other patients (Miller 1989).

Effective organization and clear and open communication about ward capacities, policies, rules, expectations, and the consequences of unacceptable behavior on the part of patients are prophylactic, to a degree. A treatment contract is a concrete antidote (Friedman 1969; Rosenbluth 1987).

Martha M. was a 45-year-old married woman with a 20-year history of migraine headaches for which she had been taking increasing doses of pain medications. At the time of her admission, her fourth for detoxification, she was taking between 50 and 60 tablets of Tylenol with codeine #4 and Percocet daily.

Ms. M. was started on an opioid detoxification regimen beginning with 30 mg of methadone per day, which was to be gradually reduced. Although she agreed to the unit rules on admission, she had great difficulty complying with them. She avoided participation in activities and refused to attend group therapy, which she viewed as meant for patients with problems unlike her own. She complained that her psychiatrist was not readily available, despite daily scheduled sessions Monday through Friday. Ms. M. also complained that reduction of the methadone dose was occurring too rapidly and spent most of her individual sessions "negotiating" the next day's dose. She saw no use in discussing any issues beyond her headaches, her need for pain medications, and the unreasonableness of the staff. On several occasions, cigarette smoke was smelled in her room. She denied smoking, but was reminded that smoking was not allowed on the unit, and if she smoked, she would be unable to remain an inpatient. Two nights later Ms. M.

was discovered smoking cigarettes smuggled into the unit by her husband, and the next morning she was discharged.

Although drug treatment is often indicated for these patients, studies have shown that personality disorders often have a negative impact on treatment response. Mood and anxiety disorders of various types have been shown to have a poorer response to pharmacologic treatment when personality disorders are comorbid (Reich and Green 1991). Therefore, an attenuated response may be all that is achievable during a relatively short inpatient stay. Some symptom relief or a degree of stability may be more realistic goals than complete symptom remission. Partial symptomatic response to medications may paradoxically represent a better outcome than if there were no potentially medication-responsive target symptoms to treat.

DISCHARGE PLANNING

Providing that the patient can be managed and helped to achieve hospitalization goals, discharge planning becomes the next hurdle. Patients may again feel threatened by the forces that led to the crisis necessitating admission and may undergo some symptomatic relapse. For example, suicidal ideation may recur. An initial discharge date may fall through. It is critical to have an established, acceptable, outpatient treatment arrangement in place before the patient is discharged. Sometimes a period of time spent in a partial day or night hospital facility will enable a person to adjust gradually to the demands of the "real" world and provide a haven in times of stress.

Amy D., a 24-year-old secretary, had been admitted to the hospital following a 2-month period during which she was, in her parents' words, "not functioning." The period began after a breakup with a man she had been seeing for a very "stormy" 3 months. Ms. D. stopped going to work, left her apartment to return to her parents' home, and spent most her time in bed with the shades drawn. When she stopped bathing, her parents arranged for hospital admission through a family friend.

A few days into her hospital stay, Ms. D. improved markedly. She was compliant with unit rules, attached herself readily to several other female patients, and seemed contented. The social worker contacted her office and found that her employer had been using office temporaries and was willing to have Ms. D. come back to work part-time. The psychiatrist advised twice-weekly outpatient therapy and half-day sessions at the day treatment program, while she adjusted again to work and independent living. Ms. D. accepted the plan, and her parents offered to support it financially.

Then a discharge date was set. Immediately, Ms. D. regressed into a tearful, withdrawn, and helpless state. She cried continuously at community meetings where her impending discharge was discussed. Other patients were up in arms that the staff would be so "cruel." Staff, in turn, explained Ms. D.'s wish to be taken care of and protected from life's vicissitudes. After two postponements of the discharge date, nursing staff physically escorted Ms. D. off the unit. She sat under a tree in the yard beneath the unit windows for about 6 hours. The next day she appeared on time at the day program. She was feeling considerably better and planned to go to work that afternoon.

CONCLUSIONS

Because the effective treatment of persons with personality disorders is necessarily a long-term project, expectations regarding the impact of a single, brief hospitalization should be modest. The object is to keep the patient alive and in relatively stable social and treatment environments, to allow the treatment to proceed. It is likely that one short hospitalization will eventually be followed by others. Long-term hospitalization may be needed by some impulsive patients who show limited capacity to cooperate with outpatient treatment but are deemed capable of benefiting from intensive therapy (Kernberg et al. 1989).

Providing an opportunity for adequate care over a sustained period appears to result in a reasonably optimistic long-term prognosis for many people with severe personality disorders (McGlashan 1986; Stone 1990). Poor prognostic signs include extreme versions of traits found in antisocial, sadistic, narcissistic, paranoid, and schizoid personality disorders. Examples include extreme hostility, contemptuousness, maliciousness, abusiveness, arrogance, lack of empathy, ruthless exploitativeness, mistrustfulness, externalization, and social detachment (Stone 1992). For those without these traits, who possess sufficient insight to internalize and take responsibility for their problems and can form a therapeutic relationship, the future need not be bleak.

REFERENCES

American Psychiatric Association: Diagnostic and Statistical Manual of Mental Disorders, 3rd Edition, Revised. Washington, DC, American Psychiatric Association, 1987

Beck AT, Freeman A: Cognitive Therapy of Personality Disorders. New York, Guilford, 1990

Benjamin LS: Diagnosis and Treatment of Personality Disorders: A Structured Approach. New York, Guilford (in press)

Clarkin JF, Marziali E, Munroe-Blum H: Group and family treatments for borderline personality disorder. Hosp Community Psychiatry 42:1038–1043, 1991

Coccaro EF, Kavoussi RJ: Biological and pharmacological aspects of borderline personality disorder. Hosp Community Psychiatry 42:1029–1033, 1991

Coccaro EF, Astill JL, Herbert JL: Fluoxetine treatment of impulsive aggression in DSM-III-R personality disorder patients. J Clin Psychopharmacol 10:373–375, 1990

Cornelius JR, Soloff PH, Perel JM, et al: Fluoxetine trial in borderline personality disorder. Psychopharmacol Bull 26:151–154, 1990

Cowdry R, Gardner DL: Pharmacotherapy of borderline personality disorder: alprazolam, carbamazepine, trifluoperazine, and tranylcypromine. Arch Gen Psychiatry 45:111–119, 1988

Friedman H: Some problems of inpatient management with borderline patients. Am J Psychiatry 126:299–304, 1969

Gardner DL, Cowdry RW: Alprazolam-induced dyscontrol in borderline personality disorder. Am J Psychiatry 142:98–100, 1985

Goldberg S, Schulz C, Schulz P, et al: Borderline and schizotypal personality disorders treated with low-dose thiothixene vs placebo. Arch Gen Psychiatry 32:680–686, 1986

Gunderson J: Borderline Personality Disorder. Washington, DC, American Psychiatric Press, 1984

Kernberg O: Borderline Conditions and Pathological Narcissism. New York, Jason Aronson, 1975

Kernberg O: Severe Personality Disorders: Psychotherapeutic Strategies. New Haven, CT, Yale University Press, 1984

Kernberg OF, Selzer MA, Koenigsberg HW, et al: Psychodynamic Psychotherapy of Borderline Patients. New York, Basic Books, 1989

Liebowitz M, Klein D: Interrelationship of hysteroid dysphoria and borderline personality disorder. Psychiatr Clin North Am 4:67–87, 1981

Linehan M: Dialectal behavior therapy for borderline personality disorder: theory and method. Bull Menninger Clin 51:261–276, 1987

Links PS, Steiner M, Bioago I, et al: Lithium therapy for borderline patients: preliminary findings. Journal of Personality Disorders 4:173–181, 1990

Markovitz PJ, Calabrese JR, Schulz SC, et al: Fluoxetine in the treatment of borderline and schizotypal personality disorders. Am J Psychiatry 148:1064–1067, 1991

McGlashan T: The Chestnut Lodge follow-up study, III: long-term outcome of borderline personalities. Arch Gen Psychiatry 43:20–30, 1986

Miller L: Inpatient management of borderline personality disorder: a review and update. Journal of Personality Disorders 3:122–134, 1989

Oldham JM, Russakoff LM: Dynamic Therapy in Brief Hospitalization. Northvale, NJ, Jason Aronson, 1987

Parsons B, Quitkin F, McGrath P, et al: Phenelzine, imipramine and placebo in borderline patients meeting criteria for atypical depression. Psychopharmacol Bull 25:524–534, 1989

Perry JC, Lavori PW, Pagano CJ, et al: Life events and recurrent depression in borderline and antisocial personality disorders. Journal of Personality Disorders 6:394–407, 1992

Reich J, Green A: Effect of personality disorders on outcome of treatment. J Nerv Ment Dis 179:74–82, 1991

Rosenbluth M: The inpatient treatment of borderline personality disorder: a critical review and discussion of aftercare implications. Can J Psychiatry 32:228–237, 1987

Rosenbluth M, Silver D: The inpatient treatment of borderline personality disorder, in Handbook of Borderline Disorders. Edited by Silver D, Rosenbluth M. Madison, CT, International Universities Press, 1992, pp 509–532

Shea MT: Standardized approaches to individual psychotherapy of patients with borderline personality disorder. Hosp Community Psychiatry 42:1034–1038, 1991

Sheard M, Marini J, Bridges C, et al: The effect of lithium on impulsive aggressive behavior in man. Am J Psychiatry 133:1409–1413, 1976

Siever LJ, Davis KL: A psychobiological perspective on the personality disorders. Am J Psychiatry 148:1647–1658, 1991

Skodol AE, Oldham JM: Assessment and diagnosis of borderline personality disorder. Hosp Community Psychiatry 42:1021–1028, 1991

Skodol AE, Buckley P, Charles E: Is there a characteristic pattern to the treatment history of clinic outpatients with borderline personality? J Nerv Ment Dis 171:405–410, 1983

Soloff P, George A, Nathan R, et al: Amitriptyline vs. haloperidol in borderlines: final outcomes and predictors of response. J Clin Psychopharmacol 9:238–246, 1989

Stone MH: The Fate of Borderline Patients. New York, Guilford, 1990

Stone MH: Treatment of severe personality disorders, in American Psychiatric Press Review of Psychiatry, Vol 11. Edited by Tasman A, Riba MB. Washington, DC, American Psychiatric Press, 1992, pp 98–115

Waldinger R, Gunderson J: Completed psychotherapies with borderline patients. Am J Psychother 38:190–201, 1984

Waldinger R, Gunderson J: Effective Psychotherapy With Borderline Patients. New York, Macmillan, 1987

Young J: Schema-Focused Cognitive Therapy for Personality Disorders. New York, Center for Cognitive Therapy, 1987

Zanarini M, Gunderson J, Frankenburg F: Cognitive features of borderline personality disorder. Am J Psychiatry 147:57–63, 1990

CHAPTER 14

Residency Training in Psychotherapy on Acute Inpatient Treatment Services

Michelle Riba, M.D.
Allan Tasman, M.D.

Although this book has focused on clinical issues regarding the use of psychotherapy in brief psychiatric hospitalization, there are a number of training and education concerns worth reviewing. *The Essentials of Accredited Residencies in Psychiatry* (American Medical Association 1989) requires a minimum of 9 months of inpatient experience, and most residents have full- or part-time inpatient responsibilities for 12 to 18 months. In the past, the controlled environment of the inpatient unit has allowed trainees to learn the skills required to conduct psychotherapy with severely ill patients, to monitor the effects of various interventions, to follow patients through the diminution or resolution of symptoms, and to apply novel treatments in refractory cases (Crowder and Jack 1988).

These objectives remain important despite recent changes in many inpatient settings that complicate the educational process. As mentioned in preceding chapters, these changes include more rapid turnover of patients, development of treatment programs requiring expertise in novel areas, and increased acuteness and severity of patient illnesses (Silver et al. 1983). Our brief discussion here highlights the psychotherapy training issues that have ensued from these changes for inpatient settings. The material is organized around supervisory issues regarding treatment setting, patient condition, trainee needs, and the supervisor's changing role.

TREATMENT SETTING

Although short-term inpatient units may differ in certain respects, they are relatively open systems regarding human traffic (Alarcon et al. 1988). More than 200 people may walk through the average inpatient unit on any given day, interacting with patients and each other (Alarcon et al. 1988). These various individuals span the entire range of health care providers, trainees, and family members. Each group of trainees has supervisors and instructors who may communicate or interact with one another. To provide optimal supervision and teaching on a given unit, it is important to understand the organization and dynamics of that particular setting.

For example, it is critical to examine unit organization in terms of power and responsibilities. Depending on the unit, duties of the attending psychiatrist may include running teams or administering the unit, making daily (or less frequent) rounds, writing notes, conferring with third-party payors, teaching and supervising trainees, reviewing charts for quality assurance, or meeting with families. This variability directly affects the type of resident supervision. For example, on some units, the attending psychiatrist makes rounds daily with trainees and helps set treatment plans. In such settings, the attendings are role models for residents and medical students in providing direct patient care. In this model, the trainee sees the attending psychiatrist interview the patient and his or her family, make clinical decisions, and interact with staff. This then can be viewed as an apprenticeship model of training.

In other treatment settings, direct patient care responsibility is mostly borne by house staff. In this model, attending psychiatrists oversee patient care from a more distant vantage point. Although there may be less patient care modeling in this setting for trainees, there are more opportunities for the trainees to assume leadership. Further, in this setting, more responsibility is placed on trainees for conveying accurate patient information to attendings. Oral presentations and written notes become more important as a means of communication.

The permanence of senior staff is also an issue. On some units, attendings are permanent staff who never rotate off to other assignments. The attending psychiatrists view their inpatient units as "home base." This feeling may convey a certain sense of stability to patients, staff, and trainees. For example, a faculty member may have treated some patients on prior admissions and can bring quick familiarity to the care of these patients. The attending may be able to communicate the patient's strengths and weaknesses to the resident, thereby quickly amplifying the resident's understanding of the case. On the other hand, this prior relationship between attendings and patients may also make it more difficult for the resident to act as the primary caregiver for the patient.

On other units, attendings rotate after a period of time. This may alleviate burnout of attending staff and allow for faculty with different expertise (e.g., psychopharmacology, psychotherapy) to bring that teaching talent to the unit. This type of faculty rotation may be destabilizing to the milieu, especially on short-term units where patient turnover is quick. However, in such settings, residents may feel more like primary therapists and not overshadowed by attendings.

The influence, then, of the attending on the short-term inpatient unit is determined by the daily time spent, the length of tenure (rotation versus permanent basis), the stature of the attending in the department (junior versus senior faculty), the amount of direct patient care, and the administrative responsibilities of the attending (clinical unit director, medical director, etc.). These issues are not only important for the attending but will also affect the resident's role and status, because some of the attending's power may be transferred onto the resident in the view of patients and staff.

The role and specific responsibilities of the trainee also may be very different depending on the treatment setting. Residents may be expected to act as primary therapists. They may also function as managers or team leaders supervising the treatment provided by other caregivers (e.g., psychologists, nurses, occupational therapists, medical students) and may provide medication backup to nonmedical therapists.

Additionally, residents may have other daily professional responsibilities apart from those on the inpatient setting, such as providing emergency room coverage, treating outpatients, attending seminars, and receiving psychotherapy supervision. As the psychiatric resident is struggling with his or her own difficult and ambiguous role and multiple tasks, he or she is also trying to be a role model for, and provide teaching and supervision to, medical students.

Because of the variability of attending and resident roles, the style, method, and content of supervision also change. On units where residents function as primary therapists, more time may be spent learning psychotherapy techniques. Where residents function as case managers, supervision may be focused on systems management, effective communication with nonmedical therapists, and psychopharmacology.

Besides understanding the responsibilities and duties of attendings and residents, it is also critical to understand the structure of the unit itself. As has been previously discussed, inpatient psychiatric units have been influenced by two models: 1) the highly structured medical model, characterized by a vertical hierarchy, strict role definitions, and well-delineated lines of authority; and 2) the therapeutic community model, which is more democratic in nature, with consensual decision making determined by multidisciplinary teams (Lofgren 1975; Starr 1982). The first model is characterized by relatively predictable roles and responsibilities. Because this medical model offers little room for change, the experience can be frustrating for residents who are inquisitive and innovative. However, it does offer an opportunity to teach about structure and the importance of boundaries. In the therapeutic community model, there is often a blurring of professional roles and boundaries, with the potential for disorganization and chaos. This model offers an opportunity to teach residents about the importance of communication and process. The supervisor's task is to help the trainee understand the prevailing model so that the treatment can be understood in the context of the unit.

The unit philosophy influences how patient care is discussed and the trainee's role in these discussions. Most units have ward rounds and some type of team meeting in which patient care is reviewed. On units organized according to the medical model, residents may be expected to run the team meetings. The resident must then learn how to conduct a well-organized meeting, setting the tone and agenda while eliciting and synthesizing information from an interdisciplinary team of professionals. On units with a strong grounding in the therapeutic community model, the resident may just be a participant in such meetings.

Whichever type of philosophy prevails, ward staffs often have well-established methods for direct and indirect communication that are not always apparent to residents who are transient members of the interdisciplinary team. Residents must be kept apprised by supervisors and other staff of these communication patterns so that they can be effective contributors to the treatment effort as well as feel welcomed and socialized to the unit. This latter point is quite important and cannot be overlooked. On the short-term unit where the staff is permanent and the resident is on the unit for a limited time, it is easy to undervalue the resident's role and bypass him or her in terms of decision making, communication, and friendship building. A well-organized orientation to the unit, clear and written position descriptions for residents, and a staff sensitive to the socialization needs of the trainee are all helpful.

The unit milieu and type of supervision provided to residents are also influenced by the diagnostic mix of the patients. It is now the accepted standard that most inpatient units treat a diverse mix of patients (Johansen 1983; Swartz et al. 1988). As a result, the demands to individualize treatment often conflict with the desire for a cohesive and unified milieu, taking into account the varying diagnostic disorders being treated. It may be difficult for the resident to clearly identify the various inpatient biological and psychotherapeutic modalities important in the treatment of such a diverse group of patients. The supervisor must help the trainee set reasonable goals and tailor treatment based on the resources of the unit and the community.

Elizabeth S., a 35-year-old single white female with a history of alcohol dependence, insulin-dependent diabetes mellitus, and borderline personality disorder, was admitted to a short-term inpatient psychiatric unit after evaluation in the emergency room. Shortly after admission, Ms. S. was found cutting herself with a razor blade, which she had managed to bring onto the unit despite being searched for weapons. She was quickly secluded and placed in restraints for safety because she was a danger to herself. She began screaming loudly, which was upsetting to both staff and other patients.

Because the PGY II resident had been responsible for the patient's admission and because the patient was causing so much "trouble," the resident believed the staff was angry at him. During morning report, the resident heard about the staff's difficult night, and he began to make plans to transfer Ms. S. to another hospital. This resident, who had just started on the inpatient unit, was unsure of his abilities. Although he had been able to establish a therapeutic alliance with Ms. S. in the emergency room, he was unsure if he could care for this medically and psychiatrically ill patient in the face of what he saw as the staff's overwhelming resentment. Because of these worries, he wanted to align himself with the staff against Ms. S. and thus began planning for her transfer. During rounds, the attending psychiatrist, with the resident, interviewed Ms. S., and provided suggestions about pharmacological treatment of her disruptive behavior, and elucidated the response by the resident and staff to Ms. S. Once Ms. S. became calm, the resident no longer thought that it was necessary to transfer her and was better able to formulate (with staff involvement) an appropriate treatment plan.

This case illustrates some of the common difficulties encountered when junior residents coordinate the treatment of severely disturbed patients on short-term inpatient units. The close supervision of the resident in this setting by the attending psychiatrist helped restore the resident's confidence, provided practical teaching on medications and psychodynamics, and helped the resident to understand his role and feelings toward Ms. S. and the staff.

ISSUES RELATED TO PATIENT CONDITION

The goals of hospitalization may vary. For some patients, management of an acute problem (e.g., violence, overwhelming stress, aggression, behavioral turmoil) provides the basis for admission and the goals for discharge. For others, an exacerbation of an ongoing condition, either a major psychiatric disorder on Axis I, a long-standing personality disorder on Axis II, or a combination of a medical disorder and psychopathology may necessitate admission. Because of this heterogeneity, it is not always easy to decide on the goals of treatment, or the types of psychotherapeutic intervention that should be emphasized.

Colin T., a 52-year-old sculptor with a history of rheumatoid arthritis, was referred to the inpatient unit by his outpatient therapist of 5 years, a prominent analyst. Mr. T. had a narcissistic personality disorder and had recently been experiencing neurovegetative symptoms of depression. Stressors included finding out he was HIV positive, being unable to create the high-quality art he had previously been able to produce, and dealing with the death of his lover.

During Mr. T.'s hospitalization, the second-year resident focused on the neurovegetative symptoms and on organic etiologies for his depression. Although his Axis I and Axis III problems were being actively treated, the manifestations of Mr. T.'s narcissistic personality and recent losses were not being addressed, because the resident became increasingly preoccupied with the medical workup and with organizing input from various consultants (i.e., infectious disease, rheumatology). The resident also worried about being compared to Mr. T.'s outpatient therapist.

The supervisor and the resident discussed the latter's avoidance of psychotherapy with Mr. T. because of competitive concerns about the outpatient therapist. In addition, supervision helped the resident prioritize the psychotherapeutic and biological issues. It was decided that the immediate psychotherapeutic goal was to help Mr. T. cope with his HIV status and to address his long-standing personality problems only as they related to his self-image.

Because inpatient lengths of stay are ever decreasing (Black and Winokur 1988), to optimally help patients, supervision must focus on setting appropriate goals for psychotherapy. Usually the daily sessions between resident and patient are short and lengths of stay are brief, so residents must learn how to move quickly from beginning to middle and then to termination phases of psychotherapy. In addition, residents must learn how to integrate psychotherapeutic inpatient interventions with outpatient therapists' goals and family and other social support issues. Residents must also learn how to integrate exploratory and supportive psychotherapeutic techniques with the overall medical and psychiatric workup.

Besides the psychotherapy and biological interventions, residents need to learn how to manage the behavior of inpatients. The regressed behavior of inpatients allows residents to see for themselves, or through the observations of other team members, how severely disturbed patients experience their internal and external worlds. Although it is difficult, understanding the patient condition is an integral part of residency education (Shershow and Savodnik 1976). Dramatic transference and countertransference feelings develop quickly and the resident may have difficulty recognizing and responding to these phenomena.

> Following a separation from her husband, Monica K., a 42-year-old lawyer, was admitted to the short-term inpatient unit for suicidal feelings and exacerbation of her obsessive-compulsive disorder. Ms. K.'s husband called and visited her often, and 2 days after admission she asked for a pass to go to dinner with him. Though the resident knew that passes were rarely granted so early in a hospitalization, she nevertheless recommended the pass.
>
> The treatment team quickly made it clear that this was not the unit's usual procedure and pointed out to the resident that Ms. K. had been admitted with suicidal feelings that had not changed significantly since admission. The resident became quite angry, said she thought there was no harm in granting the pass, and ordered it anyway. A nurse on the team called the attending psychiatrist to inform her of the situation, and the attending reviewed the case with the resident. They discussed how Ms. K.'s need for control was being reflected in the resident's over-controlled response toward the staff. The resident subsequently reversed her decision, realizing the need to keep the patient safe.

As this case points out, the resident identified with the patient and had difficulty seeing the patient's very regressed and dangerous behavior. The resident initially felt uncomfortable setting limits and did not fully appreciate the patient's or her own psychodynamic issues. Another issue raised by this case is the subject of passes on a short-term inpatient unit. Traditionally there have been well-defined systems of passes, often based on longer patient stays. For the short-term inpatient unit, there is little literature on this subject (Remeikis et al. 1988). Often little help is given to the resident concerning criteria for using passes as "therapeutic assignments"; how to document in the medical record the rationale for the pass, goals, and medications while on pass; and issues regarding third-party payment for time away from the hospital. This case points out the need to also help the resident understand the larger issue of the use of the therapeutic pass on a short-term unit. In some clinical cases, it may not be incorrect to give a pass to a patient so early into a hospitalization.

Relationships also develop between trainees and patients' families. As a result, the dynamic configuration of the patient's family network is often recapitulated on the inpatient setting. The resident's awareness of the role he or she plays in this increases his or her understanding of the patient's behavior. The short-term inpatient unit can be a useful setting for the resident to learn family therapy and family systems. However, residents may initially view their work with families as an intrusion into their already busy schedules.

> Cynthia K., a 28-year-old female with alcohol dependence, mixed personality disorder, and a history of two previous psychiatric hospitalizations in the last 2 years was readmitted to the inpatient unit following a dispute with family members with whom she lived.
>
> Ms. K.'s family had previously refused to be involved with their daughter's treatment. During previous hospitalizations, discharge plans centered on urging Ms. K. to leave the family home and move to a transitional living facility.
>
> Because the resident did not see any hope for change, he did not address family issues. With the social worker's supervision, the resident realized the sources of resistance and helped organize a plan to engage the K. family in treatment. In the family sessions, psychotherapeutic work was begun around family dynamics that adversely affected Ms. K.'s functional status.

These examples identify some of the common issues that may arise on a brief-stay inpatient unit. The supervisor needs to be aware of some trainees' tendency to overemphasize the medical management of patients to the exclusion of addressing the psychotherapeutic and psychosocial issues. The trainee needs to understand the importance of the patient's place in the family and take the time to meet with the family. This gives the trainee a unique opportunity to learn about family therapy as well as allowing the family to participate in treatment.

Treating chronically ill patients on an acute unit also forces the trainee to look at effective, brief interventions that might be more educative than exploratory. Additionally, the cases presented here raise issues regarding residents' impulses that may have functional as well as dysfunctional impact on treatment. Acknowledging this might help residents reduce their own anxiety and learn how complicated a factor emotional life is on their self-esteem. Balancing the patient's needs against the backdrop of multiple pressures on an inpatient unit always warrants review.

NEEDS OF THE TRAINEE

The PGY I or PGY II resident often looks to the inpatient psychiatry experience as a time to confirm his or her decision to specialize in psychiatry. At this early stage of training, the resident usually welcomes instruction and guidance from attending psychiatrists and finds it useful to have a concentrated exposure to the types of patients he or she will be treating throughout his or her professional career.

At the same time, the early phases of residency are quite stressful. The resident is anxious about being evaluated while still developing the skills to treat severely ill patients (Ungerleider 1965). More than 30 years ago, Halleck and Woods (1962) described the typical junior psychiatric resident in a way that is still valid today: "The two major emotional stressors of the first year concern the resident's struggle to achieve identity as a physician and psychiatrist, and the impact of the anxieties attendant upon the development of psychological-mindedness" (p. 339). The psychological resiliency demanded of the PGY I and PGY II resident is remarkable. Just as the resident is beginning to solidify his or her identity as a physician, he or she is required to acquire an identity as a psychotherapist, and to complement the identity as a physician with specialized knowledge of psychopathology (Rosnick 1987).

Emotional problems of residents have been well documented, as have the psychological effects of psychotherapy supervision (Greben 1985; Halleck and Woods 1962; Merklin and Little 1967). Residents may begin to experience anxiety or depression, increased dependence on supervisors or exaggerated efforts at independence, heightened reliance on or aggression toward other members of the treatment team, or urges to overly control or withdraw from therapeutic situations. These responses occur as residents continue with their lives outside of the inpatient unit and struggle with their own personal development. As residents cope with these emotional issues, they are assigned to short-term inpatient units that have been called "hothouse" environments because of the patients' intense and extensive access to residents throughout the workweek.

> William W., a 65-year-old man with multiple severe medical problems, was admitted to the hospital for an evaluation of recent onset of paranoid delusions. Mr. W. thought the resident was too young and inexpe-

rienced to understand his problems. On the third day of hospitalization, he became more withdrawn and asked to leave against medical advice.

The resident called the attending physician and, for the first time, related the ongoing difficulty in the treatment. During a supervisory meeting that day, the resident stated she felt she had reached the point— she was now at the end of the PGY II year—when she should have been able to handle such a patient. The resident also noted that her father had recently been diagnosed with lung carcinoma and reflected on how hectic and burdensome her own home life had become.

The supervisor noted that the resident had been focusing on Mr. W.'s paranoid delusions and the organic workup while neglecting key psychological issues. These issues included Mr. W.'s fears of illness and hospitalization, his worry about becoming demented, and the anniversary of his wife's death. All this had been "missed" by the resident. The supervisor began to work with the resident around her avoidance of some of the patient's central psychodynamic issues and an understanding of the resident's countertransference feelings. This supportive exploration fostered the development of self-reflective abilities in the resident. Using her newly acquired skills, she was able to begin to treat Mr. W. more effectively.

Appropriate methods must be sought to alleviate residents' discomfort with their new role identities as psychotherapists and to help them acquire the knowledge base that they need to understand patients and treatment options. Supervision is helpful but a formal developmental approach also must be incorporated (Mohl et al. 1990). Several approaches can be used concurrently. A practical overview course on inpatient psychotherapy should be offered early in the residency. The course should include a particular emphasis on the character disorders prevalent in hospitalized patients. Residents should also be taught basic psychotherapeutic principles and how to apply these to hospitalized patients. Early didactic experiences can help residents become more aware of their own and their patients' unconscious issues, the presence of inferred intrapsychic processes, and the phenomena of transference and countertransference (Silver et al. 1983).

Another important source of learning for residents are team meetings. There, the resident can hear the patient discussed from diverse points of view and begin to understand the complex nature of psychopathology and psychiatric treatment. In addition, the resident observes experienced team members openly acknowledging their emotional reactions toward patients, including helplessness, inadequacy, anger, and frustration. Thus, residents have the opportunity to identify with professionals who can demonstrate expertise and confidence without denying their emotions or limitations (Rosnick 1987).

ROLE OF THE SUPERVISOR

As was discussed in the section on treatment setting, the supervisor may be either the attending psychiatrist who sees patients on morning rounds or a supervisor who is solely assigned to the resident for psychotherapy supervision. In the first model, residents can often see their supervisor interview patients directly. In the second model, supervisors have information about patients only through the input of the resident. Additionally, residents may be supervised by senior residents or by the unit chief. There are therefore several supervisors who may give advice about patient care.

There are various techniques for supervision, such as three-way interviews, audio- or videotapes, and process notes (DiGiacomo 1982; Maguire et al. 1984; Oldham 1982). The use of audio- or videotape provides resident and supervisor an opportunity to discuss case material without having to rely on process notes, which may omit important information. The three-way interview can be a helpful adjunct to inpatient supervision because the supervisor evaluates the interaction between trainee and patient directly, while facilitating the communication.

Whatever the method employed, it is important for supervisors to take an active role in the treatment process, offering comments on the resident's behavior and technique and observations on how the resident appears to be feeling or reacting. The passive, remote supervisor is a thing of the past. Supervisors should be forthright and prepared to confront the resident at times. Maltsberger and Buie (1975) caution against turning the supervision into the resident's psychotherapy by exploring the personal determinants of the resident's countertransference reactions. Rather, they recommend discussing manifestations of countertransference that occur in the here and now. Often, supervisors provide healthy models for identification. Omnipotent or omniscient fantasies residents may have can be helpfully discussed using the supervisor's own experiences as a starting point.

As inpatient units change from long-term psychotherapeutically oriented settings to a focus on diagnosis, evaluation, and rapid treatment, the role of the supervisor also needs to change. Supervisors need to be active and teach how to prioritize interventions in psychotherapy, coordinate psychotherapy with other medical treatment interventions, balance exploratory with supportive psychotherapy, and integrate individual with family therapy. Similarly, the supervisor should use encouragement and suggestion with the resident as he or she works with the patient (Karasu et al. 1978). This sort of "brief and supportive" supervision provides a parallel for an important aspect of the psychotherapeutic intervention that the resident may use with the patient.

CONCLUSION

This brief discussion has highlighted some of the psychotherapy training and supervision issues on short-stay inpatient units. Supervision and teaching psychotherapy on today's inpatient units are indeed difficult, in part because the luxury of treating patients for an extended period no longer exists in that setting. Unlike a more traditional supervisory role, supervisors often provide direct patient care, supervise residents on an ad hoc basis, and fill multiple roles. At the same time, trainees must spend long hours and work quickly to understand complex clinical situations. They must also learn to work effectively with and use supervision from the multidisciplinary team to maximize sources of information.

In the past, many medical students chose psychiatry because they perceived it as one of the few remaining specialties that provided the opportunity to learn about people in depth—which takes time. Residents now often find themselves on their initial rotation on short-term inpatient units, where the impact of utilization management and other pressures to reduce length of patient stay are magnified (Riba et al. 1992). Residents may be unduly discouraged by the sense that their work is superficial and divorced from the depth of patient contact they expected.

Supervisors also see the impact of the change in psychiatry to more of a managed care model. Some believe they have little control over this process and mourn the loss of the past. This grieving process, often unacknowledged and unabated, can have a destructive impact on trainees (Riba et al. 1992).

Supervisors must help themselves and their trainees to balance the educational and clinical needs and priorities in a system that is placing time pressures on everyone—patients, families, trainees, and supervisors. Curricular changes may be needed, on aspects of psychotherapy that previously had been provided experientially. As an example, for PGY II residents, a course on "Ways of Listening Dynamically" may be more useful than teaching or speaking about psychotherapy on unit rounds.

In spite of the pressure of time, there must be ample opportunities for psychotherapy teaching and supervision. Trainees must be given clear and concise guidelines for both the biological and psychotherapeutic treatment of their patients. If a trainee seems confused or troubled, techniques such as videotapes, three-way interviews, and more frequent supervision are useful supervisory approaches. The trainee's developmental stage must also be taken into account when directing the psychotherapy supervision.

Although inpatient psychiatric units are changing in terms of lengths of stay, diagnostic mix, and types of treatment provided, clinicians must also stay vigilant about the nature and quality of psychotherapy teaching and supervision provided to residents. It is important to review various methods and organize research endeavors to make sure therapists are providing quality education and training as well as excellent clinical care. Research projects should address such questions as 1) How is patient care being affected by the changes in residency training in psychotherapy? Is patient care being improved or compromised? 2) What is the level of satisfaction of trainees and supervisors regarding psychotherapy training? What is the impact on recruitment of medical students into psychotherapy?, and finally 3) What should be the model curriculum to accompany the new inpatient psychotherapy experiences? How will such a curriculum be evaluated?

Strategies and techniques to improve the teaching and training of psychotherapy to residents on short-term units will, we hope, address some of the issues raised in this chapter. This is an important and timely topic that warrants further understanding and investigation.

References

Alarcon RD, Bancroft AA, Daniels TD: Dynamics of the inpatient psychiatric setting. Psychiatric Annals 18:102–105, 1988

American Medical Association: Essentials of accredited residencies in psychiatry, in 1989–1990 Directory of Graduate Medical Education Programs. Chicago, IL, American Medical Association, 1989, pp 105–109

Black DW, Winokur G: The changing inpatient unit: the Iowa experience. Psychiatric Annals 18:85–89, 1988

Crowder MK, Jack RA: Resident education in the inpatient setting. Psychiatric Annals 18:90–96, 1988

DiGiacomo JN: Three-way interviews and psychiatric training. Hosp Community Psychiatry 33:287–291, 1982

Greben SE: Dear Brutus: dealing with unresponsiveness through supervision. Can J Psychiatry 20(1):48–53, 1985

Halleck SL, Woods SM: Emotional problems of psychiatric residents. Psychiatry 25:339–346, 1962

Johansen KH: The impact of patients with chronic character pathology on a hospital inpatient unit. Hosp Community Psychiatry 34:842–846, 1983

Karasu TB, Rohrlich JB, Stein S: A model for individual supervision in a general hospital. Compr Psychiatry 19:323–329, 1978

Lofgren LB: Organizational design and therapeutic effect, in Group Relations Reader. Edited by Colman AD, Bexton WH. San Rafael, CA, Associates Printing, 1975, pp 185–192

Maguire GP, Goldberg DP, Hobson RF, et al: Evaluating the teaching of a method of psychotherapy. Br J Psychiatry 144:575–580, 1984

Maltsberger JT, Buie DH: The psychiatric resident, his borderline patient, and the supervisory encounter, in Borderline States in Psychiatry. Edited by Mack JE. New York, Grune & Stratton, 1975

Merklin L, Little RD: Beginning psychiatry training syndrome. Am J Psychiatry 124:193–197, 1967

Mohl PC, Lomax J, Tasman A, et al: Psychotherapy training for the psychiatrist of the future. Am J Psychiatry 147:7–13, 1990

Oldham JM: The use of silent observers as an adjunct to short-term inpatient group psychotherapy. Int J Group Psychother 32:469–480, 1982

Remeikis G, Wise TN, Mann LS, et al: Use of passes on a general hospital psychiatric unit. Hosp Community Psychiatry 39:988–989, 1988

Riba M, Greenfeld D, Glazer WM: Utilization management and psychiatric education: problems and opportunities. Psychiatric Annals 22:378–383, 1992

Rosnick L: Use of a long-term inpatient unit as a site for learning psychotherapy. Psychiatr Clin North Am 10:309–323, 1987

Shershow JD, Savodnik I: Regression in the service of residency education. Arch Gen Psychiatry 33:1266–1970, 1976

Silver D, Book HE, Hamilton JE, et al: Psychotherapy and the inpatient unit: a unique learning experience. Am J Psychother 37:121–128, 1983

Starr P: The Social Transformation of American Medicine. New York, Basic Books, 1982

Swartz MS, Hargett AB, Fraker WW, et al: The inpatient milieu: organizational and functional principles. Psychiatric Annals 18:80–84, 1988

Ungerleider JT: That most difficult year. Am J Psychiatry 122:542–545, 1965

Afterword

Ellen Leibenluft, M.D.

How can inpatient psychotherapists respond to the realities of modern hospital practice? Each of the chapters in this book describes one facet of how the therapist can adapt his or her goals and techniques to treat seriously ill patients effectively in the limited time available. The preface and Dr. Tasman's chapter on milieu therapy (Chapter 1) argue that traditional models of inpatient treatment can be modified to remain useful in the current economic and social climate. Specifically, Dr. Tasman suggests that the traditional therapeutic community model can be adapted to serve important self-regulatory functions for regressed patients on the modern short-term unit. Drs. Silver and Goldberg (Chapter 2) state that somatic and psychological treatments can have complementary therapeutic effects and outline the issues that arise (and the techniques one can apply) when integrating psychotherapy with biological treatments. Dr. Adler (Chapter 3) also teaches us about integrating therapies—in this instance, inpatient with outpatient individual psychotherapy. In addition, Dr. Adler emphasizes the unique potential of the inpatient setting to serve as the site for a thorough and comprehensive evaluation of the patient's clinical status, relevant psychodynamics, and therapeutic needs.

In his chapter on inpatient family psychotherapy, Dr. Cole (Chapter 4) outlines the use of a psychoeducational, nonjudgmental approach to engage patients' families in the therapeutic process. Dr. Kibel (Chapter 5) describes how a well-run group psychotherapy program can increase the effectiveness of the entire inpatient milieu. In Chapter 6, the final chapter in Section I, Dr. Thase describes a highly structured cognitive and behavioral approach that can complement other approaches to the treatment of severely depressed inpatients.

Whereas Section I outlines general principles for each of the major inpatient modalities, Section II describes the application of these principles to the treatment of patients in particular diagnostic and demographic groups. There are some common threads between the guidelines provided by Drs. Cournos and Horwath for treating chronically mentally ill patients (Chapter 7) and Drs. Borg and Frances's description of inpatient treatment for alcoholic patients (Chapter 8). In both instances, the therapist's greatest challenge is to establish a therapeutic alliance with the patient and define appropriate treatment goals. Furthermore, both populations benefit from a particularly flexible, comprehensive team approach.

Next, Drs. Rothschild and Green describe how to integrate medical and psychiatric approaches in the treatment of patients with eating disorders (Chapter 9) or with concurrent psychiatric and medical illnesses (Chapter 10). In this context, Dr. Green describes the techniques of medical psychotherapy. Drs. Slomowitz and Bienenfeld then note the importance of a developmental perspective in treating adolescent (Chapter 11) and geriatric (Chapter 12) inpatients. Both describe useful techniques for engaging patients who are not psychologically minded and discuss the special management issues that arise for each population (e.g., integrating school with the psychiatric treatment of adolescents, treating the demented geriatric patient). In Chapter 13, Drs. Skodol and Oldham address the special problems presented by time-limited treatment of patients with severe personality disorders. Finally, Drs. Riba and Tasman (Chapter 14) discuss the implications of the recent changes in inpatient practice for the training of psychiatric residents.

Each of these authors sees his or her approach as one part of a comprehensive treatment plan; the whole is more than the sum of its parts. With all inpatients, no matter what their diagnosis or clinical situation, the therapy should progress in an orderly fashion throughout the hospitalization. The initial evaluation must be rapid and yield specific goals for the hospitalization. Medication and targeted behavioral techniques should be used to ameliorate the acute symptoms that necessitated hospitalization. From the psychodynamic perspective, the emphasis should be on supportive techniques, with more exploratory work occurring as tolerated. Family and other members of the support system should be included in the therapeutic process throughout the hospitalization— from the beginning, when they help to define goals by identifying precipitating stresses, to the end, when they are centrally involved in discharge planning. Where medical consultants are indicated, their input must be integrated with that of the treatment team.

The inpatient therapist (and his or her patients) cannot afford the luxury of a narrow philosophy or a limited range of skills. However, although flexibility and a broad scope of talents provide an opportunity for therapeutic success, they also pose the danger of fragmentation. The chaotic atmosphere of the average inpatient unit derives not only from the intensity of the patients' psychopathology, but also from the many urgent and often conflicting demands made on the staff. Therefore, the inpatient unit must have a strong leader who accepts responsibility for decision making but is able to work in a collaborative fashion. The unit chief bears the ultimate responsibility for combining disparate therapeutic approaches into a coherent, workable treatment plan. Without effective leadership, the inpatient staff will suffer undue stress, and their therapeutic effectiveness will be diminished. However, the degree to which the unit chief is able to mobilize his or her staff depends to some extent on their number, the adequacy of their training, and the support that the chief receives from the institution to which the unit belongs. If the unit has weak leadership, untenable clinical demands, and/or inadequate staff or physical plant, the already considerable difficulties inherent in treating seriously ill patients quickly will be magnified, and the unit's ability to treat patients effectively will be compromised.

In addition, the unit chief must manage the interface between the unit and managed care companies. This includes ensuring that staff conceptualize and document the necessity for the suggested treatment plan, communicating the plan and its appropriateness to outside reviewers, and addressing the staff's frustration about limited (and often inadequate) funding. At times the inpatient staff may be asked to discharge patients when they believe it is not clinically appropriate; the unit chief must ultimately decide whether discharge is in the patient's best interest.

Will psychotherapy survive to be a vital part of inpatient treatment in the future? Indeed, will inpatient units themselves survive, or will they be replaced by partial hospital programs, perhaps complemented by supervised housing arrangements? Will the average length of inpatient stay continue to decrease, or has it reached its lowest possible level? We would argue that, no matter what form care delivery takes in the future, the nature of our patients' problems will require that psychiatrists and other mental health professionals be proficient in "talking therapies" with seriously ill patients in crisis who require rapid intervention and multimodal, comprehensive care. Indeed, many of the general principles and therapeutic techniques described in these chapters could be applied in other settings.

In conclusion, the practice of psychotherapy on the inpatient unit requires an eclectic and energetic approach. Only by drawing on a variety of resources and approaches, and blending them into a plan tailored to meet the needs of an individual patient, can therapists begin to meet the challenges of caring for hospitalized patients.

Index

*Page numbers printed in **boldface** type refer to tables or figures.*